Drugs in Sport

Drugs in Sport

Second edition

Edited by

David R. Mottram

School of Pharmacy
Liverpool John Moores University
Liverpool, UK

E & FN SPON
An Imprint of Chapman & Hall

London · Glasgow · Weinheim · New York · Tokyo · Melbourne · Madras

Published by E & FN Spon, an imprint of Chapman & Hall, 2–6 Boundary Row, London SE1 8HN, UK

Chapman & Hall 2–6 Boundary Row, London SE1 8HN, UK

Blackie Academic & Professional, Wester Cleddens Road, Bishopbriggs, Glasgow G64 2NZ, UK

Chapman & Hall GmbH, Pappelallee 3, 69469 Weinheim, Germany

Chapman & Hall USA, 115 Fifth Avenue, New York, NY 10003, USA

Chapman & Hall Japan, ITP-Japan, Kyowa Building, 3F, 2-2-1 Hirakawacho, Chiyoda-ku, Tokyo 102, Japan

Chapman & Hall Australia, 102 Dodds Street, South Melbourne, Victoria 3205, Australia

Chapman & Hall India, R. Seshadri, 32 Second Main Road, CIT East, Madras 600 035, India

First edition 1988

Reprinted 1993

Second edition 1996

© 1996 E & FN Spon

Typeset in 10/12 pt Palatino by Mews Photosetting, Beckenham, Kent

Printed in Great Britain by Hartnolls Ltd, Bodmin, Cornwall

ISBN 0 419 18890 8

The views expressed in Chapters 2 and 9 do not necessarily accord with those of the Sports Council.

The term 'athlete' applies generically to those competing in sport rather than specifically to the sport of athletics.

A catalogue record for this book is available from the British Library

Library of Congress Catalog Card Number: 95-74645

∞ Printed on permanent acid-free text paper, manufactured in accordance with ANSI/NISO Z39.48-1992 and ANSI/NISO Z39.48-1984 (Permanence of Paper).

Contents

Contributors

David J. Armstrong
Peter Elliott
Alan George
David R. Mottram

The above contributors are currently affiliated to

School of Pharmacy
Liverpool John Moores University
Byrom Street
Liverpool L3 3AF
UK

Thomas Reilly is affiliated to

Centre for Sports and Exercise Sciences
School of Human Sciences
Liverpool John Moores University
Byrom Street
Liverpool L3 3AF
UK

Michele Verroken is Head of Doping Control

The Sports Council
Walkden House
3–10 Melton Street
London NW1 2EB
UK

Foreword

So much has been written about the subject of drugs in sport it is sometimes difficult to know what is truth and what is rumour. There is no doubt that drugs have been used by sportsmen and women; the reasons why may be many and various. If the high profile doping cases have taught us anything, it is that the issue of drugs and sport is not straightforward. The science behind the analysis, behind the motivation to use substances to improve performance and behind the use of drugs for medical or other purposes is complex. Too often there is an assumption of cheating. However the doping regulations control a range of substances from medicines to steroids; their effects on the body are different, their effect on sport generally is almost indescribable. Performance-enhancing drugs have no place in true sporting competition. In fact the use of any drug has to be carefully considered given the intensity of competing and training.

Drugs in Sport provides a comprehensive resource and reference book to assist students' understanding of the issues. I am sure it will make a valuable contribution to the debate as an informative and interesting guide.

Sally Gunnell.

Glossary of terms

Absorption The process through which a drug passes from its site of administration into the blood.

Addison's disease A disorder caused by degeneration of the adrenal cortex resulting in impairment of sodium reabsorption from the urine.

Adrenal glands The two glands which comprise an outer cortex which produces the mineralocorticoid and glucocorticoid hormones and the inner medulla which produces the hormone adrenaline.

Adrenaline A hormone released from the adrenal medulla under conditions of stress; sometimes referred to as epinephrine.

Adrenoceptors Receptors (subclassified alpha and beta) through which adrenaline, noradrenaline and sympathomimetic drugs exert their effects.

Agonist A drug that interacts with receptors to produce a response in a tissue or organ.

Agranulocytosis The destruction of granulocytes (blood cells) often induced by drugs. The condition responds to treatment by corticosteroids.

Allergy A hypersensitivity reaction in which antibodies are produced in response to food, drugs or environmental antigens (allergens) to which they have previously been exposed.

Anabolic steroid A hormone or drug which produces retention of nitrogen, potassium and phosphate, increases protein synthesis and decreases amino acid breakdown.

Anaerobic metabolism Biochemical reactions which occur when oxygen supply to cells is lacking.

Analgesic drug A drug which can relieve pain. Generally they are subclassified as narcotic analgesics, e.g. morphine or non-narcotic analgesics, e.g. aspirin.

Anaphylaxis An immediate hypersensitivity reaction, following administration of a drug or other agent, in an individual who has previously been exposed to the drug and who has produced antibodies to that drug. It is characterized by increased vascular permeability and bronchoconstriction.

Androgen A steroidal drug which promotes the development of male secondary sexual characteristics.

Anorectic agent A drug which suppresses appetite through an action in the central nervous system.

Antagonist drug A drug that occupies receptors without producing a response but prevents the action of an endogenous substance or an agonist drug.

Antihistamine drug An antagonist drug which stops the action of histamine and therefore is used in the treatment of hay fever.

Antihypertensive drug A drug which lowers abnormally high blood pressure.

Anti-inflammatory drug A drug that reduces the symptoms of inflammation and includes glucocorticosteroids and non-steroidal anti-inflammatory drugs, such as aspirin.

Antipyretic drug A drug which can reduce an elevated body temperature.

Antitussive drug A drug which suppresses coughing either by a local soothing effect or by depressing the cough centre in the central nervous system.

Atherosclerosis The accumulation of lipid deposits such as cholesterol and triacylglycerol on the walls of arteries. These fatty plaques can lead to a narrowing of arteries and therefore ischaemia or can encourage the formation of a thrombus (blood clot).

Atopy The acquisition of sensitivity to various environmental substances, such as pollen and house dust, thereby rendering the individual allergic to those substances.

Atrophy A wasting away or decrease in size of a mature tissue.

Axon A projection of nerve cell bodies which conduct impulses to the target tissue.

Beta blocker An antagonist of the beta group of adrenoceptors with a wide variety of clinical uses, principally in treating angina and hypertension.

Blind or double-blind trial A method for testing the effectiveness of a drug on a group of subjects where the subjects alone (blind) or the subjects and evaluators (double-blind) are prevented from knowing whether the active drug or a placebo has been administered.

Blood–brain barrier The cells of the capillaries in the brain which impede the access of certain substances in the blood from reaching the brain.

Bronchodilator drug A drug which relaxes the smooth muscle in the respiratory tract thereby dilating the airways. Many bronchodilators are agonists on $beta_2$ adrenoceptors.

Capillaries Blood vessels whose walls are a single layer of cells thick, through which water and solutes exchange between the blood and the tissue fluid.

Cardiac output The volume of blood per minute ejected from the left ventricle of the heart.

Cardiac rate The number of times the heart beats each minute. The normal resting heart rate is around 60 beats per minute.

Cardioselective beta blockers Antagonists of beta adrenoceptors which have a selective action on the $beta_1$ adrenoceptors, a major site of which is the cardiac muscle in the heart.

Cerebrovascular accident An alternative term for a stroke. This occurs when an area of the brain is deprived of oxygen either through a rupture or spasm of an artery.

Chemotaxis Chemically mediated attraction of leucocytes to a site of injury.

Cholinergic neurones Nerve fibres that release acetylcholine from their nerve terminals.

Claudication Pain caused by temporary constriction of blood vessels supplying the skeletal muscle.

Co-enzyme A biochemical which is needed by an enzyme to catalyse other biochemical reactions in the body.

Coronary heart disease Malfunction of the heart caused by occlusion of the artery supplying the heart muscle.

Coronary occlusion Obstruction of the arteries supplying heart muscle, either through vasoconstriction or a mechanical obstruction such as an atheromatous plaque or blood clot.

Cumulation The process by which the blood levels of a drug build up, thereby increasing its therapeutic and toxic effects.

Diabetes mellitus A disorder of carbohydrate metabolism, characterized by an increased blood sugar level, caused by decreased insulin activity.

Diuresis Increased output of urine which may be induced by disease or the action of drugs.

Dose regime The amount of drug taken, expressed in terms of the quantity of drug and the frequency at which it is taken.

Drug allergy A reaction to a drug which involves the production of antibodies when first exposed to the drug.

Drug dependence A compulsion to take a drug on a continuous basis, both to experience its psychic effects and to avoid the adverse physical effects experienced when the drug is withdrawn.

Drug idiosyncrasy A genetically determined abnormal reactivity to a drug.

Drug metabolism The chemical alteration of drug molecules by the body to aid in the detoxification and excretion of the drug.

Dyscrasia A morbid condition of the blood or fluids of the body.

Electroencephalogram (EEG) A recording of the electrical potential changes occurring in the brain.

Electromyography The measurement of muscular contraction using needle electrodes inserted into the muscle.

Endogenous biochemical A chemical substance, such as a hormone or neurotransmitter, which is found naturally in the body.

Epileptogenic effect An effect likely to lead to the symptoms of epilepsy.

Epinephrine *see* Adrenaline.

Epiphyses The articular end structures of long bones.

Ergogenic aids Agents which are used in an attempt to increase the capacity to work.

Erythropoiesis The process by which bone marrow produces new red blood cells.

European Antidoping Charter for Sport Recommendations adopted by the Committee of Ministers of the Council of Europe in 1984 for the control of drugs in sport.

Generic name The official name of the active drug within a medicine. Different manufacturers of a drug may use their own proprietary or brand name to describe the drug.

Glomeruli The units within the kidney where filtration of the blood takes place.

Glucocorticosteroids Steroid hormones and drugs which affect carbohydrate metabolism more than electrolyte and water balance (cf. mineralocorticoids). They can be used as anti-inflammatory drugs.

Glycogenolysis The breakdown of the storage material, glycogen, into the energy source glucose. Glycogenolysis is a major function of adrenaline.

Hepatic circulation The arteries, capillaries and veins carrying blood to and from the liver.

Hormones Endogenous biochemical messengers that are released from endocrine glands directly into the bloodstream. They interact with specific receptors on their target tissues.

Hyperpnoea An increase in the rate and depth of respiration.

Hyperpyrexia Increase in body temperature.

Hypertrophy An increase in tissue size due to an increase in the size of functional cells without an increase in the number of cells.

Hypokalaemia A condition in which there is a profound lowering of potassium levels in the extracellular fluid.

Iatrogenic disease Originally the term for physician-caused disease. Now it applies to side-effects of drugs caused by inappropriate prescribing or administration of drugs.

Interstitial fluid The water and solute contents of the fluid found between cells of tissues.

Intracellular fluid The water and solute contents of the fluid found within cells.

Ischaemic pain Pain within a tissue induced by reduced blood flow to that tissue.

Isometric contraction Contraction of skeletal (striated) muscle in which the muscle develops tension but does not alter in length.

Isotonic contraction Contraction of skeletal muscle in which the muscle shortens under a constant load, such as occurs during walking, running or lifting.

Kinins Endogenous polypeptides (e.g. kallidin, bradykinin, angiotensin and substance P) which have a marked pharmacological effect on smooth muscle.

Leucocytes White blood cells, comprising several different types with differing functions.

Ligand An atom or molecule (including drugs) that interacts with a larger molecule, at a specific (receptor) site.

Lipolysis The breakdown of fats into free fatty acids.

Mast cells Large cells containing histamine and other substances which are released during allergic responses.

Medicine A preparation containing one or more drugs designed for use as a therapeutic agent.

Metabolite The chemical produced by the metabolic transformation of a drug or other substance.

Mineralocorticoid A steroid hormone which has a selective action on electrolyte and water balance.

Monoamine oxidase A major metabolizing enzyme responsible for the breakdown of monoamines such as adrenaline and noradrenaline.

Mydriasis Contraction of the iris in the eye leading to an increased pupil size.

Myocardium The cardiac muscle which makes up the walls of the heart.

Narcolepsy A disorder characterized by periodic attacks of an overwhelming desire to sleep.

Narcotic analgesic A drug that induces a state of reversible depression of the central nervous system (narcosis) as well as producing pain relief (analgesia). Most narcotic analgesics are related to morphine.

Nasal decongestant A drug (usually a sympathomimetic) which reduces the mucus secretion in the nasal passages, normally by vasoconstriction in the nasal mucosa.

Nebulizer therapy A method of drug administration in which the drug, dissolved in a solution, is vaporized and the vapour inhaled. This method is primarily used for bronchodilator drugs.

Necrosis Tissue death.

Neurotransmitter A biochemical agent released from nerve endings to transmit a response to another cell.

Non-steroidal anti-inflammatory drug A drug, such as aspirin or indomethacin, the structure of which is not based on a steroid nucleus and which is able to control the inflammatory response within tissues.

Noradrenaline The neurotransmitter in certain sympathetic and central nerves. Sometimes referred to as norepinephrine.

Oedema Tissue swelling due to accumulation of fluid in the interstitial spaces.

Osteoporosis A condition in which bone tissue becomes demineralized.

Over-the-counter medicines Drugs which can be purchased directly from a pharmacy or drug store without a medical practitioner's prescription.

Paranoia A mental disorder characterized by persistent delusions, particularly of persecution or power.

Pepsin A digestive enzyme, secreted in the stomach, that hydrolyses proteins into smaller peptide fractions.

Phagocytosis The ingestion of bacteria or other foreign particles by cells, usually a type of white blood cell.

Pharmacokinetics A study of the absorption, distribution and excretion of drugs using mathematical parameters to measure time courses.

Pharmacology The study of the modes of action, uses and side-effects of drugs.

Placebo A substance which is pharmacologically inactive and which is usually used to compare the effects with an active drug in blind or double-blind trials.

Plasma proteins Proteins (albumin and globulins) which circulate in the plasma of blood. Many drugs are capable of binding to these proteins, thereby reducing their availability as therapeutic agents.

Prepubertal male A male who has not yet reached the age at which he is capable of adult sexual functions.

Prescription only medicine A therapeutic agent which can only be obtained on the written authority (prescription) of a medical or dental practitioner.

Prostaglandins A group of chemical agents found in the body that have a wide variety of actions, some of which are involved in inflammation.

Psychomotor stimulant drug A drug which can reduce fatigue and elevate mood. They are also referred to as psychostimulants, psychoanaleptics, psychoactivators and psychotonics.

Pulmonary emphysema A chronic lung disease in which the walls of adjacent alveoli and bronchioles degenerate, forming cavities in the lung tissue.

Purulent secretion A secretion (e.g. nasal) containing a bacterial infection.

Receptor An area on a macromolecule through which endogenous biochemicals or drugs can interact to produce a cellular response.

Respiratory quotient A parameter used to indicate the nutrient molecules being metabolized within the body. It can be determined by dividing the amount of carbon dioxide produced by the amount of oxygen consumed. On a balanced diet, the respiratory quotient should approximate to 0.85.

Re-uptake The mechanism by which neurotransmitters, released from nerve terminals, are taken back into the nerve ending for storage and re-release.

Rheumatic fever Damage to valves of the heart caused by a streptococcal bacterial infection. It is an autoimmune response to the streptococcal toxin.

Rheumatoid arthritis An autoimmune disease principally affecting joints, characterized by pain, inflammation and stiffness.

Rhinitis Inflammation of the mucous membrane within the nose, resulting in increased mucus secretion. Rhinitis may be caused by infection or an allergic response.

Salicylates Drugs that are chemically related to salicylic acid. They possess anti-inflammatory, antipyretic and analgesic activity.

Sedative drug A drug which can calm an anxious person without inducing sleep.

Selectivity The ability of a drug to exert a greater effect on a particular population of receptors due to its chemical structure. This property reduces the incidence of side-effects.

Serotonin A neurotransmitter substance, also known as 5-hydroxytryptamine.

Spermatogenesis The production of sperm cells from spermatogonia or germ cells within the seminiferous tubules of the testes.

Stroke volume The amount of blood pumped by the ventricles with each beat of the heart.

Sympathomimetic drug A drug which mimics some or all of the effects produced by stimulation of the sympathetic nervous system. The effects it produces depend upon the adrenoceptors through which it interacts.

Synapse The narrow gap between the nerve terminal and its target cell into which the neurotransmitter is released.

Tachycardia A rate of beating of the heart above the normal rate.

Tachyphylaxis A rapid decrease in the effect of a drug as the dosage is repeated. It is probably caused by desensitization of receptors.

Therapeutic effect The desired response of a drug taken to treat or cure a disease.

Tolerance The effect whereby increasing doses of a drug have to be given to maintain the desired effect.

Urticaria A localized rash on the skin, usually due to an allergic reaction.

Vascular permeability The passage of fluid and solutes across the membranes of blood vessels.

Vasoconstriction The reduction in the diameter of blood vessels produced by contraction of the smooth muscle in the walls.

Vasodilation Relaxation of vascular smooth muscle leading to an increase in the diameter of blood vessels, resulting in a fall in blood pressure.

Withdrawal syndrome The physical response of an individual who is deprived of a drug on which he or she has become physically dependent.

What is a drug? 1

David R. Mottram

1.1 DEFINITION OF A DRUG

(Drugs are chemical substances which, by interaction with biological targets, can alter the biochemical systems of the body.) The branch of science investigating drug action is known as pharmacology. These interactions may be mediated through a variety of target tissues within the body: effects on cardiac muscle by drugs such as ephedrine can lead to an increase in the force and rate of beating of the heart; stimulation of nerve endings in the central nervous system by drugs such as amphetamine can produce changes in mood and behaviour; interaction with metabolic processes can be used in the treatment of disorders such as diabetes.

(It is important to remember that drugs are designed to rectify imbalances of biochemical systems which have been induced by disease.) They are not primarily designed to affect biochemical systems in healthy subjects. Therefore the use of drugs to bring about a physiological response that may enhance performance in sport may be totally inappropriate.)

1.2 DEVELOPMENT OF NEW DRUGS

Some drugs are still derived from natural sources. For example the morphine group of drugs is extracted from the fruiting head of the opium poppy (*Papaver somniferum*) and digoxin is derived from the foxglove plant (*Digitalis purpurea*). However, the majority of drugs are produced through chemical synthesis. The pharmaceutical industry is one of the largest and most successful international organizations. Companies are continually

Drugs in Sport, 2nd edn. Edited by David R. Mottram. Published in 1996 by E & FN Spon, London. ISBN 0 419 18890 8

striving, through research and development, to produce new drugs. The process is complex and time-consuming, as outlined in Figure 1.1.

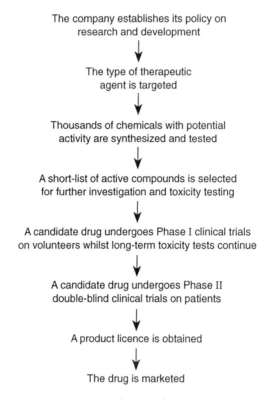

The company establishes its policy on
research and development

↓

The type of therapeutic
agent is targeted

↓

Thousands of chemicals with potential
activity are synthesized and tested

↓

A short-list of active compounds is selected
for further investigation and toxicity testing

↓

A candidate drug undergoes Phase I clinical trials
on volunteers whilst long-term toxicity tests continue

↓

A candidate drug undergoes Phase II
double-blind clinical trials on patients

↓

A product licence is obtained

↓

The drug is marketed

Figure 1.1 The development stages of a new drug.

This development procedure is monitored by government agencies who evaluate the data on the activity and safety of new drugs before the company is awarded a product licence. In the USA, the agency is the Food and Drug Administration (FDA), in the UK it is the Committee on Safety of Medicines (CSM). Agencies do not always agree, therefore a drug may have a product licence in one country but not in another. The product licence states for what therapeutic purpose(s) the drug may be used, which, again, may vary from one country to another. The development of new drugs can take between 10 and 12 years, at a cost of 150 to 250 million dollars.

1.3 DRUGS AND THEIR TARGETS

Ideally a drug should interact with a single target to produce the desired effect within the body. However all drugs possess varying degrees of side-effects, largely dependent on the extent to which they interact with sites other than their primary target. During their development, drugs undergo a rigorous evaluation in an endeavour to achieve maximum selectivity. The aim of selectivity is to increase the drug's ability to interact with those sites responsible for inducing the desired therapeutic effect, whilst reducing the drug's tendency to interact with secondary target sites responsible for producing its side-effects.

The sites through which most drug molecules interact are known as receptors. These receptors are normally specific areas within the structure of cells. They may be located intracellularly, but most receptor sites are found on cell membranes. Receptors are present within cells to enable naturally occurring substances, such as neurotransmitters, to induce their biochemical and physiological functions within the body.

The interaction between a drug (ligand) and a receptor is the first step in a series of events which eventually leads to a biological effect. This process is illustrated in Figure 1.2.

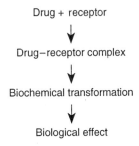

Figure 1.2 The drug–receptor process.

The drug–receptor interaction can therefore be thought of as a trigger mechanism.

There are many different receptor sites within the body, each of which possesses its own specific arrangement of recognition sites. Drugs are designed to interact with the recognition sites of particular receptors, thereby inducing an effect in the tissue within which the receptors lie. The more closely a drug can fit into its recognition site, the greater the triggering response and, therefore, the greater the potency of the drug on that tissue. In designing drugs it is sometimes necessary to sacrifice some degree of potency on the target receptor site in order to decrease the drug's ability to interact on other receptors. A tendency towards the therapeutic effect and away from side-effects is thereby achieved, thus producing a greater degree of selectivity.

1.4 AGONISTS AND ANTAGONISTS

A drug which mimics the action of an endogenous biochemical substance (i.e. one which occurs naturally in the body) is said to be an agonist. Another group of drugs used in therapeutics is known as the antagonists. They also have the ability to interact with receptor sites but, unlike agonists, do not trigger the series of events leading to a response. Their pharmacological effect is produced by preventing the body's own biochemical agents from interacting with the receptors and therefore inhibiting particular physiological processes. This is illustrated in Figure 1.3, where the agonist fits closely into the receptor, induces a biochemical transformation and therefore produces an effect. The antagonist does not have all the characteristics required to produce a biochemical transformation and cannot therefore produce an effect. It does, however, inhibit the agonist from interacting with the receptor.

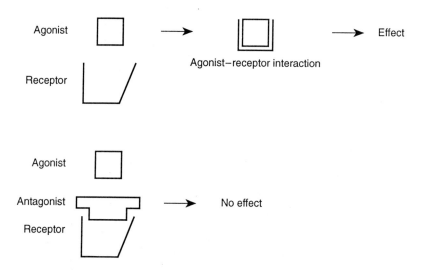

Figure 1.3 Diagrammatic representation of how an agonist drug can interact with a receptor to produce an effect, whilst an antagonist drug can interfere with this interaction.

A typical example of this can be seen with the group of drugs known as the beta blockers. They exert their pharmacological and therapeutic effects by occupying beta receptors without stimulating a response, but, by so doing, they prevent the neurotransmitter, noradrenaline and the hormone, adrenaline, from interacting with these receptors. One of the physiological functions mediated by noradrenaline and adrenaline through beta receptors is to increase heart rate in response to exercise or stress; therefore the administration of a beta blocker antagonizes this effect, thereby maintaining a lower heart rate under stress conditions.

The principle of drug selectivity applies equally to agonists and antagonists. Research into drug–receptor interactions has led to a greater understanding of receptor structure and function, consequently, the original concepts of receptors have had to be modified. There are now many examples of receptor subclassification, allowing for a greater degree of selectivity in drug design.

This can be illustrated by looking at the effect of adrenaline (epinephrine) on adrenergic receptors. We know that there are at least four subclasses of adrenergic receptors, known as alpha$_1$ (α_1), alpha$_2$ (α_2), beta$_1$ (β_1) and beta$_2$ (β_2). Adrenaline can interact with all of these receptors producing a variety of physiological effects, some of which are shown in Figure 1.4. In recent years, a drug called salbutamol has been developed which has a selective effect on beta$_2$ receptors. It will, therefore, produce bronchodilation without the other effects associated with adrenaline. As such, it is a first-line drug in the treatment of asthma. The selective nature of salbutamol is recognized by the International Olympic Committee (IOC) who permit its use in sport, whilst other less selective sympathomimetics are banned.

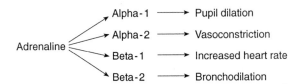

Figure 1.4   Some physiological effects of adrenaline mediated through the four classes of adrenergic receptors.

1.5 DRUG TOXICITY

It is important to remember that all drugs, even the most selective, produce toxic side-effects, though some of these may be deemed acceptable to a patient when weighed against the beneficial therapeutic effects of the drug. However, no such counterbalance exists for individuals taking drugs for non-therapeutic purposes where toxic side-effects can only be perceived as detrimental to health. Some side-effects occur at therapeutic dose levels, whilst other side-effects are experienced only at higher dose levels. It should be remembered that, in many instances, athletes are taking drugs in doses far in excess of those required for therapeutic purposes, and in so doing increase the risk of experiencing toxic side-effects.

1.5.1 FACTORS AFFECTING DRUG RESPONSES

For a drug to exert its effect it must reach its site of action. This will involve its passage from the site of administration to the cells of the target tissue or organ. The principal factors which can influence this process are the absorption, distribution, metabolism and elimination of the drug. Consideration of these factors is known as the pharmacokinetics of drug action.

Absorption

The absorption of a drug is, in part, dependent upon its route of administration. Many drugs can be applied topically for a localized response. This may take the form of applying a cream, ointment or lotion to an area of skin for treatment of abrasions, lesions, infections or other such dermatological conditions. Topical applications may also involve applying drops to the eye or the nose.

Drugs administered by a topical route are not normally absorbed into the body to the same extent as drugs administered orally. Consequently, some drugs, such as corticosteroids, are subject to certain restrictions with regard to their route of administration. They are allowed if applied topically but are subject to written notification if administered by injection or by inhalation.

Most drugs must enter the bloodstream in order to reach their site of action, and the most common route of administration for this purpose is orally, in either liquid or tablet form. Where a drug is required to act more rapidly, or is susceptible to breakdown in the gastrointestinal tract, the preferred route of administration is by injection. There are a number of routes through which drugs are injected, the main ones being subcutaneous (under the skin), intramuscular (into a muscle), intravenous (directly into the bloodstream via a vein) and intra-articular (into a joint).

Distribution

By whatever route the drug is administered a significant proportion of it will reach the bloodstream. Most drugs are then dissolved in the water phase of the blood plasma. Within this phase, some of the drug molecules may be bound to proteins and thus may not be freely diffusible out of the plasma. This will affect the amount of drug reaching its target cells. Plasma protein binding is but one factor in the complicated equation of drug distribution. As a general rule, the amount of drug reaching the tissue where it exerts its effect is a small part of the total drug in the body. Most of the drug remains in solution within the various fluid compartments of the body.

The principal fluid compartments are the plasma, the interstitial spaces between the cell, and the fluid within the cells of the body (intracellular fluid). These compartments are separated by capillary walls and cell membranes respectively. Therefore, drugs which can pass through the capillary wall but are unable to cross cell membranes are distributed in the extracellular space, and those drugs which permeate all membranes are found within the total body water.

Very few molecules, with the exception of proteins, are unable to cross capillary walls; hence, most drugs, except those which bind extensively to plasma protein, can be found outside the plasma. For a drug to be able to penetrate cell membranes it must be lipid soluble as well as water soluble. The majority of drugs are lipid soluble and are therefore distributed widely throughout the total body water. Drugs which are not lipid soluble are unable to penetrate the cells of the gastrointestinal tract and are therefore poorly absorbed orally. Such drugs must be administered by injection.

An additional obstruction to the passage of drugs occurs at the so-called 'blood–brain barrier' which comprises a layer of cells covering the capillary walls of the vessels supplying the brain. This barrier effectively excludes molecules which are poorly lipid soluble. The blood–brain barrier is an important factor to be considered in designing drugs, since a drug's ability to cross this barrier can influence its balance of therapeutic and toxic effects.

Metabolism

The body has a very efficient system for transforming chemicals into safer molecules which can then be excreted by the various routes of elimination. This process is known as metabolism, and many drugs which enter the circulation undergo metabolic change.

There are several enzyme systems which are responsible for producing metabolic transformations. These enzymes are principally located in the cells of the liver but may also be found in other cells. They produce simple chemical alteration of drug molecules by processes such as oxidation, reduction, hydrolysis, acetylation, alkylation, dealkylation and conjugation.

The consequences of drug metabolism may be seen in a number of ways:

- An active drug is changed into an inactive compound. This is a common metabolic process and is largely responsible for the termination of the activity of a drug.

- An active drug can be metabolized into another active compound. The metabolite may have the same pharmacological action as the parent drug, or it may differ in terms of higher or lower potency or a different pharmacological effect.

- An active drug can be changed into a toxic metabolite.

- An inactive drug can be converted into pharmacologically active metabolites. This mechanism can occasionally be used for beneficial purposes where a drug is susceptible to rapid breakdown before it reaches its site of action. In this case, a 'prodrug' can be synthesized which is resistant to breakdown, but which will be metabolized to the active drug on arrival at its target tissue.

Generally speaking, metabolism of drugs results in the conversion of lipid-soluble drugs into more water-soluble metabolites. This change affects distribution, in that less lipid-soluble compounds are unable to penetrate cell membranes. The kidneys are able to excrete water-soluble compounds more readily than lipid-soluble molecules, since the latter can be reabsorbed in the kidney tubules and therefore re-enter the plasma.

Metabolism is a very important factor in determining a drug's activity, since it can alter the drug's intrinsic activity, its distribution and therefore its ability to reach its site of action, and its rate of elimination from the body. The testing procedures in doping control detect both the parent drug and its metabolite(s) where appropriate.

Excretion

There are many routes through which drugs can be eliminated from the body. They may be excreted through salivary glands, sweat glands, pulmonary epithelium and mammary glands. Excretion via the faeces may take place either by passage from the blood into the colon or through secretion with the bile.

The most important route for drug excretion, however, is through the kidneys into the urine. Most drugs and their metabolites are small molecules which are water soluble and, as such, can be easily filtered through the capillaries within the glomeruli of the kidneys. Having been filtered out from the plasma, the molecules may be reabsorbed, to a greater or lesser extent, from the renal tubules. This will depend on their lipid/water partition coefficients, and on whether there is a specific membrane carrier transport system for the particular molecule. The net effect, in all cases, is that a constant fraction of the drug is eliminated at each passage of the blood through the kidney filtration system. The drug and/or its metabolites are then voided with the urine. It is for this reason that urine sampling is, currently, the principal method used in dope testing. The methods available for detecting drugs and their metabolites are extremely sensitive and capable of determining both the nature and the concentration of the drug/metabolite present.

Pharmacological means have been used in an attempt to mask drug-taking activities. These have included the concomitant use of drugs such as probenecid, whose therapeutic use is in the treatment of gout. Probenecid has also been used for many years in combination with certain antibiotics, as it will delay the excretion of these antibiotics and therefore prolong their antibacterial effect within the body. This property of probenecid has been used by competitors to try to delay the excretion of banned drugs such as anabolic steroids and thereby avoid detection. However, this effect is not absolute, and the testing procedures are sophisticated enough to detect minute quantities of drugs in the urine. In addition, probenecid itself has been on the IOC list of banned substances since 1987. As a result of all this, masking agents such as probenecid nowadays rarely feature in the lists of substances found to have been used.

Effect of exercise on pharmacokinetics

Under most circumstances, exercise does not affect the pharmacokinetics of drug action. During severe or prolonged exercise blood flow within the body will be altered, with a decrease in blood supply to the gastrointestinal tract and to the kidneys. However, there is little documentary evidence to suggest that such changes significantly affect the pharmacokinetics of the majority of drugs.

1.6 SIDE-EFFECTS OF DRUGS

There are many different receptor sites throughout the body through which drugs can interact and produce pharmacological effects. The same receptor may be found in several different tissues and organs within the body. It is not surprising, therefore, that drugs exhibit a multiplicity of actions. Usually a drug is prescribed for the purposes of producing its most pharmacologically active response, which is its desired or therapeutic effect. Responses other than this are usually unwanted and are referred to as side-effects. For example sufferers from hay fever are frequently prescribed antihistamine drugs whose therapeutic effect is to prevent histamine, which is responsible for many of the symptoms associated with hay fever, from occupying the receptor sites through which it exerts its effect. Therapeutically, antihistamines relieve the symptoms of hay fever principally associated with the respiratory tract and the eyes. However, antihistamines can also cross the blood–brain barrier where they occupy receptors in the central nervous system, resulting in a central depressant effect which manifests itself as drowsiness. This is obviously an undesirable side-effect of antihistamines, and patients receiving these drugs are advised not to drive a vehicle or operate machinery. Under different circumstances, however, this central depressant effect of antihistamines has been turned to therapeutic advantage, where such drugs can be administered to calm an excited or feverish child and to promote sleep.

In another example, opiate drugs, such as morphine, have a potent analgesic action which is their primary therapeutic effect. They also produce constipation and respiratory depression as side-effects. Even this effect of inducing constipation has been used to therapeutic advantage in that diphenoxylate, a member of the narcotic analgesic group of drugs, is used as an antidiarrhoeal agent. Being a relatively mild member of this class of drugs, it is excluded from the IOC list of banned substances. Morphine is also present in some antidiarrhoeal preparations and is included in the IOC list. These side-effects of drugs can vary from mild untoward effects which, though unpleasant, can be tolerated, through to effects which are positively deleterious to health and can be described as toxic. It is very difficult to draw a line between these two extremes. In general, the distinction between a desirable (therapeutic) effect and a toxic effect is as much quantitative as qualitative, and every drug is potentially toxic if administered in high enough doses. **A completely non-toxic drug does not exist.**

Drug toxicity can, to a large extent, be predictable. The toxic side-effects of drugs are usually well documented as a result of extensive toxicity studies during the development of the drug and from adverse reaction reporting once the drug is on the market. These predictable toxic effects are more pronounced when the drug is taken in overdose. This could occur intentionally (suicide, murder) or accidentally. Accidental overdose may result from children mistaking drugs for sweets; iatrogenic (physician produced) toxicity, resulting from incorrect dosing of patients; and patient-induced toxicity when the patient does not comply with the prescribed method of treatment. Accidental toxicity can easily occur with anybody who self-medicates without appreciating the full implications of their actions. The naive philosophy that if one tablet produces a particular desired effect then three tablets must be three times as good frequently prevails in these circumstances.

In addition to predictable toxicity, there are a number of ways in which non-predictable toxicity can occur following the administration of therapeutic or even sub-therapeutic doses of drugs. An example of this is **idiosyncrasy**, where a drug produces an unusual reaction within an individual. This effect is normally genetically determined and is often due to a biochemical deficiency, resulting in an over-reaction to the drug. This may be due to the patient's inability to metabolize the drug.

A second type of non-predictable toxicity is **drug allergy**. This is an acquired, qualitatively altered reaction of the body to a drug. It differs from normal toxicity to drugs in that the patient will only exhibit the reaction if they have been previously exposed to the drug or a closely related chemical. This initial exposure to the drug, or its metabolite, sensitizes the patient by inducing an allergic response. The drug combines with a protein within the body to produce an antigen, which, in turn, leads to the formation of other proteins called antibodies. This reaction in itself does not induce toxic effects. However, subsequent exposure to the drug will initiate an antigen–antibody reaction. This allergic reaction can manifest itself in a variety of ways. An acute reaction is known as anaphylaxis and normally occurs within 1 hour of taking the drug. This response frequently involves the respiratory and cardiovascular systems and is often fatal. Subacute allergic reactions usually occur between 1 and 24 hours after the drug is taken, and the most common manifestations involve skin reactions, blood dyscrasias, fever and dysfunctions of the respiratory, kidney, liver and cardiovascular systems. Examples of drugs known to produce such allergic responses are aspirin and some antibiotics including penicillins and cephalosporins. Delayed allergic reactions may occur in some cases: this is known as serum sickness syndrome and occurs several days after the drug has been administered.

1.7 COMPLEX DRUG REACTIONS

In addition to the side-effects associated with drugs, there are other complex reactions which may occur. These are particularly likely to happen during long-term usage of a drug or where more than one drug is being taken simultaneously.

The dose regime for a drug is chosen with the objective of maintaining a therapeutic dose level within the body. This regime is determined by two factors: the potency of the drug, which indicates the concentration required at each administration, and the rate of metabolism and excretion of the drug, which dictates how frequently the dose has to be taken. If the frequency of administration exceeds the elimination rate of a drug, then that drug will cumulate in the body, thereby increasing the likelihood of toxicity reactions. The reason for a slow elimination may be related to a slow metabolism, a strong tendency to plasma protein binding or an inhibition of excretion, such as occurs in patients with kidney disease.

Sometimes the drug itself is not cumulative, but its effect is. An example of this can be seen when a drug inhibits an enzyme system. The drug may be present in the body for only a short period of time, but the cumulative inhibition of the enzyme, each time the drug is taken, may exceed the rate at which the enzyme system can be regenerated for normal function.

The opposite response to cumulation is seen in patients with drug resistance. This drug resistance may be genetically inherited or acquired. The former type of resistance is not common in humans, though it is an increasing problem in antibacterial therapy where pathogenic microbes can develop genetic changes in their structure or biochemistry which renders them resistant to antibiotic drugs. Acquired resistance to drugs, also known as tolerance, can develop with repeated administration of a drug. Where tolerance occurs, more drug is needed to produce the same pharmacological response. A typical example is the group of narcotic analgesics, which includes morphine and heroin. Regular use of these drugs invariably leads to the necessity for increased doses in order to maintain the central euphoric effect. There are several mechanisms responsible for acquired resistance.

Decreased intestinal absorption can develop with repeated use of a drug. It has been observed that chronic alcoholics absorb less alcohol from the gastrointestinal tract. Increased elimination of drugs, either through enhanced metabolism or a more rapid excretion rate, can induce tolerance. In the case of increased metabolism, chemically related substances may induce cross-tolerance to each other.

A very rapidly developing tolerance is known as **tachyphylaxis** and is seen when a drug is repeatedly administered with a decreasing response to each administration. This is usually caused by a slow rate of detachment of the drug from its receptor sites, so that subsequent doses of the drug are unable to form the drug–receptor complexes which are required to produce an effect. Alternatively, the drug may exert its response through the release of an endogenous mediator whose stores become rapidly depleted with consecutive doses of the drug. Amphetamines produce this effect through release of the neurotransmitter, noradrenaline (norepinephrine). A consequence of regular amphetamine use, leading to tachyphylaxis, is a sleep deficit which must be met in order to replenish stores of noradrenaline.

There are several instances where the apparent tolerance to drugs cannot be explained in such simple terms and where other factors are evidently involved. A number of drugs acting on the central nervous system, particularly the group known as the narcotic analgesics, produce tolerance which is accompanied by **physical dependence**. This is a state in which an abrupt termination of the administration of the drug produces a series of unpleasant symptoms known as the abstinence syndrome. These symptoms are rapidly reversed after the re-administration of the drug. A further manifestation of this problem involves psychogenic dependence, in which the drug taker experiences an irreversible craving, or compulsion, to take the drug for pleasure or for relief of discomfort.

Where more than one drug is being taken, there is a possibility for a **drug interaction** to occur. Less commonly, drugs may interact with certain foodstuffs, particularly milk products in which the calcium can bind to certain drugs and limit their absorption. The anti-epileptic drug, phenytoin, and the tetracycline group of antibiotics are prone to this interaction. The interactions are, in the main, well documented. Their effects can range from minor toxicity to potential fatality. Such interactions may occur at the site of absorption, where one agent may increase or decrease the rate or extent of absorption of the other. Alternatively, drug interactions may affect the distribution, metabolism or excretion of the interacting drugs. These types of interaction are known as pharmacokinetic drug interactions. For example barbiturates are enzyme inducers, and thereby increase the metabolism of other drugs and reduce their therapeutic effect. A second type is pharmacodynamic drug interaction, where one drug can affect the response of another drug at its site of action. In this category, diuretics can increase the risk of kidney damage due to non-steroidal anti-inflammatory drugs.

1.8 DRUGS AND THE LAW

The manufacture and supply of drugs is subject to legal control. This legislation may vary from country to country but the principles are the same.

1.8.1 THE MANUFACTURE OF DRUGS

Any company or individual who wishes to manufacture a drug or medicine must comply with the strict rules and regulations which ensure comprehensive testing of a new drug for its therapeutic activity, toxicity and quality assurance. The new drug, formulated as a medicine, may then be licensed for specific therapeutic purposes.

1.8.2 THE SUPPLY OF MEDICINES

Medicines may be obtained through receipt of a prescription from a medical practitioner or by purchase **over the counter (OTC)**, normally from a pharmacy. The law of the country dictates which medicines may be purchased and which can only be obtained through a prescription. In general, these laws are similar from country to country, but exceptions do occur. This may lead athletes to travel abroad specifically to purchase a drug which is only available on prescription in their own country. Doctors may normally only prescribe drugs or medicines to patients for their licensed therapeutic use. Patients can obtain these **prescription only medicines (POMs)** from medical practitioners in a hospital, clinic or community practice. Prescriptions are then dispensed by a pharmacist or, in some cases, by a dispensing doctor. Once the prescription has been dispensed, the medicine becomes the property of the patient.

OTC medicines are available for purchase by the general public, without a prescription. These medicines are normally only available from a pharmacy although some medicines, such as aspirin, may be obtained in small pack sizes from other retail outlets. OTC drugs pose particular problems for athletes, since a number of drugs subject to IOC regulations are available in OTC preparations. Some examples are given in Table 1.1. It is the responsibility of the athlete to ensure that they are not taking a banned substance, therefore advice from a pharmacist should be sought when an OTC medicine is purchased.

Table 1.1 Drugs present in OTC medicines which are subject to IOC regulations

Drug	Present in certain medicines for:
Ephedrine	Coughs and colds
Pseudoephedrine	Hay fever
Phenylpropanolamine	Hay fever
Phenylephrine	Hay fever
Morphine	Diarrhoea
Codeine	Coughs and colds
	Diarrhoea
	Headache

In March 1993, the IOC removed codeine from the list of banned narcotic analgesics and permitted its use for therapeutic purposes. If selected for testing, treatment of a medical condition using codeine should be declared. In September 1994, the IOC allowed two further narcotic analgesics, dihydrocodeine and dextromethorphan, for therapeutic use.

Controlled drugs (**CDs**) are those drugs with addictive properties which are normally subject to further legal restrictions. In most countries, CDs include narcotic analgesics, amphetamines, cocaine and marijuana. For these drugs, the law states that it is illegal to possess such drugs, except where the user is a registered addict and has obtained their drug legally on prescription. In some countries, consideration is being given to include anabolic steroids as a class of CDs, as a further deterrent to their misuse in sport.

1.9 DIETARY SUPPLEMENTS

In an attempt to enhance performance through ergogenic aids, without contravening IOC doping control regulations, many athletes have turned to 'natural' products and nutritional supplements. It is a widely held view that, by using such supplements, performance will be enhanced through replacement of the body's biochemical stores or by modification of the processes involved in weight control and energy function.

Nutritional supplements include vitamins, minerals, carbohydrate, protein and various extracts from plant sources. Many of these products are promoted as having ergogenic properties. Such claims are rarely substantiated by sound scientific data in peer-reviewed journals. Additionally, there is a commonly held view that 'natural' products are, by definition, free of toxic side-effects. This is clearly a misconception, particularly when it is remembered that in the early days of pharmacological science all drugs were derived from plant and animal sources and that many of these derivatives are amongst the most toxic chemicals known to man, for example strychnine, morphine, botulinum toxin, digitalis and atropine.

1.9.1 VITAMINS

Vitamins are frequently taken by athletes on the supposition that they are experiencing a vitamin deficiency due to exercise and training regimes. However, Cotter (1988) has suggested that there is little evidence to suggest that exercise would necessitate vitamin supplementation.

In terms of using vitamin supplements as ergogenic aids, the B-complex vitamins have been taken because they are co-enzymes in the processes of red blood cell production and in the metabolism of fats and carbohydrates. Vitamin C is reputed to aid in the wound-healing process, and vitamin E has been claimed to increase aerobic capacity. All these claims for ergogenic properties of vitamins have been discussed by Barone (1988) but, in general, there is little evidence available to substantiate these claims.

Vitamins, taken in excess, are toxic. This applies particularly to the fat-soluble vitamins (A, D, E and K) which are stored in the body and which can therefore accumulate. Even the water-soluble vitamins (B and C) can produce toxic effects when taken in excess (Hecker, 1987).

In general, a balanced diet will provide the necessary nutritional requirements of vitamins. Vitamin supplements are only of benefit where there is a clear deficiency, such as occurs with an exceptional nutritional intake (Wadler and Hainlain, 1989).

1.9.2 PROTEINS AND AMINO ACIDS

Protein and amino acid supplements are frequently used by athletes, particularly where muscle development is of prime importance. Protein is obviously an essential component of a balanced diet, but there is no experimental evidence to show that protein supplementation enhances metabolic activity or leads to increased muscle mass (Wilmore and Freund, 1986; Hecker, 1987).

Excessive intake of protein can produce toxic effects, due to over-production of urea with a concomitant loss of water, leading to dehydration with a risk to the competitor of muscle cramp and an impairment of body temperature regulation.

The amino acids, arginine and ornithine, have been shown to stimulate the release of growth hormone (Bucci, 1989). Such an effect requires intravenous infusion of the amino acids. A similar effect, following oral administration of arginine or ornithine, has not been established.

Furthermore, the literature does not support the idea that growth hormone releasers have an ergogenic effect (Beltz and Doering, 1993).

1.9.3 GINSENG

Ginseng is a herbal preparation comprising a complex mixture of glycosides, known as ginsenosides. There are many varieties of plant from which ginsenosides are extracted and multiple preparations within which they are presented. No two preparations will therefore contain the same combination and dose of ginsenosides.

Ginseng has been used for thousands of years, particularly by the Chinese, and many claims have been made as to its therapeutic value. Few scientific experiments have been reported with regard to its performance-enhancing properties. Teves, Wright and Welch (1983) failed to find any statistically significant difference in maximum aerobic capacity, heart rate or time to exhaustion during a comparative controlled trial on a small group of marathon runners.

Several disparate side-effects have been described (Seigel, 1979) as being common with long-term use of ginseng.

1.9.4 CARNITINE

Carnitine is synthesized in the kidneys and liver. It can be obtained through the diet from animal sources. Carnitine deficiency is extremely rare. It is required for the oxidation of long-chain fatty acids, and athletes have used its supplementation in the diet to promote fat loss and to enhance aerobic and anaerobic capacity (Beltz and Doering, 1993). A review by Cerretelli and Marconi (1990) was unable to show any beneficial effects on performance as a result of carnitine supplementation. At the dose ranges used, no reports of toxicity due to carnitine were described.

1.10 REFERENCES

Barone, S. (1988) Vitamins and athletes, in *Drugs, Athletes and Physical Performance,* (ed. J.A. Thomas), Plenum, New York, pp. 1–9.

Beltz, S.D. and Doering, P. L. (1993) Efficacy of nutritional supplements used by athletes. *Clinical Pharmacy,* **12**, 900–908.

Bucci, L.R. (1989) Nutritional ergogenic aids, in *Nutrition in Exercise and Sport,* (eds I. Wolinsky and J.F. Hickson), Boca Raton, Florida, pp. 107–84.

Cerretelli, P. and Marconi, C. (1990) L-carnitine supplementation in humans: the effects on physical performance. *Int. J. Sports Med.,* **11**, 1–14.

Cotter, R. (1988) Nutrition, fluid balance and physical performance, in *Drugs, Athletes and Physical Performance,* (ed. J.A. Thomas), Plenum, New York, pp. 31–40.

Hecker, A.L. (1987) Nutrition and physical performance, in *Drugs and Performance in*

Sports, (ed. R.H. Strauss), Saunders, Philadelphia, pp. 23–52.

Siegel, R.K. (1979) Ginseng abuse syndrome: problems with the panacea. *JAMA*, **241**, 1614–15.

Teves, J.E., Wright, J.E. and Welch, M.J. (1983) Effects of ginseng on repeated bouts of exhaustive exercise. *Med. Sci. Sports Exerc.*, **15**, 162.

Wadler, G.I. and Hainlain, B. (1989) *Drugs and the Athlete*, Davis, Philadelphia.

Wilmore, J.H. and Freund, B.J. (1986) Nutritional enhancement of athletic performance, in *Nutrition and Exercise*, (ed. M. Winick), Wiley, New York, pp. 67–97.

Drug use and abuse in sport

2

Michele Verroken

2.1 HISTORICAL PERSPECTIVE

The extensive use of medicinal products for the alleviation of the symptoms of disease can be traced back to the Greek physician, Galen, in the third century BC. Interestingly, it was Galen who reported that Ancient Greek athletes used stimulants to enhance their physical performance. At the Ancient Olympic Games, athletes had special diets and were reported to have taken various substances to improve their physical capabilities. The winner of the sprint at the Olympic Games of 668 BC was said to have used a special diet of dried figs! (Finlay and Plecket, 1976.)

The Ancient Egyptians used a drink made from the hooves of asses, which had been ground and boiled in oil, then flavoured with rose petals and rose hips, to improve their performance. In Roman times, gladiators used stimulants to maintain energy levels after injury. Similar behaviour by medieval knights has also been noted (Donohoe and Johnson, 1986). In fact, throughout history there are examples that athletes have sought a magic potion to give them that extra edge, to help them take a short cut to achieving a good performance or to enable them to compete under circumstances when otherwise it might not have been possible, such as injury or illness.

In the nineteenth century, swimmers in the Amsterdam canal races were thought to have used some form of stimulant, as were cyclists in the endurance events. Caffeine, cocaine, strychnine, ether, alcohol and oxygen were reported to have been used alone and in combination (Goldman, 1992). Probably the first reported drug-related death in sport was the cyclist, Arthur Linton, in 1968, who was reportedly administered strychnine by his coach. Although later reports suggest that Linton died of typhoid fever, his coach had been banned from the sport, presumably for his part in the doping. Another British athlete, Thomas Hicks, came

Drugs in Sport, 2nd edn. Edited by David R. Mottram. Published in 1996 by E & FN Spon, London. ISBN 0 419 18890 8

close to death after winning the 1904 Olympic Marathon in St Louis, USA, following the use of strychnine and brandy. His life was probably saved by the actions of doctors at the finish.

The use of drugs was not only restricted to humans – horses were also found to have been doped. The intention was not always to improve performance but to 'nobble' the opposition. Doping of horses was prohibited in 1903; however it was not until saliva testing was used effectively in 1910 that horse doping could be proven.

Up to the middle of this century, there was little documentary evidence available to substantiate the hypothesis that drugs have been used in sport. Whilst there were no control mechanisms in place in sport, in Britain the Dangerous Drugs Act was introduced in 1920 to restrict the availability of cocaine and opium to prescription only. Similar legislation has been introduced in other countries. Perhaps the dearth of evidence for the abuse of drugs in sport up to the Second World War is reflective of the paucity of substances available, coupled with their low potency, when compared with the powerful chemicals of today. Moreover, sport itself had a lower profile. Around the time of the Second World War, the development of amphetamine-like substances reached a peak. These drugs were administered to combat troops in order to enhance their mental awareness and to delay the onset of fatigue. Not surprisingly, in the 1940s and 1950s, amphetamines became the drugs of choice for athletes, particularly in sports such as cycling, where the stimulant effects were perceived to be beneficial to enhancing sporting performance.

Deaths of sportsmen from amphetamine abuse in the 1960s demonstrated how widespread drug abuse had become. At the 1960 Rome Olympics, the cyclist Knud Jensen died on the opening day of the Games as he competed in the 100 km team time trial. Two team mates were also taken to hospital. The post mortem revealed traces of amphetamine and nicotinyl nitrate in Jensen's blood. In 1967, the death of the British cyclist, Tommy Simpson, during the Tour de France was televised across the world. Weeks later, it was revealed that traces of amphetamine, methylamphetamine and cognac were found in Simpson's body. Amphetamines were also found in the pocket of his jersey and his luggage. Two other deaths in cycling and football were recorded in the next year. Further evidence of the increase in amphetamine abuse came from the admission by the British athlete, Alan Simpson, that he had used them during the 1966 Commonwealth Games.

The phenomenon of drug use in sport must be seen in parallel with two other factors. Firstly, the 1960s heralded a more liberal approach to experimentation in drug taking in society in general, particularly amongst the followers of pop music. Secondly, and of far greater significance, a 'pharmacological revolution' began in the 1960s. The search by pharmaceutical companies for more potent, more selective and less toxic drugs resulted in a vast array of powerful agents capable of altering many biochemical, physiological and psychological functions in the body. Not surprisingly some athletes saw, in these chemical agents, a means of enhancing performance beyond anything that they could achieve by hard work and rigorous training. Moreover, there was a greater menu of choice for athletes. They could simply select the most specific drugs to meet their particular needs for improving performance.

Originally, athletes used amphetamines and other stimulants, mainly on the day of or during performance. There was growing evidence that these drugs might be linked with sudden collapse or death, usually from cardiac or respiratory arrest, particularly during competition, yet the long-term side-effects on the body were regarded as minor. By comparison, the drugs which emerged in the 1950s amongst body-builders in America and later amongst track and field athletes and weightlifters, the anabolic steroids, were a different story. These drugs, used in an attempt to increase size and strength, are also known to cause significant side-effects. The advantage these drugs offered was their usefulness to an athlete in training, in preparation for a competition. Training, whilst taking steroids, could be intensified, so the user benefited from increased aggression and seemed to recover from fatigue more quickly. This was especially important in the early days of testing programmes to control the use of drugs, which focused on testing in competition.

Drug misuse today has increased in sophistication; athletes are seeking out ways to improve performance using the most advanced technology. The former coach to Ben Johnson, Charlie Francis, wrote: 'There are thousands of possible synthetic permutations of the testosterone molecule. The great majority of these steroids remain an unexplored frontier ... private laboratories stand ready to synthesise any number of these steroids and keep the athletes ahead of the game' (Francis, 1990).

Unfortunately, evidence for the performance-enhancing properties of drugs is sparse. It has not been possible to undertake controlled trials, where drugs could be evaluated on large groups of individuals and compared with a placebo, preferably on a double-blind basis, where neither the tester nor the individuals being tested are aware of whether they are taking the drug or the placebo. This approach would have been similar to that adopted by drug companies in order to establish whether new drugs are effective therapeutic agents. Clearly there are logistical and ethical reasons why such trials could not take place. Consequently, much of the rationale behind drug taking in sport is based on hypothetical performance-enhancing properties, speculation, misinformation from 'underground' booklets and sheer ignorance.

In addition, little cognizance is taken of the side-effects associated with drugs, and the potential adverse effect these may have on performance. Statistics published by the International Olympic Committee (IOC) accredited laboratories since 1986 (obtained from testing programmes throughout the world) indicate that anabolic steroids are the most frequently detected substance, consistently representing a significant percentage of the total findings.

Table 2.1 Percentage detection levels of stimulants and anabolic steroids in IOC accredited laboratories

	1986	1987	1988	1989	1990	1991
Stimulant findings (%)	26.3	31.8	31	40.4	32.9	22
Anabolic steroid findings (%)	65.3	55.4	58.5	48.6	56	55

Source: IOC Laboratory Statistics.

2.2 DEFINITION OF DOPING

The origin of the word doping is interesting. Dop referred to a stimulant drink used in tribal ceremonies in South Africa around the eighteenth century. Dop first appeared in an English dictionary in 1889; it was described as a narcotic potion for racehorses to reduce their performance. Contemporary use has extended the definition to include the improvement of performance. As practice has developed, the definition also refers to maintenance of performance and manipulation of the testing procedures by the use of doping classes or methods.

So the word 'doping' is now used to describe not only the misuse of drugs by sportsmen and women, but also the use of other methods of improving performance or of attempting to manipulate the test. This definition is not without controversy. There are many different ways in which athletes attempt to improve their performance, for example altitude training, diet, biomechanical analysis and psychological preparation. However, these techniques are generally accepted as part of an athlete's training and preparation regime.

The doping definition of the IOC (IOC, 1990) is based on the banning of pharmacological classes. Rule 29A of the Olympic Charter states: 'Doping is forbidden. The IOC Medical Commission shall prepare a list of prohibited classes of drugs and of banned procedures'. Further explanation of this approach is given in the introductory paragraph to the published list. 'The definition has the advantage that new drugs, some of which may be especially designed for doping purposes, are also banned.'

This definition demonstrates the concern for the increasing sophistication in chemical technology, as athletes and their scientists seek chemical agents to improve performance, but which may not yet be covered by current regulations; a veritable competition between the testing regime and some athletes.

The doping definition given in the IOC Medical Code of September 1994 reflects the growing complexity of the issue, particularly in respect of the increasing number of legal challenges to doping offences. Doping contravenes the ethics both of sport and medical science. The IOC Medical Commission bans: (1) the administration of substances belonging to selected classes of pharmacological agents; and (2) the use of various doping methods.

A comparison of initial attempts to define doping illustrates the difficulties of reflecting practice in words. An early definition from the International Amateur Athletic Federation (IAAF) referred to:

> The administration of, or use by a competing athlete of any substance foreign to the body or any physiological substance taken in abnormal quantity or taken by an abnormal route of entry into the body with the sole intention of increasing in an artificial and unfair manner his/her performance in competition. When necessity demands medical treatment with any substance which, because of its nature, dosage or application is able to boost the athlete's performance in competition in an artificial and unfair manner, this too is regarded as doping (IAAF, 1982, Rule 144).

This definition could be challenged on many points; that not all substances are foreign to the body; the issue of intention and the link with performance improvement.

Legal challenges have encouraged the progress of a definition of doping, and most sports federations have adopted an absolute offence approach. The more recent definition of the IAAF states:

> Doping is strictly forbidden and is an offence under IAAF rules. An offence of doping takes place when either
>
> 1. a prohibited substance is found to be present within an athlete's body tissue or fluids; or
> 2. an athlete takes advantage of a prohibited technique; or
> 3. an athlete admits having used or taken advantage of a prohibited substance or prohibited technique.
>
> (IAAF Handbook, 1992–1993, Rule 55)

Further explanations refer to metabolites of a prohibited substance and to a more detailed definition of prohibited techniques, including blood doping and use of substances to alter the integrity and validity of urine samples used in doping control. Ancillary offences, such as failure or refusal to submit to doping control, are indicated, as is assisting or inciting others to use a prohibited substance or technique.

Already the definition has been extended, not only to take account of a move from the analysis of urine to blood or other body tissues, but also to supporting evidence of doping, admission, supply and not submitting to a test. The British Athletic Federation have also tackled the issue of availability for testing by including a regulation about notification of a contact address if an athlete is absent from the address for a period of five days or longer. This in itself may be regarded as a doping offence, and, whilst it seems far removed from the misuse of drugs, it is further evidence of the need to reflect practice in the rules and procedures that control doping in sport.

One of the problems with a definition based upon a list of substances is that not all sports may adopt the same classification. The offence of doping may vary between sports. This situation occurred during the 1988 Tour de France, when the Spanish cyclist Pedro Delgardo tested positive for a substance banned by the IOC. However, because this substance was not banned by the International Cycling Union, no penalty could be imposed. Defining doping as the use of prohibited substances places great emphasis on the role of a drug-testing programme to detect banned substances. However, as discussed in the next section, not all substances listed as banned are or were detectable. This is particularly relevant to endogenous substances where a natural 'acceptable' level has not been established. There are also complications with substances permitted by specified routes of administration (e.g. inhalation, topical or local injection), as the detection of the substance and investigation into its presence are separate stages in the disciplinary process.

2.3 A REVIEW OF THE IOC LIST OF DOPING CLASSES AND METHODS

Doping classes

Since the IOC list of doping classes was first published in 1967, it has evolved gradually to its present form. Five doping classes are now recognized by the IOC, although in 1992 the list had grown to six classes. The first IOC list included stimulants and narcotic analgesics. Anabolic steroids were first banned in 1974 by the IOC Medical Commission when the technology to detect these substances became available. Although the addition of anabolic steroids to the list recognized their potential for abuse by athletes, testing was based at competitions, so the regime of drug use was not effectively addressed. The introduction of out-of-competition testing acknowledged the use of anabolic steroids in training.

A detection method for testosterone was introduced at the 1982 Commonwealth Games in Brisbane. The inclusion of this substance in the IOC list in 1983 was significant as it was the first endogenous or naturally produced steroid to be banned. Up to that time banned substances were foreign to the body. Scientists were faced with the problem of determining limits for the concentration of a natural substance in the body, beyond which it could be determined doping had taken place. Detection of testosterone (T) was based upon a comparison of hormones in the body: luteinizing hormone (LH) secreted by the pituitary gland and epitestosterone (E) secreted by the testes. Originally the ratio for testosterone to epitestosterone (T/E) determination was set at 6:1; however, in 1992 the IOC introduced evaluation criteria for T/E ratios above 6 and below 10. If the ratio exceeded 6 to 1, further investigations were recommended, including a review of previous tests, endocrinological investigations and longitudinal testing over several months. A doping offence would be reported, unless it could be determined that the ratio was due to a physiological or pathological condition. A ratio that exceeded 10 would be regarded as a doping offence. In 1994, the upper category was removed from the IOC's list of doping classes and all T/E ratios above 6 were recommended for further investigation.

A quantitative test for the stimulant, caffeine, was introduced at the Olympic Games in Sarajevo and Los Angeles in 1984. The concentration level was originally set at 15 micrograms per ml. This was reduced to 12 micrograms per ml in 1988.

In 1985, the IOC added the classes of beta blockers and diuretics to the list. For the first time, the IOC acknowledged the need for greater sports specificity in the application of the doping classes. Supporting information for the class of beta blockers referred to the 'misuse of beta blockers in some sports where physical activity is of no or little importance'. This was unlikely to include endurance events. Some international federations adopted the IOC's list, but took an opportunity to apply the doping classes more specifically to their sport and set aside the inclusion of all the doping classes. Thus not all sports have included beta blockers and/or diuretics in their regulations. In 1993, the IOC moved beta blockers from the main section of doping classes to the 'Classes of Drugs Subject to Certain Restrictions', indicating that they should be tested for only in those sports where they are likely to enhance performance.

Probenecid and other masking agents were added in 1987, together with human chorionic gonadotrophin (hCG). Growth hormone (GH) and other peptide hormones were included in the 1989 list under the new class of peptide hormones. This class also includes corticotrophin and erythropoietin. The development of recombinant technology has increased the availability of GH in synthetic form.

The evolution of the list is clearly indicative of the increasing sophistication of techniques to improve performance and a growing concern to regulate in the absence of unequivocal detection methods. The classifications have also been broadened by the inclusion of the term 'and related compounds' to the list of examples of each class.

Doping methods

Blood doping was banned in 1985, although no detection method existed at that time. Its inclusion came about as a result of admissions of blood doping from long-distance runners and latterly from members of the US cycling team. Evidence emerged that US cyclists had received blood transfusions two days prior to the start of the Los Angeles Olympics. A detection method was not available, so early offences of blood doping rested on admissions from athletes. Only recently has the testing procedure in some sports been extended to allow for the collection of blood samples (urine samples are also collected from athletes). The first blood testing was carried out at the 1988 World Ski Championship and continued in a limited way in skiing and track and field athletics. Blood testing at the Olympic Games was first carried out during the Winter Olympic Games in Lillehammer in 1994. The samples are investigated for evidence of homologous blood cells, i.e. blood other than the athlete's own. Current scientific knowledge is insufficient to confirm the use of autologous (same) blood, although scientists have made advances in detecting refrigerator-stored blood (Birkeland, 1994).

Pharmacological, chemical and physical manipulation was also added to the list in 1985 in an attempt to control the growing trend of deception that had entered into the procedure. Anecdotal evidence of urine substitution, catheterization and, in some cases, actually having the sample provided by impostors threatened the effectiveness of the testing system. Athletes also tried to use substances to inhibit renal excretion of anabolic steroids, such as probenecid, and to titrate testosterone/epitestosterone levels in the body. Where evidence of these manipulation techniques emerged, the classification of doping methods enabled the sports authorities to act. Significantly, very few cases of manipulation are ever confirmed as doping offences, indicating perhaps the difficulty of presenting evidence. The most well-known case to have been heard was that involving Katrin Krabbe, Silke Muller and Grit Breuer, whose urine samples, provided during a training session in South Africa, bore such a similarity it led to the allegation that they had been provided by the same person. Evidence brought forward at the disciplinary hearing in London, in June 1992, concluded that the samples probably had been provided by the same individual and that an opportunity had existed for the athletes to catheterize urine from another person prior to the sample collection. The alleged offences could not be pursued as the doping regulations of the German Athletic Federation did not provide the authority to collect samples out of competition abroad (IAAF, 1992).

Classes of drugs subject to certain restrictions

In addition to the doping classes and methods noted above, there are restrictions on specific pharmacological classes in certain sports. The responsibility is with the international federation to determine whether controls on these substances are necessary. Within this group, alcohol and marijuana are prohibited. Alcohol may be tested for by breath or blood testing; actual levels may vary between sports which restrict the use of alcohol. Control of the abuse of alcohol has taken on a different dimension with the timing of breath testing prior to a competition in order that offenders may be withdrawn. One sport, volleyball, has extended testing to include the match officials, to control the use of alcohol which might impair decision making.

Injectable local anaesthetics and corticosteroids are permitted under restricted conditions, and only if medically justified.

Summary

Sport has now inherited a substantial list of prohibited substances that reflects, in part, the practices of athletes, but also the concerns of pharmacologists that loopholes might exist in the regulations that would allow athletes to design their own doping substances. There is considerable debate amongst the medical profession and sporting fraternity as to whether some of the drugs should remain on the list. However, the justification for inclusion of substances is not simply based on their potential for performance enhancement. Unfortunately, the list of doping classes has also become a reference point for those considering using drugs to improve performance, without any real understanding of why they are prohibited or what their effects are.

There is ongoing debate about the increased use of asthma inhalers by competitors, the concern being whether this is justified by a medical condition or perceived as an aid to performance or recovery.

The mere presence of one of the banned drugs or their metabolites in a urine sample collected as part of an authorized testing programme may constitute an offence. In the case of caffeine and testosterone, a quantitative analysis of the urine is required. This will determine whether the drug is present in the urine in quantities significantly greater than those 'normally' found in urine. More recently, the legal process in certain sports has imposed a sanction at the 'A' sample report stage.

Initially, the IOC list only included drugs for which a specific, conclusive testing procedure was available. However, in recent years blood doping and peptide hormones have been included, for which confirmatory tests were unavailable. Research into definitive detection methods is ongoing and likely to catch athletes unaware. The use of blood rather than urine sampling would significantly assist testing of these substances; however there are ethical, legal, procedural and medical issues to be resolved before this form of testing becomes more widely accepted and useful. Donike *et al.* (1994) have suggested that, 'blood sampling is less meaningful when performed after a competition; blood sampling should be performed before competition and in the training periods'. If this hypothesis is proven, this will have a huge impact on the organization of testing.

International Olympic Committee Medical Commission
List of doping classes and methods (1994)

I   Doping classes
      A   Stimulants
      B   Narcotics
      C   Anabolic agents
      D   Diuretics
      E   Peptide and glycoprotein hormones and analogues

II   Doping methods
      A   Blood doping
      B   Pharmacological, chemical and physical manipulation

III   Classes of drugs subject to certain restrictions
      A   Alcohol
      B   Marijuana
      C   Local anaesthetics
      D   Corticosteroids
      E   Beta blockers

In response to changing trends in the misuse of drugs in sport, the IOC periodically revise the list of doping classes and methods. Unfortunately there is no strict timetable for this, which can cause some delay in the implementation of revised regulations. In anticipation of potential challenges to the testing programmes, particularly at major games, sports organizations are beginning to establish their own timetables. For example the Commonwealth Games Federation is operating from a list of doping classes which has been in place 3 months before the Games begin. This will stop late additions, particularly those involving therapeutic medications, catching athletes unaware.

For each of the classes of drugs, the IOC lists examples of the drugs which fall within that group. The lists are not comprehensive and include the phrase 'and related substances'. The term describes drugs which are related to that class by their pharmacological actions and/or chemical structure. This phrase was added to the 1993 IOC list. The principal reason for giving such a broad definition is to ensure that any new drug which is introduced on to the market and which belongs to a prohibited class is automatically included in the list. This avoids the need for a continual update of the lists and prevents an athlete from claiming that the substance they have taken is not covered by the regulations.

The drugs are listed under their generic name, which identifies the particular chemical substance(s) the drug contains. However the same drug may be manufactured and sold by several different drug companies throughout the world, and each company will use its own commercial name to describe that drug; for example the analgesic paracetamol (generic name) can be bought under the commercial names Panadol, Disprol and Paldesic. Paracetamol is permitted under current doping regulations.

The situation is further complicated where, as frequently occurs, a drug is combined with other drugs within a medication. This commonly occurs with the sympathomimetics combined with other substances in cough remedies, and there are many examples of where the second substance is prohibited. Paracetamol is often combined with caffeine and codeine, although the latter is now permitted for therapeutic use.

2.4 THE RATIONALE FOR DRUG MISUSE IN SPORT

> Have we … lost track of what athletic competition is about? Is there too much emphasis by the public and by the media on the winning of a gold medal in Olympic competition as the only achievement worthy of recognition?
>
> (*Dubin, 1990*)

The substances which have been prohibited or restricted for sportsmen and sportswomen are only a minority of the number of drugs and medications available. The reasons why they may be misused by athletes are many and various, but the justification for controlling the use of drugs is simply explained: 'The use of doping agents in sport is both unhealthy and contrary to the ethics of sport' (IOC, 1990).

There may be many reasons why an athlete uses drugs. If the motivation is performance enhancement, the type of drug used will depend on its pharmacological action and the sporting activity the athlete is involved in. Other reasons may be injury or illness or perhaps for social reasons, e.g. relaxation. To understand why athletes may use prohibited or restricted substances, the effects and perceived benefits to athletes of doping substances are explained in the following section. However, there are athletes who combine substances in an attempt to increase their effects or to counter side-effects.

Stimulants

By comparison with other classes of drugs, stimulants have probably been misused in sport over the longest period of time. Their main purpose has been to improve performance by the general action of stimulation of the central nervous system. Athletes may use stimulants to reduce tiredness, and to increase alertness, competitiveness and aggression. They are considered to have a performance-enhancing effect on endurance events as well as on explosive power activities, because of an increased capacity to exercise strenuously and a reduction in sensitivity to pain. Probably one of the earliest reasons for the use of stimulants was to help athletes through 'the pain barrier'. Stimulants are more likely to be used on the day of a competition; however, it seems likely that athletes now consider the use of stimulants in training to allow the intensity of the training session to be increased. There is little scientific evidence available to suggest that stimulants do improve performance *per se*. Voy (1991) comments that 'lack of concrete evidence to verify or nullify the claims of drug effects on performance is a problem characteristic of almost every drug abused in sport'.

As stimulants could increase an athlete's aggression towards other competitors or officials, there are potential dangers involved in their misuse in contact sports. The stimulant class includes psychomotor stimulants, sympathomimetics and miscellaneous central nervous system stimulants. Examples of this class include caffeine, the amphetamines, ephedrine and cocaine.

Caffeine is the pharmacologically active substance which occurs in social drinks such as tea, coffee and cola. The amount which normally occurs varies according to the type of drink and the way it has been prepared. Relatively high doses are needed to reduce fatigue and the side-effects of tremor may be detrimental. According to one study, doses of about 1000 mg would be needed to produce caffeine levels exceeding 12 mcg/ml in the urine, the current quantitative level set by the IOC (van der Merwe, Muller and Muller, 1988). Concentrations found in tea and coffee are, on average, 50–80 mg and 80–150 mg respectively. In addition, caffeine is a constituent of some medications such as cold preparations and migraine treatment, usually in quantities of less than 100 mg per dose. Caffeine produces a mild central stimulation, similar to amphetamine, reducing fatigue, and increasing concentration and arousal. Physiological effects include increased heart rate and output, and increased metabolic rate and urine production. High doses can cause anxiety, insomnia and nervousness.

Amphetamines are a controlled drug in many countries; in the UK they are covered under the Misuse of Drugs Act 1971. Although they have been prescribed as appetite suppressants and for the treatment of narcolepsy, amphetamines, in increasing doses, are known to produce dependence. Athletes have probably used amphetamines to sharpen reflexes, reduce tiredness and increase euphoria. However competitors have also died as a result of amphetamine misuse, as they raise blood pressure which, with increased physical activity and peripheral vasoconstriction, makes it difficult for the body to cool down. If the body overheats and is unable to cool down, it dehydrates and blood circulation decreases. The heart and other organs are unable to work normally.

The sympathomimetic drug, ephedrine, has been used in cold treatments and originally in bronchodilation for asthmatics, but it is now regarded as less suitable for use as a bronchodilator, having been linked with cardiac arrhythmias. Ephedrine is likely to be misused for its euphoric effect, but could also be used inadvertently as an over-the-counter (OTC) medication to treat cold or influenza symptoms. Because of the possibility that inadvertent use could be argued, it is likely that athletes would try to misuse ephedrine to obtain an amphetamine-like euphoria.

Cocaine has been used in a variety of treatments for many years; it even appeared as an original ingredient in Coca Cola until it was removed in 1903. Its therapeutic indication is as a local anaesthetic, though it is likely to be misused for its euphoric effects and feeling of decreased fatigue. Moreover, it has the potential for use as a recreational drug arising from the lifestyle some athletes engage in. Cocaine has been directly linked to the deaths of US basketball player Len Bias and American footballer Don Rogers. In sprint-trained athletes, cocaine is thought to increase heat and lactic acid formation, which, coupled with the vasoconstriction effect, contributes to fatal cardiac damage (Cooper, 1986).

One of the more controversial group of stimulants is the beta$_2$ agonists which are frequently used in medicine as an anti-asthmatic treatment. Up to 1993, the IOC permitted the following beta$_2$ agonists by inhalation only: bitolterol, orciprenaline, rimiterol, salbutamol and terbutaline.

In 1993, this group was reduced to two beta$_2$ agonists: salbutamol and terbutaline. Concerns about the potential mild anabolic effects, and of misuse of beta$_2$ agonists by inhalation, have led to a tightening of the regulations. The IOC have now created a special section for this particular group of drugs under the class of Anabolic Agents.

Sports are also beginning to regulate for potential misuse of asthma inhalers in a different and more applicable way. Rumours circulated that use of asthma inhalers just prior to competing would improve performance. This appeared to have gained credence amongst competitive swimmers, who believed that use of an inhaler would enable them to take in more air before diving into the water, to stay underwater for longer and therefore to experience less resistance. Reduction of resistance might provide the split-second advantage needed to win. To counter this, the governing body has ruled that an athlete must move away from the pool-side to receive treatment and to allow time for recovery. Similar action is being considered by other sports.

Narcotic analgesics

Pain relief was one of the earliest medical uses of drugs. Narcotic analgesics act on the brain to reduce the amount of pain felt from injury or illness. In sports, the use of powerful pain-killing drugs might enable athletes to exert themselves beyond their normal pain threshold. There are considerable dangers in this to the health of the individual athlete, who may try to compete or train despite an existing serious injury which could lead to further injury, permanent damage or to physical dependence on the drugs themselves.

Narcotic analgesics have strong addictive properties and, as such, are tightly controlled by legislation in most countries. The IOC regulations apply specifically to the opiate analgesics, including derivatives such as morphine, heroin, pethidine and dextropropoxyphene. Particular mention is made in the IOC regulations of those substances which are permitted: dextromethorphan, pholcodine and diphenoxylate. One of the milder forms, codeine, was previously prohibited for use. Codeine is widely available in a variety of medicines, analgesics, diarrhoea suppressants, cough mixtures and cold remedies, over the counter. The level of codeine present in these medicines is too low to induce the serious adverse effects associated with narcotic analgesics, but its availability may have caused difficulties in self-medication without contravening doping regulations.

In 1993, the IOC removed codeine from the list of examples of prohibited substances, and initially indicated that it was now permitted for therapeutic use. (A revised version of the IOC list which appeared later in the year did not contain this advice.) Whilst this move is likely to be welcomed by athletes, it does, however, cause difficulties for testing, since codeine is metabolized to morphine, amongst other substances, in the body. Not all sports federations had agreed with the IOC's previous ruling prohibiting codeine; track and field athletics, for example, had similarly permitted the therapeutic use of codeine. In terms of treatments for pain, non-steroidal anti-inflammatory drugs, such as aspirin, remain permitted.

Anabolic agents

In March 1993, the IOC changed its classification of Anabolic Steroids to Anabolic Agents and created two subgroups: Androgenic Anabolic Steroids and Other Anabolic Agents and Beta$_2$ Agonists (e.g. clenbuterol).

This realignment of anabolic agents within a broader group was a further clarification of the IOC's position in respect of clenbuterol. In particular, a rather acrimonious and lengthy debate followed reports of clenbuterol use by British athletes prior to the Barcelona Olympics and the classification of clenbuterol as an anabolic agent as well as a stimulant. The reports, having arisen from out-of-competition testing which concentrates primarily upon anabolic agents, masking agents and peptide hormones, have been challenged by the competitors concerned, and the matter remains unresolved.

Clenbuterol has been shown in animal studies to increase skeletal muscle mass and reduce body fat (Matlin *et al.*, 1987). It is described in the *Underground Steroid Handbook* (Duchaine, 1992) as 'the hottest drug on the steroid black market ... It has changed body building forever'. Reports of the presence of clenbuterol in athletes' urine, particularly when the substance is not licensed for legal therapeutic use in the country of the athletes concerned, or is available only on prescription yet no prescription has been written for the competitor, is growing evidence of the misuse of the substance.

The trend away from the relatively short-term use of stimulants towards longer-term administration of androgenic anabolic steroids (AAS), aimed at increasing performance by modifying muscle size or nature, marks a serious departure into planned and organized drug misuse. The steroid drugs currently in use are largely chemically derived alternatives to naturally occurring testosterone. Contrary to popular belief, oral administration of AAS is more dangerous than injection of these drugs. Oral forms have to be broken down in the liver first, creating risks of liver damage, such as cholestasis. Orally active AAS, such as stanozolol (Winstrol) are water soluble and are likely to have a shorter clearance time in the body, making their use more popular amongst athletes subject to drug testing. However, clearance times are also likely to be dose related and are difficult to calculate with any certainty.

Injectable forms, e.g. nandrolone (Deca-Durabolin), are oil-based and fat soluble, making their release into the body system slower, as fat stores are broken down. This action is more effective when used in conjunction with intensive weight-training programmes. However, the slow release does mean it may take longer, i.e. months, to clear the system. Testosterone derivatives (or esters) are active when taken orally or injected (examples include testosterone propionate). Detecting synthetic testosterone use involves the establishment of the ratio between testosterone and epitestosterone.

The use of AAS by athletes has become widespread, in particular in strength, power , body-building and stamina activities. Whilst the precise reason for using AAS in certain sports is to increase muscle development, there is no strong evidence to show that AAS exert a direct growth-promoting effect on muscles, the exception here would be in female athletes and pre-pubescent males (Yesalis, 1993).

Attempts to interfere with the ageing process have been made since the first use of 'monkey glands' 100 years ago. Emphasis has mainly been on the male sex hormones, e.g. testosterone, and their ability to improve the quality of life. The protein-building properties of anabolic steroids had led to the hope that they might be more widely useful in medicine, but this has not been realized due to the adverse side-effects reported. The side-effects associated with AAS are extremely serious, particularly the consequences of long-term or high dosage. Regrettably, these side-effects do not seem to have deterred athletes, in particular body-builders, from misusing steroids (and other drugs to counter some of the side-effects). Anabolic steroids are discussed in greater detail in a subsequent chapter; the following summarizes some of the main reasons why athletes would use them and why there are concerns about their use.

The side-effects associated with these drugs are extremely serious, particularly the consequences of their long-term use. Dr Robert Voy warned that, 'there is absolutely no anabolic–androgenic steroid that affects an athlete anabolically without also affecting him or her androgenically ... There isn't an anabolic–androgenic steroid an athlete can take to increase muscle mass, endurance or speed without risking dangerous hormonal side-effects' (Voy, 1991).

To overcome the difficulties of administering testosterone orally, manufacturers of the chemically derived versions attempted to separate the androgenic properties (masculinization in females, acne, suppression of testicular function) from the anabolic effects of increased muscle mass and body weight, positive nitrogen balance and the general feeling of well-being. This complete separation has not proved possible, so athletes who wish to use these drugs have to accept the androgenic and anabolic effects. The oil-based esters are reported to have the least dangerous side-effects of the three forms of steroids because they do not have to be broken down in the liver first (Yesalis, 1993). Use of steroid drugs alone will not improve performance. An athlete would require a high protein intake and intensive training if gains in performance are to be achieved. Research suggests that physical performance is enhanced in a limited way, for example as increased strength but not endurance (Haupt and Rovere, 1984). However, another effect of androgens in the body is to stimulate the production of endogenous erythropoietin, which would lead to an increase in the number and stability of red blood cells (Royal Society of New Zealand, 1990).

It is in the two groups of individuals who are most likely to derive benefit from muscular development that the greatest risk of toxic side-effects occurs. Females will undergo masculinization, resulting in hair growth on the face and body, irreversible voice changes and serious disturbances to the menstrual cycle. Adolescent males may experience stunting of growth. All users are likely to experience severe acne on the face and body. In males, depending on the types and doses, the side-effects may include gynaecomastia, heart disease, hypertension, liver toxicity and premature baldness.

Users seem likely to ignore these side-effects, particularly as they may not be obviously apparent. The side-effects which are more serious and

potentially fatal are side-effects such as atherosclerosis and fluid retention, both of which may lead to cardiovascular problems and the
increased risk of developing cancer of the liver and kidney. Another
important point to remember is that some reported adverse side-effects
may coincide with other factors. Body-builders, for example, use a wide
variety of other drugs to achieve their body image, such as diuretics,
insulin, thyroid hormone and growth hormone, in addition to steroids.
They also ingest many nutritional supplements and sports supplements
which are unregulated and may contain contraindicated substances.
Yesalis suggests that some of the effects (e.g. thrombotic stroke) may be
uniquely related to the extraordinary doses used by athletes. In fact, he
indicates that for some the only limit seems to be cost and availability of
the drugs (Yesalis, 1993).

Unfortunately, the reputation of anabolic steroids as performance-
enhancing drugs has achieved a considerable level of notoriety
amongst athletes, whilst the adverse effects, being more long term,
have been ignored. It is debatable whether an extensive programme of
education and information to warn users of the consequences of AAS
use in a non-therapeutic manner would bring about a change in behaviour and attitude. Angela Issajenko, Olympic silver medallist,
confessed to taking anabolic steroids, hCG and testosterone (BBC,
1989.)

> I came to the conclusion that people I'd competed with in Moscow
> were also on anabolics so I decided that was the way to go. People
> are not concerned with the side-effects, or so-called side-effects, with
> anabolic use. They don't believe it. First and foremost, what comes
> to mind is this is going to help me be the best in the world. Whatever
> comes later, comes later.

Charlie Francis, Ben Johnson's former coach, speaking at the Dubin
Inquiry (Dubin, 1990) stated: 'It's pretty clear that steroids are worth the
price of a metre at the highest levels of sport' (BBC, 1989).

The introduction of an out-of-competition testing programme has
added a potential deterrent to steroid use for those subject to a testing
programme; however the programme is not implemented on any large
scale world-wide and certainly lacks the necessary coordination.

Diuretics

Diuretics have the pharmacological effect of elimination of fluid from the
body. As such, they have a medical use in removing excess fluid due to
heart failure and, in lower doses, in reducing blood pressure. These drugs
may, however, be misused by sportsmen and sportswomen for three main
reasons. Firstly, they may be taken to effect acute reduction of weight to

meet weight-class limits. In this respect they may offer a potential advantage in sports such as boxing, judo or weightlifting where competition is in weight categories. Secondly, diuretics may be used to overcome fluid retention induced by AAS. This could be useful to body-builders trying to obtain a 'cut' look. Thirdly, athletes may use diuretics to modify the excretion rate of urine and to alter urinary concentrations of prohibited drugs. An athlete likely to be selected for drug testing might attempt to increase the volume of urine and so dilute the doping agent or its metabolites in the urine. The sophistication of detection techniques means that this form of manipulation is unlikely to be effective (Delbeke and Debackere, 1986).

Diuretics are controlled in competition because of their weight reduction potential. Out of competition, there is careful monitoring of their use as a manipulation technique. Before, during and after exercise, athletes should take in considerable amounts of fluid. Competitors who misuse diuretics could suffer from dehydration; insufficient fluid in the body may cause faintness, muscle cramps, headaches and nausea. Losing too much water could also cause the kidneys and heart to stop working.

There may also be some additional benefits to the use of some diuretics, which might support a claim of therapeutic use. The systemic diuretic, acetazolamide, appears to reduce mountain sickness and improve exercise performance at high altitude (Bradwell et al., 1986). Research suggests it can also produce an alkaline urine and so decrease the urinary output of some drugs for short periods of time; however, drugs are excreted in the urine for longer.

Probenecid has also been used by athletes in an attempt to mask the presence of drugs or their metabolites because of its ability to alter the excretion rate of acidic metabolites. Use of probenecid first came to light in the Delgardo affair; suspicions were alerted when a treatment for gout appeared in the urine of a seemingly healthy, active cyclist in competition. Subsequently, probenecid itself has been banned. The combination of gas chromatography and mass spectrometry in the analytical procedure ensure that probenecid use no longer prevents detection (Royal Society of New Zealand, 1990).

Peptide hormones and analogues

The increasing availability of hormone substances has led to greater use by athletes. Moreover, the difficulties in detecting levels of abuse make them an attractive drug for athletes subject to testing. Corticotrophin (ACTH) increases adrenal corticosteroid levels in the body. The powerful anti-inflammatory action of corticosteroids may be a useful aid to recovery from injury. Athletes might also seek the testicular stimulatory function of the gonadotrophins as a way to counter AAS effects.

Growth hormone would be used, presumably, for its anabolic properties to increase size, strength or ultimate height, depending on the age of the user. As an injectable drug, there are risks associated with shared needles and syringes. Prior to the availability of synthetic growth hormone, use of cadaver pituitary gland infected with the Creutzfeldt-Jakob virus might have led to the development of Creutzfeldt-Jakob disease. Athletes are also using amino acid supplements in an attempt to stimulate their own growth hormone production; this is not currently prohibited.

Erythropoietin is a peptide hormone which has been reported to have been used by athletes. Usually released from the kidney, it has recently become more readily available due to recombinant DNA technology. Erythropoietin is the major hormone regulator of red blood cell production, used in medicine in cases of kidney failure. The long-term effects of use in medicine or misuse in sport are unknown; however, overload of the cardiovascular system is likely where there is no medical need.

Blood doping

Blood doping is a unique form of performance enhancement, as it does not involve the administration of drugs. Red blood cells or blood products containing red blood cells are administered intravenously in an attempt to gain unfair advantage in competition. The intravenous administration of red blood cells (either from the same individual or from a different but blood-type matched person) would increase the oxygen carrying capacity of the blood. Competitors in endurance activities, such as marathon and long-distance running, cycling and skiing, might use blood doping to increase the oxygen-carrying capacity of the blood. Similar effects are reported from training at altitude.

Blood doping carries considerable risk to the athlete. Injection of an additional volume of blood can overload the cardiovascular system and induce metabolic shock. The use of an athlete's own blood can be safer in terms of cross-infection; however, adverse effects can be compounded if blood from a second individual is used. There may be a potentially fatal haemolytic reaction with kidney failure which can result from mismatched blood or allergic reaction. There is also an increased risk of contracting infectious diseases, such as AIDS or viral hepatitis. An alternative method of increasing blood haemoglobin and haematocrit is the use of erythropoietin.

Beta blockers and other drugs with sedative action

Amongst the range of drugs which may be misused are those whose actions are the opposite to the stimulant drugs. Certain sports, such as archery and shooting, require a steady action and an ability to control movements.

If an athlete was seeking a drug which might help to improve performance, where a steady action was required, beta blockers have the potential to enhance this type of performance. By moderating the cardiac output and muscle blood flow caused by the nervous system's response to stress and arousal, beta blockers would generally reduce ability to perform strenuous physical sports. However, one of the side-effects noted in the treatment of cardiac arrhythmia was an ability to reduce muscle tremor. This would be of benefit in accuracy events and those where extraneous movement had to be kept under control.

The inclusion of beta blockers in the list of doping classes has not been without controversy. Their primary therapeutic use is in diseases of the cardiovascular system, due to their actions in reducing heart rate and cardiac output. This sedating effect can be useful. Side-effects of misuse include glycogenolysis and low blood pressure, which may lead to male impotence and gastrointestinal upset. However, other side-effects, such as cold hands and sleep disturbances, may militate against their use in sport (Goldman, 1992).

It is significant that early attempts to monitor the use of beta blockers were made by requiring a declaration of the medications and a doctor's certificate stating the reasons why they were required. At the 1984 Los Angeles Olympics, team doctors came forward with certificates to cover the whole team. The inclusion of beta blockers on the list of doping classes in 1985 was only one method to control their misuse. Officials in the sport of modern pentathlon tried to amend the competition timetable to hold the shooting event on the same day as the cross-country event. It was hoped that although beta blockers might be an advantage for the shooting event, they would be a positive disadvantage for running. In response, athletes simply moved to beta blockers with a shorter life, which were metabolized before the running event began (Donohoe and Johnson, 1986).

Fears that beta blockers may be misused in professional snooker have led to their inclusion on the list, but, under pressure to address cases of medical need, the World Professional Billiards and Snooker Association has taken the unusual step of permitting, under certain circumstances and with prior permission, the use of cardioselective beta blockers for a heart condition. Applications for consent may require an independent medical examination and presentation of the full medical history. The introduction of this procedure reflects a growing trend towards acceptance of therapeutic drugs but a need to maintain control over potential misuse.

Beta blockers were moved to the 'Classes of Drugs Subject to Certain Restrictions' section of the IOC list in 1993, to indicate their specific application to certain sports. The IOC has also listed those Olympic sports where this restriction would be applicable (archery, shooting, biathlon, modern pentathlon, bobsleigh, diving, luge and ski-jumping). Recent debate as to whether beta blockers are prohibited for the sport of bowls has been inconclusive. However, the international federation decided that beta blockers should not be prohibited at the 1994 Commonwealth Games. Modern pentathlon has also controlled the misuse of other sedative drugs, such as barbiturates, benzodiazepines and antihistamines with sedative properties. More recently, the International Federation for Archery (FITA) has also introduced tighter controls on these drugs.

Obviously there are difficulties in trying to separate therapeutic use from misuse. With the increasing emphasis on scientific support for athletes, it is now possible to control anxiety without the use of drugs by calling on mental rehearsal and relaxation techniques (Williams, 1983).

Local anaesthetics

Local anaesthetics are permitted provided their use is medically justified and if the route of administration is either local or intra-articular. Cocaine is not permitted. In an attempt to control the misuse of local anaesthetics, details of the diagnosis, dose and route of administration must be submitted, in writing, to the IOC Medical Commission or the Sports Federation. Local anaesthetics may be used to treat local injury but their use to block pain to enable an athlete to continue participating beyond the normal pain barrier is to be deprecated. There is a high risk of greater injury if the body's normal pain threshold is masked.

Corticosteroids

Corticosteroids are potent anti-inflammatory substances. In their naturally occurring form, they are released by the adrenal gland during stress activity. The synthetically produced versions are used in medicine as analgesics and anti-inflammatories. In addition, corticosteroids are used in the treatment of asthma, a disease characterized by an inflammation of the respiratory tract. Athletes seeking to open up the airways or, in larger doses, to mask injury or to increase training ability might misuse corticosteroids. They should not be confused with anabolic steroids. Serious toxic effects can occur if corticosteroid use is prolonged or under inadequate medical control. Topical administration of corticosteroids is used in medicine wherever possible in preference to systemic treatment as adverse side-effects are less likely.

Originally the IOC attempted to restrict their use in competition by requiring a declaration from doctors. However, because it became known that corticosteroids were being used non-therapeutically by the oral, rectal, intramuscular and even the intravenous route in some sports, stronger measures were introduced. The use of corticosteroids is now prohibited except for topical use (aural, ophthalmological and dermato-logical), inhalation therapy (asthma, allergic rhinitis) and local or intra-articular injections. Written notification must be given to the IOC Medical Commission or the Sports Federation.

Alcohol

For most sports, the use of alcohol would be detrimental to performance, so it is logical that alcohol falls into the category of 'Classes of Drugs Subject to Certain Restrictions'. In low doses, alcohol (or ethanol) has some sedative effects. Higher doses can cause poor coordination, reduced reaction time and mental confusion. As a potential doping substance to reduce anxiety, the dose would have to be carefully controlled. In sports such as archery or shooting, the use of alcohol may stabilize tremor but could adversely affect reaction time and reduce the steadiness of the arm when aiming. Because of the degree of euphoria alcohol can produce, it might also be used to overcome nervousness in other sports such as motor racing. Alcohol is also restricted for referees and umpires at international volleyball competitions.

Pharmacological, chemical or physical manipulation

As the testing programmes to control the use of doping substances have increased in sophistication, one response from athletes has been to try to manipulate the test in some way; the purpose being to invalidate the sample given or to secure the collection of a clean sample. Athletes are reported to have used other substances, like vinegar, in an attempt to influence the quality of the urine, although there is no scientific justifi-cation for this. More often an athlete would try to provide a clean urine sample (which had been obtained from another person) during the pro-cedure. The clean sample is then secreted around the body or catheterized into the bladder and voided in place of the athlete's own urine. Tightening of the collection procedures, particularly in relation to the time between notification and collection of the sample, have helped to control this prac-tice. The validity of collection procedures may also be challenged by an individual who masquerades as the athlete by presenting for testing. Checks on the identity of the athlete and confirmation by official docu-mentation are the only way to control this. Other forms of physical manip-ulation involve collusion between the athletes and the officials in the safe custody of the samples, the analysis of the samples at a laboratory or the manipulation of results when this is not subject to independent monitoring. Rumours of these forms of manipulation were noted in several govern-mental and Sports Federation inquiries into drug abuse in sport (Dubin, 1990; Senate Standing Commmittee, 1989 and 1990; Coni Report, 1988;

Moynihan and Coe, 1987 and Voy, 1991). Evidence of state-controlled drug-taking programmes, with and without the knowledge of the participants, has emerged from former Eastern European countries.

Summary

It is sometimes difficult to justify scientifically why a substance has been included in the list of doping classes; it is not always for performance-enhancement reasons. The main objective of doping control is to control cheating, but there is also a concern to protect the health of the athlete. More recently this has been extended to protect the image of sport from the 'social drugs culture'. However, one of the complexities is that, in the minds of some athletes, drugs do work, that to win you need to take drugs and that everyone is doing it. A further complication is the tendency for athletes to engage in polypharmacy and supplementation, emphasizing the belief that there are substances which will improve performance and that more is better. How much is a placebo effect or an ergogenic aid is difficult to determine.

2.5 THE USE OF DRUGS IN SPORT

Although there may be many reasons why sportsmen and women use drugs, four main reasons can be identified:

- legitimate therapeutic use;
- performance continuation;
- recreational/social use;
- performance enhancement.

Inevitably, clear distinctions cannot always be made between these uses. This may have implications for the detection of drugs which have been taken at a time when an athlete is involved in competition. It would be easy to say that athletes should avoid taking drugs, for any reason, particularly at the time of a competition. However, there are many circumstances when drug taking is advisable, if not imperative, for the general health and well-being of the athlete. Therefore it would be prudent for athletes to consider the specific need for taking drugs and the full implications of their action.

Legitimate therapeutic use of drugs

Like any other person, an athlete is liable to suffer from a major or minor ailment that requires treatment with drugs. A typical example might involve a bacterial or fungal infection of a tissue necessitating the use of an antibiotic or antifungal agent. How many sportsmen or sportswomen have experienced athlete's foot? Apart from the slight risk of side-effects due to the drug's action, it is difficult to perceive how such a treatment would affect an athlete's performance. A less common but more serious medical condition would be epilepsy or diabetes. Under these circumstances, it would be inconceivable for an athlete to consider participating in sport without regular treatment with drugs. A similar situation arises with athletes with disabilities; in these sports, at national and international level, drug use and potential misuse is strictly controlled.

For many minor illnesses, from which we all suffer from time to time, such as coughs, colds, gastrointestinal upsets and hay fever, it is possible to obtain medications without visiting the doctor. There are a wide range of preparations available for the treatment of minor illnesses which can be purchased from a pharmacy without the need for a doctor's prescription. The drugs contained in these OTC medications are relatively less potent than those available on prescription. Banned substances are not only contained in medicines which may be prescribed by doctors. Athletes should carefully scrutinize the label on any medication or substance which is being taken, to ensure that a banned substance is not included in the medicine. Examples of such substances include the psychomotor stimulant, caffeine; and the sympathomimetic amines, ephedrine, pseudoephedrine, phenylpropanolamine and phenylephrine. Though dose levels are low in OTC medications, the sophisticated methods used for the analysis of urine are capable of detecting these drugs or their metabolites. It is also in the athlete's interest, in the event of visiting a medical practitioner, to discuss the nature of any drug treatment, to avoid the prescribing of prohibited substances wherever possible. As with any medical condition requiring treatment, a decision needs to be taken as to whether the athlete is fit to continue in competition.

In the UK, the Sports Council has produced a leaflet entitled 'Guide to Allowable Medications'. This list contains examples of medications which are available on prescription and those available for purchase over the counter.

Performance continuation

Sportsmen and sportswomen frequently experience injuries involving muscles, ligaments and tendons. Provided that the injury is not too serious, it is common for the athlete to take palliative treatment in the form of analgesic and anti-inflammatory drugs. This enables the athlete to continue to train and even compete during the period of recovery from the injury. The wisdom of such action is perhaps open to question, but the use of analgesics under these circumstances is unlikely to confer an unfair advantage. It might however cause further injury. The doping regulations restrict the type of analgesics which can be used and control the administration of corticosteroids by injection. In weighing up the consequences of giving a pain-killing injection, a doctor would probably take into account the time available before the athlete is in competition, the type of injury and cause of the pain, and the site of the injury. In contrast, an athlete is more likely to be thinking about the effort which has been expended in reaching this stage – the remaining opportunities, the rewards from sponsors, the acclaim from family and friends – therefore often the risks of treatment are inadequately reviewed.

Evidence given by athletes to the Dubin Inquiry (1990) led to the conclusion that 'cheating in sport ... is partially a reflection of today's society. Drugs and the undisciplined pursuit of wealth and fame at any cost now threaten our very social fabric'. Permitted drug treatments to alleviate the symptoms of minor ailments such as sore throats, colds and stomach upsets can be seen as simply allowing the athlete to continue performing during a temporary period of ill-health or injury.

Recreation/social use

Increasingly, the drugs of abuse or 'street drugs' are being taken for 'recreational' purposes. These may range from the relatively soft drugs, such as marijuana, to the hard, addictive drugs, such as the narcotic analgesics related to heroin and morphine and the psychomotor stimulants such as cocaine.

Marijuana (cannabis) is a drug derived from the hemp plant which is normally taken by inhalation in the form of a cigarette ('joint') but can be taken orally. The precise mode of action of cannabis is not fully understood, but the effects produced are principally euphoria and elation accompanied by a loss of perception of time and space. Conflicting opinions exist about the dangers associated with prolonged use of cannabis. There is evidence that short-term recall memory can be impaired and that permanent brain damage may be induced. Marijuana can adversely affect psychomotor functions, and these effects may last up to 24 hours following its use (Haupt, 1989). Although unlikely to be used as a performance-enhancing substance in sport, there is concern that marijuana could be used as part of the lifestyle of a sportsman or woman. Controls have been introduced in motorized sports, and a number of professional sports, such as association football and rugby league, have regulated against its use in order to preserve the reputation of the sport and the health of players. It has, however, been suggested that marijuana may be used to reduce apprehension and to steady the nerves.

The narcotic analgesics are readily absorbed when taken orally, by injection or by inhalation. They are potent drugs whose effects are primarily on the central nervous system. They depress certain centres of the brain, resulting in reduced powers of concentration, fear and anxiety. Prolonged pain, more so than acute pain, is reduced. Some centres of the brain, such as the vomiting centre and those associated with salivation, sweating and bronchial secretion, are initially stimulated, though they become depressed on continued use of the drugs. The respiratory and cough centres are depressed. Respiration becomes slow, deepens and may be periodic in nature. Death as a result of overdose of narcotic analgesics normally occurs through respiratory depression. Characteristic side-effects of narcotic analgesics include constricted pupil size, dry mouth, heaviness of the limbs, skin itchiness, suppression of hunger and constipation. Athletes are in danger of addiction to the analgesics they use in an attempt to mask injury during training or competition.

The recent discovery of opiate receptors within the brain has helped in the understanding of the mode of action of morphine, heroin and other related opiates in the relief of pain. They appear to be mimicking the effect of certain endogenous opiates, known as endorphins and enkephalins which are thought to control pain.

Narcotic analgesics are renowned for their ability to cause tolerance and dependence in the regular user. Tolerance to the drugs occurs over a period of time and increasing dose levels are needed to produce the same pharmacological effect. Dependence on narcotic analgesics leads to physical withdrawal symptoms. Symptoms normally begin with sweating, yawning and running of the eyes and nose. These are followed by a period of restlessness which leads to insomnia, nausea, vomiting and diarrhoea. This is accompanied by dilation of the pupils, muscular cramp and a 'goose flesh' feeling of the skin commonly referred to as 'cold turkey'. Relief from the physical withdrawal symptoms of narcotic analgesics can be achieved by the re-administration of these drugs, hence the difficulty that addicts experience in trying to terminate their dependence on narcotic analgesics.

Though taken for recreational purposes, the effects of these drugs may well be manifested in the field of sport. Some sporting events even take place in an environment where alcohol is freely available, both through the spectator and the performer. In other instances, recreational drugs may have been taken with no intent to alter performance but the repercussions for the drug taker or his fellow competitors could be significant, especially where aggressive instincts are altered (Voy, 1991).

Perhaps the most widely used recreational drug is caffeine which is present in many of the beverages that we consume daily, including tea, coffee, colas and other soft drinks. At the levels at which caffeine is normally consumed, its pharmacological effects are minimal. However, attempts have been made to use caffeine as a doping agent by taking supplements in the form of tablets, injections or suppositories. This has necessitated the introduction into the doping control regulations of an upper limit of 12 mcg/ml for caffeine present in urine samples. In general, all recreational drugs are subject to doping control either by the IOC or by specific sports federations.

Performance-enhancing drugs

This particular area of drug use is potentially the most serious threat to the credibility of competitive sport and has become subject to doping control regulations. It concerns the deliberate, illegitimate use of drugs in an attempt to gain an unfair advantage over fellow competitors.

It would be appropriate, at this point, to provide a definition of a performance-enhancing drug. Unfortunately a precise definition is extremely difficult to formulate for a number of reasons:

1. A particular drug which may be considered performance enhancing in one sport may well be deleterious to performance in another sport. Drugs with a sedative action, such as alcohol and beta blockers, would be considered useful in events such as rifle shooting, where a reduced heart rate and steady stance are important. However, these drugs would be counterproductive, if not dangerous, in most other sports.
2. Should performance-enhancing drugs be defined by the fact that they are 'synthetic' or 'unnatural' substances to the body? This type of definition would exclude testosterone and other naturally occurring peptide hormones which are used for illicit purposes. 'Blood doping', the method by which competitors store quantities of their own or other blood in a frozen state and reinfuse it prior to competing in an attempt to increase oxygen-carrying capacity, would also be excluded by such a definition.
3. Should substances used in special diets, such as vitamin supplements, be classed as performance-enhancing drugs? There is a heavy reliance upon sophisticated dietary and training programmes to obtain the winning edge. Some so-called vitamin preparations and nutritional supplements may contain banned substances. There is no legal requirement for manufacturers to list all the contents of food supplements. To avoid any potential conflict with the doping regulations, these supplements are best avoided. Despite warnings, athletes are still being caught having used herbal preparations; in particular athletes are advised to avoid products containing the naturally occurring plant Ma Huang (Chinese ephedra) as this plant contains the stimulant substance, ephedrine. (Sports Council Information Booklet No. 2, 1993.)

   Certainly, other naturally occurring substances, such as creatine and L-carnitine, have been widely used in the expectation that they would enhance performance.

Creatine is an amino acid, present in skeletal muscle. Taking dietary supplements of creatine will add to the whole body creatine pool, but the saturation point is soon achieved. Thereafter, dietary creatine is simply excreted. Approximately half of the endogenous creatine is in the form of phosphocreatine. The development of muscle fatigue during exercise is associated with the depletion of muscle phosphocreatine stores. This results in an inability to re-synthesize ATP at the normal rate, therefore the force of muscle contraction is reduced. Creatine ingestion will not increase the maximal force or power that an individual can produce, but will improve the ability to maintain performance close to maximum as exercise continues. Parallels to the use of creatine have been drawn with carbohydrate loading (Greenhaff, 1993).

L-carnitine, another endogenous biochemical, is involved in the transport of long-chain fatty acids into mitochondria for the production of energy. It is therefore postulated that ingesting more L-carnitine will lead to more fat being burned to supply energy. However, most placebo-controlled trials have failed to demonstrate any improvement in maximal oxygen uptake or endurance performance in response to oral L-carnitine (Brown, 1993).

4. Perhaps the greatest difficulty in precisely defining performance-enhancing drugs concerns the prescribing and use of drugs which can be perceived as possessing performance-enhancing properties but which are used for legitimate therapeutic purposes. This problem is readily illustrated when considering athletes who suffer from asthma. One of the most important classes of drugs used for their treatment is the group of bronchodilators, many of which are sympathomimetics and therefore the subject of doping control. Since asthmatic attacks are frequently associated with stress, of which competitive exercise is an extreme case, then this obviously produces severe problems for the asthmatic if they are to avoid transgressing the doping control regulations. Selected bronchodilator sympathomimetics are allowed under doping control regulations.

Definitions may actually obscure the fundamental principle, as explained by Sir Arthur Porritt, first Chairman of the IOC Medical Commission. 'To define doping is, if not impossible, at best extremely difficult, and yet everyone who takes part in competitive sport or who administers it knows exactly what it means. The definition lies not in words but in integrity of character' (Porritt, 1965). In essence, it encompasses the principle of cheating, defined in the anti-doping regulations of individual sports. The issue of performance enhancement is one which will retain media attention at major sporting events.

2.6 THE CONTROL OF DRUG MISUSE IN SPORT

Most individuals and organizations involved in sport condemn the misuse of drugs. However it is not sufficient merely to express condemnation of drug misuse, it is necessary to take steps to prevent such abuse and to take sanctions against those who are found to have misused drugs in sport. To this end, the IOC and sports federations at international and national level require athletes to undergo testing to establish whether an individual has been involved in drug misuse. Testing programmes were originally based at competitions, but, as has already been explained, testing organized in this way did not address the regime of drug misuse. The extension of testing out of competition goes some way to counter the use of drugs in training which are then stopped a short time before competition when testing would be almost certain. The athlete retains most of the effects of the drugs but avoids detection. Such is the sophistication of the drugs now in use that a continuous testing programme has become the only way to control the misuse of drugs.

At competitions, athletes are usually selected at random, by place or by lane. In addition, world, area and national record breakers may be tested. Competition testing consists of the full range of substances; conversely, out-of-competition testing focuses on the anabolic agents, peptide hormones and masking agents. Out-of-competition testing programmes concentrate on athletes in representative teams and in the top-ranking tables. In team sports, it is possible to organize testing at squad training sessions. For individual activities, such as track and field athletics, swimming and weightlifting, testing may take place at any time, at the athlete's home, place of work or training venue. This type of testing is not appropriate for all sports.

In most countries, the responsibility for organizing testing lies with the governing bodies of individual sports. There is, however, a growing trend towards the establishment of national anti-doping bodies which can deliver a testing service which is independent of sports and of a consistent standard. Criticisms of the sports-led testing programmes were levelled in a number of government reports on drug misuse in sport and, in particular, by key individuals in the anti-doping movement. One of these individuals, Dr Robert Voy, formerly Chief Medical Officer for the United States Olympic Committee observed:

> There is simply too much money involved in international sports today. One needs to understand that the officials in charge of operating sport at the amateur level need world-class performances to keep their businesses rolling forward. The sad truth is that people don't pay to watch losers, and corporations don't sponsor teams that can't bring home the gold. The athletes and officials realise this, so they're willing to do whatever it takes to win. And sometimes that means turning their backs on the drug problem.

(Voy, 1991)

In the UK, the national organization for doping control is the Sports Council. Governing bodies are required to submit details of their competitive and training calendars and of nationally ranked competitors as a condition of grant and services they receive from the Sports Council. The service is also available to non-grant aided sports with adequate regulations. A charge is made to these bodies. Samples are collected in accordance with IOC and international federation procedures and analysis takes place at an IOC accredited laboratory. Similar national anti-doping organizations are found elsewhere in the world. In Australia, New Zealand and France these organizations have been established by legislation. In Canada, Sweden and Norway, the commitment of government to include anti-doping programmes as an integral part of state financial support for sport has led to the setting up of organizations which have responsibility for anti-doping.

Accreditation of laboratories is dependent upon adequate facilities and expertise being available at the laboratory, both in terms of the range and capability of the analytical equipment and the capacity of the laboratory for testing the numbers of samples required for a comprehensive control programme. For major sporting events, it is sometimes necessary to assemble a drug-testing laboratory specifically for that event. Procedures for doping control are dealt with in a subsequent chapter.

The emergence of a range of organizations with an interest in the testing of athletes does give rise to possible duplication, unless the testing programmes are coordinated. Athletes may be tested by the national federation and international federation as well as a national agency or legislative body. Regrettably this does mean that athletes themselves are likely to become victims of a lack of harmonization, which might also allow loopholes to occur. For example some testing procedures (such as testosterone/epitestosterone) require a longitudinal study of the analytical findings. Vital information may be dispersed between several organizations, and it could be some time before steroid profiling or testosterone/epitestosterone ratios can be monitored. As a result of the duplication of testing programmes, athletes may be confused by the different types of collection equipment in use.

One of the failures of the testing programme in effectively controlling drug misuse is the focus only on the athlete who has been found to have used performance-enhancing drugs. No further investigation is made into the circumstances which led to the athlete using drugs and whether responsibility should be attached to any other person or organization.

2.7 ATTITUDES TOWARDS DRUGS IN SPORT

'The overwhelming majority of athletes I know would do anything and take anything, short of killing themselves, to improve athletic performance.'

These are the words of Harold Connolly, 1956 Olympic hammer-throw champion, testifying to a United States Senate Committee in 1973.

There are many reasons why an athlete may take a drug, other than for legitimate therapeutic purposes. Previous experiences, at school or college, may prompt further experimentation with drugs within a sporting context. This approach may easily be fuelled by an athlete reading about drugs and their effects in popular magazines or even in serious scientific journals. Unfortunately, too many people involved in sport, at all levels, are prepared to speculate through television, newspapers or other media on the problem of drug abuse in sport. Too often these unsubstantiated reports lead to accusations and counter-accusations between those involved in the practice and administration of sport. Such activities do little to enhance the reputation of sport and inevitably lead to confusion in the minds of the majority of sportsmen and women who do not take 'performance-enhancing' drugs. This uncertainty presents the greatest danger to those younger athletes who either become disenchanted with their chosen sport or are misled into believing that drug taking has become a necessary part of the route to sporting success.

Other athletes may experience pressure from peer groups, particularly fellow athletes from their own or other sports. This pressure may result from a desire to conform with the 'in-crowd'. Alternatively, it may be a fear of competing, on unequal terms, with athletes who are suspected of taking drugs. Peer pressure may also be exerted through fellow athletes encouraging an individual to participate in drug taking. Certainly drugs have become readily available and black-market prices ensure that drug peddlers can make a handsome profit at the expense of athletes.

A different type of psychological pressure may be involved in another group of athletes. For these athletes, drug taking may be the last resort for the improvement of performance, having reached their apparent limit of capability by conventional methods of training.

The motivating factors for drug misuse do not necessarily lie in the hands of the athlete. It is an unfortunate fact that certain athletes are coerced into taking drugs by someone in authority. This person may be their coach, trainer or team doctor. The directive may even have originated from a country's governing body. Such pressures are obviously extremely difficult to resist, particularly where team selection is at stake. Whilst the majority of athletes, coaches, medical practitioners and others involved in sport do not favour the use of performance-enhancing drugs, in practice the pressures of competition may compel them to take a more pragmatic approach to drug taking. The denial of drug taking is a common feature amongst alcohol and drug abusers and further hinders any attempt at tackling the problem. Potentially more damaging is the type of athlete who openly admits to taking drugs and by so doing provides a model for the younger, more impressionable athletes to follow.

The blame for taking drugs does not, of course, always lie entirely with the athlete. There is often a body of so-called 'enablers', such as friends, family, coaches, and so on, who either actively encourage the athlete to participate in drug taking or vehemently shield the user from the need to deal with the problem. The reasons for this attitude are not always clear but in most cases involve self-interest. Conversely, those closely associated with the athlete may be unaware of their drug-abusing habits. This may, to a large extent, be due to a lack of knowledge and understanding of the drugs used and of their pharmacological effects.

It is clear that the majority of those involved in sport, both administrators and participants, are against the misuse of drugs in sport. It is equally clear that there is too little understanding of both the motivating factors that lead an athlete to take drugs and the effects that those drugs can induce. It is vital that a wider knowledge of drugs and their adverse effects is achieved, so that the current problem of drug abuse in sport can be contained and that future generations can be educated and persuaded against such misuse.

2.8 ETHICAL ISSUES ASSOCIATED WITH DRUG USE IN SPORT

The use of doping agents in sport is both unhealthy and contrary to the ethics of sport. ... It is necessary to protect the physical and spiritual health of athletes, the values of fair play and of competition, the integrity and unity of sport, and the rights of those who take part in it at whatever level.

(IOC, 1990)

Drug use in sport is contrary to the very principles upon which sport is based. Sport is considered as character building, teaching 'the virtues of dedication, perseverance, endurance and self-discipline' (Dubin, 1990). If, as Justice Dubin observes: 'Sport helps us to learn from defeat as much as from victory, and team sports foster a spirit of co-operation and interdependence ... import(ing) something of moral and social values and ... integrating us as individuals, to bring about a healthy, integrated society', then drug abuse would have no place in sport. Justice Dubin goes on to ask: 'How has it come about, then, that many athletes have resorted to cheating? Why are the rules that govern sport often regarded as obstacles to be overcome or circumvented rather than as regulations designed to create equality of competitive opportunity and to define the parameters of the sport?'.

Using drugs in sport for the purpose of gaining an unfair advantage presents an ethical dilemma for athletes, coaches, doctors and officials. It is clearly cheating; moreover it may put the health of the athlete at risk. Furthermore, it may also be calculated cheating, when quantities and substances are carefully monitored in an attempt to cheat the rules on drug testing. It has been argued that the ethical dilemma has emerged for many reasons:

- media pressure to win;
- prevalent attitude that doping is necessary to be successful;
- public expectations about national competitiveness;
- huge financial rewards of winning;
- desire to be the best in the world;
- performance-linked payments to athletes from governments and/or sponsors;
- coaching which emphasizes winning as the only goal;
- unethical practices condoned by national and international sports federations;
- competitive character of the athlete;
- infallibility of the medical profession to cure and improve performance;
- psychological belief in aids to performance – the 'magic pill';
- development of spectator sport;
- crowded competition calendar.

The majority of these reasons were cited in the Dubin Inquiry itself, as explanations were sought for the context in which five Canadian athletes (four weightlifters and a track and field athlete) came to be disqualified for anabolic steroid use at the Seoul Olympics.

René Maheu (1978) has noted that development of spectator sport has turned attention away from the moral value of sport for the individual towards its entertainment potential: 'The success of spectator sport and the importance it has come to assume in everyday life are unfortunately too often exploited for purposes alien or even opposed to sport – commercialism, chauvinism and politics – which corrupt and deform it'.

Dubin, however, whilst acknowledging the existence of all the influences and their undoubted effects which might lead to drug misuse in sport, argued, firstly, that there can be no justification for athletes to cheat in order to win; and secondly, that the pressures and temptations are the same for all athletes, yet most show greater character and do not succumb. He concluded the problem is not educational, economic or social but, essentially, a moral problem.

The sporting context is seen to have been replaced by a competition between doctors and biochemists on the one side and the regulating authorities on the other. The athlete becomes the puppet of this technology, health risks are simply ignored, and other competitors cannot participate in the competition unless they, too, are prepared to use substances to improve performance. In an era where genetic and chemical manipulation has become commonplace, it is hardly surprising that some athletes no longer rely on their natural abilities and skills.

In 1892 at a conference at the Sorbonne, Baron de Coubertin, founder of the modern Olympics said: 'Before all things it is necessary that we should preserve in sport these characteristics of nobility and chivalry which have distinguished it in the past, so that it may continue to play the same part in the education of the peoples of today as it played so admirably in the days of Ancient Greece'. This may have been so at the turn of the century and the emergence of the modern day Olympic Games, but in present-day sport, the pressures on all concerned are immense. An athlete is faced with the pressures of winning, of competing and of meeting the expectations of the coach, team-mates, family and friends. Coaches are under pressure to produce the winning combination, coping with fitness levels and making demands on individual competitors, all of which may give the wrong signals in respect of drug misuse. Doctors may be faced with the dilemma of prescribing drugs for athletes and monitoring their effects as a safe way of containing drug misuse rather than knowing an athlete will seek black-market sources and advice. The doping regulations may also apply to others who assist or incite an athlete to commit a doping offence.

Occasionally, criticisms of the drug-testing procedure itself are made, in particular the suggestion of invasion of privacy and impropriety in observing a person urinating. It is suggested that athletes are looking forward to the advent of blood testing as a sophisticated progression towards comprehensive doping control. However, it is likely to be some time before scientists are willing to move from urine analysis because of the range of substances which can be detected. Blood testing offers a limited opportunity for detection of prohibited substances at present (Donike et al., 1994).

There is also another perspective, that of what constitutes drug misuse. Some banned substances, such as testosterone, actually originate in the body, and it is an excessive level which has been deemed to be a doping offence. Critics would argue this level has been arbitrarily set (Voy, 1991). Although research is ongoing, the change in definition of an offence involving testosterone/epitestosterone ratios illustrates that the debate is also ongoing. Other substances, such as ephedrine and caffeine, commonly occur in OTC medications, herbal preparations and even in social drinks. Do they actually improve performance? There is no doubt that athletes are prepared to make use of these substances to assist their performance. In terms of drugs with a therapeutic purpose, such as beta blockers and beta$_2$ agonists, there is also considerable abuse by athletes who have no therapeutic indication. Given this array of drug misuse by sportsmen and women, it is hardly surprising that anti-doping rules have been introduced.

The definition of doping has to begin somewhere. The time may have come for the critics and the sports regulators to work together to achieve a practical set of rules, a realistic competitive calendar, an efficient support system and greater controls on the commercialization of sport. Elite athletes have become the focus of a considerable amount of media attention, with stories about their injuries and illnesses filling column inches. Moreover, speculation and reporting about the lifestyle of professional athletes has given rise to an image totally out of step with the dedication, training and motivation required to survive the sporting calendar. In many sports, increasing commercialism has seen a price put on an athlete's head; some cope better with this than others.

2.9 AN INTERNATIONAL POLICY PERSPECTIVE

Drug use and abuse by athletes has now become a frequent feature of sport. Initially, sport attempted to put its own house in order, but there was concern that the commitment required to achieve effective controls was lacking. Testing was limited to major competitions such as the Olympic Games and world championships. Some international sports federations introduced regulations and testing in a limited way. The IOC created a reference list of prohibited substances and proceeded to amend it to reflect doping practices. Testing programmes rested on accurate analysis. Laboratories were accredited by the IAAF and the IOC to undertake analysis of urine samples from athletes. However, the limitations and potential conflicts of interest which developed in the testing programmes began to compel others to take an interest in the control of drugs in sport.

Interestingly, governments became the other key players in the fight against doping. Sport is played on a national level throughout the world. The Council of Europe Committee of Ministers adopted a resolution on doping in 1967, the first international text of its kind. The resolution stressed the moral and ethical principles at stake for sport, and the health dangers for athletes. The resolution explicitly referred to doping as cheating. Governments were recommended to persuade sports organizations to take the necessary steps to have proper and adequate regulations and to penalize offenders. Finally, the resolution recommended governments to take action themselves if the sports organizations did not act sufficiently within 3 years.

Having monitored the situation for 11 years, sports ministers adopted a further resolution in 1978, which called for governments to provide a coordinated policy and an overall framework in which the doping controls of sports organizations could take place. A European Charter, a statement of principles, anti-doping strategies and policies was adopted in 1984. It is significant that the Chairman of the drafting group was the Chairman of the IOC Medical Commission, Prince Alexandre de Merode, and that the Charter received support from international sports organizations. However it was obvious that sport alone would be unable to contain the problem.

Anxious to keep up the momentum, the Council of Europe Committee of Ministers pressed for testing out of competition, without prior warning to the athlete. Ministers also sought to secure a commitment to international harmonization, not only amongst sports but also amongst countries. Ministers agreed to the drafting of an anti-doping Convention which would be binding on governments. To date, some 25 countries are committed to the Convention's principles, including four non-European countries. The key significance of this document was the recognition of political will to address the problem of doping. The Convention also provides a number of common standards – legislative, financial, technical and educational – for implementation by all the bodies concerned with the state, by governments themselves and by governments in support of sports organizations. It will be interesting to see whether the first of these, urine sample collection procedures, will be adopted by sports organizations. The standards being agreed through the Convention are being embraced by the national anti-doping organizations which are emerging, supported by government and/or national sports organizations. In some countries these have been established by legislation.

Cooperation between international and national sports federations and the newly created national anti-doping organizations could provide one of the strongest deterrents to drug misuse. However, the authority of international sports federations and of national legislation can sometimes lie uneasily together. Some sports have interpreted the intervention of governments in anti-doping matters as threatening their independence and challenging their abilities to undertake urine samples. As the majority of testing and, certainly, of laboratory expertise is government funded, a mutually supportive relationship between sports organizations and governments will be crucial to the ongoing success of anti-doping activities.

Recognition of the need for a symbiotic relationship between sports organizations and governments was noted in the IOC/IF Agreement against Doping in Sport, in June 1993. In seeking ways to 'intensify the prevention of, education and fight against doping in sport', the IOC and international sports federations agreed to 'develop the cooperation between the IOC, The International Sports Federations, the National Olympic Committees, the National Federations and the governmental or other organisations concerned in order to combat the trafficking of doping substances'. Interestingly, international sports federations were invited 'to adopt each year, as a basic minimum document, the list of banned classes and methods established by the IOC Medical Commission and to undertake the appropriate controls for each sport'. The identification of roles may be illustrative of underlying concerns by sport that it is not totally in control of anti-doping programmes.

It is significant that the IOC's own role indirectly extends outside the Olympic Games through the accreditation of laboratories, the establishment of the list of doping classes, a financial assistance programme for international federations who need help to intensify their anti-doping controls and encouragement to Olympic sports to comply with the principles of the agreement.

If drug use and abuse in sport is to be treated seriously, it will require consolidated action, a joint commitment by sport, governments and others. In the words of Justice Dubin: 'The resolution of this problem cannot simply be left to those who govern sport nationally and internationally'.

2.10 REFERENCES

Amateur Athletic Association (1988) *The Coni Report*, September, London, England.

Birkeland, K. (1994) Towards blood sampling in doping control – the road ahead, in *Blood Samples in Doping Control*, (eds P. Hemmersbach and K. Birkeland) On Demand Publishing, Oslo.

Bradwell, A.R., Dykes, P.W., Coote, J.H., Forster, P.J.E., Milles, J.J., Chesner, I., Richardson, J.V. (1986) Effect of acetazolamide on exercise performance and muscle mass at high altitude. *Lancet*, 1 part 2, 1001–5.

British Broadcasting Corporation (1989) *On the Line*, BBC2 production.

Brown, M. (1993) Performance enhancement. *Coaching Focus*, No. 23, 5–6.

Cooper, N. (1986) Cocaine is a loaded gun. *Newsweek*, July 7.

Delbeke, F.T. and Debackere, M. (1986) The influence of diuretics on the excretion and metabolism of doping agents. *Drug Res.*, **36**, 134–7, 1413–16.

Donike, M., Geyer, H., Gotzmann, A., Horning, St., (1994) Blood analysis in doping control – advantages and disadvantages, in *Blood Samples in Doping Control*, (eds P. Hemmersbach and K. Birkeland) On Demand Publishing, Oslo.

Donohoe, T. and Johnson, N. (1986) *Foul Play? Drug Abuse in Sport*, Blackwell, Oxford.

Dubin, C.L. (1990) *Commission of Inquiry into the Use of Drugs and Banned Practices Intended to Increase Athletic Performance*, Canadian Government Publishing Center, Ottawa.

Duchaine, D. (1992) *Underground Steroid Handbook*. Power Distributors, Venice, California, USA.

Finlay, M. and Plecket, H. (1976) *The Olympic Games: The First Hundred Years*, Chatto and Windus, London.

Francis, C. (1990) *Speed Trap*, Lesters, Orpen, Dennys, Toronto, Canada.

Goldman, B. (1992) *Death in the Locker Room/Drugs and Sport*, Elite Sports Medicine Publications, Illinois.

Greenhaff, P. (1993) Update – creatine ingestion and exercise performance. *Coaching Focus*, No. 23, 3–4.

Haupt, H. (1989) Drugs in athletics. *Clin. in Sports Med.*, **8**, (3), 146–9.

Haupt, H.A. and Rovere, G.D. (1984) Anabolic steroids: a review of the literature. *Am .Sports Med.*, **12**, 469–84.

IAAF (1982) IAAF Doping Control Regulations and Guidelines, London.

IAAF (1992) IAAF Arbitration Panel Statement, June, London.

International Olympic Committee (1990) International Olympic Charter against Doping in Sport, Medical Commission, internal communication.

IOC (1994) Doping Classes and Methods of the International Olympic Committee. IOC, Lausanne, September.

IOC/IF Agreement against Doping in Sport, Medical Commission, internal communication, June 1993.

Maheu, R. (1978) L'éducation et le sport, in *Sport, A Prison of Measured Time*, (ed. J.M. Brohm), InkLinks, London.

Matlin, C., Delday, M., Hay, S. *et al.* (1987) The effect of the anabolic agent, clenbuterol, on the overloaded rat skeletal muscle. *Bioscience* reports, **7**, 143–8.

Moynihan, C. and Coe, S. (1987) *The Misuse of Drugs in Sport*, Department of the Environment, London.

Porritt, A. (1965) Doping. *Journal of Sports Medicine and Physical Fitness*, **5**.

Royal Society of New Zealand (1990) *Drugs and Medicines in Sport*, Thomas Publications, Wellington.

Senate Standing Committee on Environment, Recreation and the Arts, Australia (1989) *Drugs in Sport*. Interim Report (The Black Report), Australian Government Publishing Service, Canberra.

Senate Standing Committee on Environment, Recreation and the Arts, Australia (1990) *Drugs in sport*. Second Report (The Black Report), Australian Government Publishing Service, Canberra.

Sports Council (1993) *Doping Control Information Booklet No. 2, IOC Doping Classes*, the Sports Council, London.

van der Merwe, P.J., Muller, F.R. and Muller, F.O. (1988) Caffeine in sport: urinary excretion of caffeine in healthy volunteers after intake of common caffeine containing beverages. *South African Medical Journal*, 74, 163–4.

Voy, R. (1991) *Drugs, Sport and Politics*, Human Kinetics Publishers, Illinois, USA.

Williams, M.H. (1983) *Ergogenic Aids and Sport*, Human Kinetics Publishers, Illinois, USA.

Yesalis, C.E. (1993) *Anabolic Steroids in Sport and Exercise*, Human Kinetics Publishers, Illinois, USA.

2.11 FURTHER READING

Hemery, D. (1991) *Sporting Excellence*, Collins Willow, London.

Hemmersbach, P. and Birkeland, K.I. (eds) (1994) *Blood Samples in Doping Control*, On Demand Publishing, Oslo.

Radford, P. (1992) The fight against doping in sport: the last five years. *Sport and Leisure*, May/June.

Sports Council (1993) Doping Control Information Booklet No. 4, Guide to Allowable Medications, Sports Council, London.

Sympathomimetic amines and their antagonists

3

David J. Armstrong

3.1 SUMMARY

The sympathetic nervous system (SNS) controls many aspects of bodily function, including cardiac function, blood pressure, airways diameter and the somatic manifestations of anxiety. Consequently, drugs which either mimic or block the SNS have considerable potential for abuse. The commonest therapeutic uses of sympathomimetic drugs are in the treatment of asthma and coughs and colds. The possible stimulation of both the cardiovascular system and the central nervous system (CNS) by some drugs in this class has led to their being banned by the International Olympic Committee (IOC). Beta adrenoceptor blocking drugs (antagonists) are widely used to treat high blood pressure and angina pectoris. It is important that patients who are receiving these drugs understand the effects they have upon performance and tolerance of exercise. Beta blockers reduce the symptoms of anxiety which are mediated by the SNS, e.g. muscle tremor. The potential for abuse exists in those activities in which fine motor control is more important than oxygen utilization, e.g. snooker, shooting and archery. Alpha adrenoceptor antagonists, though commonly prescribed for the treatment of hypertension, are not the subject of abuse in sport.

Sympathomimetic amines are exogenous drugs which mimic the effects of noradrenaline and adrenaline which in turn are the naturally occurring (endogenous) agonists of the SNS. Antagonists are drugs which block the effects of the agonists.

3.2 ANATOMY AND PHYSIOLOGY OF THE AUTONOMIC NERVOUS SYSTEM (ANS)

The ANS is divided into the parasympathetic and sympathetic branches. The parasympathetic nervous system (PNS) is that branch of the ANS

Drugs in Sport, 2nd edn. Edited by David R. Mottram. Published in 1996 by E & FN Spon, London. ISBN 0 419 18890 8

which is responsible for controlling many bodily functions under normal resting conditions. The SNS is that branch of the ANS which prepares the body for what is often referred to as the fight/flight or fright response, i.e. it increases cardiac activity, dilates the airways and increases blood sugar concentrations but slows down digestion and the passage of food through the gastrointestinal tract.

The SNS consists of parts of the brainstem and the spinal cord, certain nerves arising from the spinal cord and the adrenal glands. Because the sympathetic nerves arise principally from the thoracic and lumbar regions of the spinal cord, this branch of the ANS is referred to as the thoraco-lumbar division of the ANS. The nerves of the PNS arise from the brain-stem and the sacral region of the spinal cord and it is referred to, there-fore, as the craniosacral division of the ANS.

The sympathetic nerves do not go directly from the spinal cord to the target glands or effectors, e.g. the heart and lungs, etc. Instead they make synapses with a second order of neurones in structures known as ganglia, which lie adjacent to the spinal cord and which form the paravertebral chain. Nerves between the spinal cord and the glanglia are pre-ganglionic nerves and those between ganglia and the effectors are post-ganglionic. The junctions between neurones and between neurones and effectors are synapses. The neurotransmitter released by the pre-ganglionic nerve fibres is acetylcholine, consideration of which is beyond the scope of this chapter. The neurotransmitter released by the post-ganglionic nerves of the SNS is noradrenaline (Figure 3.1). The effects of noradrenaline are supplemented by adrenaline which is released from the chromaffin cells in the medullae of the adrenal glands. Noradrenaline and adrenaline exert different effects on the body because they affect different receptors on cells in tissues and organs (Table 3.1).

The classification of adrenoceptors was first defined by Alhquist in 1948. Adrenoceptors are defined on the basis of those drugs that stimulate them, i.e. agonists, and those drugs that block or antagonize them, i.e. antagonists. Alpha receptors are those that demonstrate

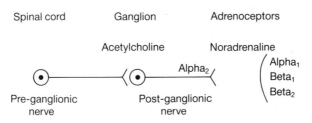

Figure 3.1 The distribution of pre- and post-synaptic adrenoceptors.

the following sensitivity to agonists: adrenaline > noradrenaline >> isoprenaline (a synthetic sympathomimetic drug). Beta receptors demonstrate a different sensitivity: isoprenaline > adrenaline > noradrenaline.

Table 3.1 The effects of the sympathetic nervous system

Effector	Receptor	Response
Heart		
S-A node	$Beta_1$	↑ Heart rate
Ventricles	$Beta_1$	↑ Force of concentration
Lungs		
Bronchial muscle	$Alpha_1$	Contraction
Bronchial muscle	$Beta_2$	Relaxation
Blood vessels		
Coronary	$Alpha_1$	Constriction
	$Beta_2$	Dilation
Skeletal muscle	$Alpha_1$	Constriction
	$Beta_2$	Dilation
Skin	$Alpha_1$	Constriction
Renal	$Alpha_1$	Constriction
GIT		
Motility	$Beta_1$	↓ Contraction
Liver	$Beta_2$	Glycogenolysis
Pancreas	$Alpha_1$	↓ Insulin
	$Beta_2$	↑ Insulin
Adipose tissue	$Beta_2$	Lipolysis
Eye		
Radial muscle of iris	$Alpha_1$	Contraction (mydriasis)
Ciliary muscle	$Beta_2$	Relaxation for distant vision

Classification of adrenoceptors has been extended to two sub-types of both alpha and beta adrenoceptors based upon sensitivity to selective agonists:

Receptor	Location	Agonist
Alpha$_1$	Post-synaptic alpha receptors	Phenylephrine
Alpha$_2$	Pre-synaptic alpha receptors	Clonidine
Beta$_1$	Post-synaptic beta receptors	Noradrenaline
Beta$_2$	Post-synaptic beta receptors	Salbutamol

The adrenoceptors subserve different functions, depending upon their location – stimulation of alpha$_1$ receptors causes vasoconstriction; alpha$_2$ receptors inhibit the release of noradrenaline from post-ganglionic sympathetic nerves; beta$_1$ receptors increase the rate and force of contraction of heart muscle; stimulation of beta$_2$ receptors causes bronchodilation.

3.3 ADRENERGIC AGONISTS

3.3.1 ENDOGENOUS AGONISTS

Adrenaline (epinephrine) is the hormone released from the adrenal medullae during stress. It stimulates alpha$_1$, alpha$_2$, beta$_1$ and beta$_2$ receptors. Beta$_1$ receptor stimulation increases heart rate and myocardial contractility and hence increases cardiac output. Stimulation of alpha$_1$ receptors causes vasoconstriction and raises systolic arterial blood pressure. Stimulation of beta$_2$ receptors in blood vessels in skeletal muscle causes vasodilation and may decrease peripheral resistance and hence cause a fall in diastolic blood pressure. Neurogenic vasodilation during exercise will be supplemented by humoral vasodilation in exercising muscles. The magnitude of this response is directly related to the exercising muscle mass. Adrenaline also increases respiratory rate, tidal volume and hence minute ventilation. It is an effective, rapidly acting bronchodilator (15 minutes) through stimulation of beta$_2$ receptors. The duration of action is between 60 and 90 minutes after either subcutaneous injection or inhalation from a pressurized aerosol.

Noradrenaline (norepinephrine) is the neurotransmitter at sympathetic nerve endings. It has similar effects to adrenaline on beta$_1$ receptors in the heart. However, it is a less potent agonist of alpha receptors and has little effect on beta$_2$ receptors. It is contraindicated for the treatment of asthma. It increases peripheral vascular resistance, systolic and diastolic arterial blood pressures and cardiac output. It is banned by the IOC although it is rarely used therapeutically.

3.3.2 SYMPATHOMIMETIC AMINES

These are manufactured drugs which mimic the actions of the SNS, primarily through stimulating one or more adrenoceptors. Examples include ephedrine and isoprenaline. Unlike adrenaline and isoprenaline, ephedrine is active orally. It has high bioavailability and 10 times the duration of action of adrenaline. It is less likely to cause tachycardia but causes greater CNS stimulation than adrenaline. Ephedrine is only a weak bronchodilator. Its primary mode of action is the release of stored catecholamines, i.e. adrenaline and noradrenaline. It is commonly used as a topical nasal decongestant and is included in numerous cough and cold remedies. It is banned by the IOC because of its cardiac stimulant and amphetamine-like CNS stimulant activity.

Isoprenaline is a potent beta receptor agonist that has little effect upon alpha receptors. When applied as an aerosol, it is a potent bronchodilator. Indeed, it was the original beta agonist to be used as a topical bronchodilator. It also serves as the best example of the problems inherent in the use of a non-selective beta agonist. Although stimulation of $beta_2$ receptors causes bronchodilation, simultaneous stimulation of $beta_1$ receptors increases heart rate to potentially dangerous levels. Since an asthmatic attack causes great anxiety, heart rate will already be elevated by increased SNS activity and the circumstances are ideal for the induction of cardiac arrhythmia. Indeed, following the introduction of isoprenaline in the 1960s, there was a significant increase in the incidence of fatal cardiac arrhythmias in those asthmatics treated with inhaled isoprenaline. Whether this was due to incorrect use/abuse of the drug or to the inherent problems of a non-selective beta agonist has been the subject of much inconclusive debate. Like adrenaline and ephedrine, the use of isoprenaline in competition is banned by the IOC.

Sympathomimetic amines have many therapeutic indications, including asthma, cough and cold remedies, cardiopulmonary resuscitation, anaphylactic shock, cardiogenic shock, heart block, drug overdoses which cause hypotension, local anaesthetic preparations and topical nasal decongestants (British National Formulary (BNF), 1995). Perhaps those therapeutic uses which are more likely to pose problems to the sportsperson are the treatments of asthma and of coughs and colds.

Asthma

Asthma is a disease which is characterized by widespread narrowing of the peripheral airways which, in the early stages, can be paroxysmal and reversible. There are numerous causes of asthma, e.g. allergy, drugs, occupational pollution, emotion, stress and viral infection of the upper respiratory tract (URT). Exercise can also be a trigger factor for an asthmatic attack. Asthma was formerly classified as either extrinsic or intrinsic depending upon the presence or absence of a positive skin-prick test. However, that distinction has fallen into disrepute because it had little or no relevance to treatment of the disease. Instead, treatment is now based upon the understanding that asthma is a chronic inflammatory disease of the airways. The underlying inflammatory process can be demonstrated by biopsy during both remission and relapse from symptoms. It is characterized by desquamation of the epithelial lining of the airways, infiltration of the airway lining by pro-inflammatory cells (particularly eosinophils), oedema of the airway lining, increased secretion of viscous mucus and hypertrophy of airway smooth muscle. Acute symptoms are evoked by bronchoconstriction.

Prophylactic therapy (prevention of an attack)

1. Avoidance of allergens or 'trigger factors'. If the asthmatic can be shown to be hypersensitive to either an inhaled or an ingested allergen, then exposure should be reduced to an absolute minimum. This will help to reduce the frequency of the attacks.
2. Sodium cromoglycate (SCG). This is one of the safest drugs of any class. Administration is by inhalation of dry powder, by aerosol or nebulizer. The only common side-effect is generation of a cough by inhalation of the dry powder. This can be circumvented either by aerosol, if the patient can use one correctly; by prior administration of a beta$_2$ agonist or, most simply, by drinking a little water after administration of the drug. It is effective in 40–50% of children but relatively ineffective in adults. The mode of action is controversial. The classical explanation is that SCG stabilizes the membrane of mast cells and prevents the release of the mediators of inflammation and bronchoconstriction. However, at least 39 other mast-cell stabilizers have been ineffective in the treatment of asthma. There is an increasing volume of evidence which suggests that the anti-inflammatory activity of SCG may be attributable to inhibition of airway sensory receptors, and hence of neurogenic inflammation of the airways. It must be emphasized to the patient that SCG prevents airway inflammation but does not cause bronchodilation of constricted airways. Consequently, it will not relieve the symptoms of an attack. SCG should be used continually to prevent attacks and not to relieve symptoms of an established attack. If this is not explained to patients then they may dismiss the drug as being ineffective. The duration of action is 2–4 hours. Nedocromil sodium, a derivative of SCG, has a similar profile of activity but a longer duration of action (6–12 hours). SCG has no effect on the cardiovascular system and is of no ergogenic value. It should be used from Step 2 onwards of the British Thoracic Society (BTS) guidelines (1993) for the treatment of asthma. Its use is permitted by the IOC.

3. Steroids. Glucocorticosteroids are the mainstay of the treatment of chronic asthma in both children and adults. They are also a quintessential component of the emergency treatment of asthma in both children and adults. At the molecular level they increase the synthesis of anti-inflammatory mediators. Therapeutically, they decrease the swelling and oedema of the inflamed bronchial mucosa , mucus secretion and airway hypersensitivity, whilst increasing the sensitivity to beta$_2$ agonists. Steroids may be administered orally, by injection or by inhalation. Oral and intravenous steroids produce many unwanted side-effects. Inhaled steroids (betamethasone, beclamethasone and budesonide) can be used to replace oral steroids in many asthmatics and are without systemic side-effects in therapeutic doses. They are, therefore, the formulation of choice for administration of steroids. Inhaled/topical steroids do not have a positive ergogenic effect and are permitted by the IOC. The glucocorticoid group of steroid hormones has different effects from those of the anabolic steroids which are discussed in Chapter 7.

Bronchodilator therapy (relief of symptoms)

There are three groups of drugs which are used to relax the constricted airways of the asthmatic during an attack; therefore these drugs are used to treat the symptoms of asthma, rather than to prevent an attack from occurring.

1. Selective beta$_2$ adrenoceptor agonists
The first beta agonist to be used in the treatment of asthma was isoprenaline. The increase in asthma mortality which paralleled the introduction of isoprenaline prompted the development of a new generation of selective beta$_2$ agonists for use as bronchodilators. Those available on prescription in the UK are listed in Table 3.2.

Table 3.2 Selective beta$_2$ adrenoceptor agonists

Salbutamol (Ventolin)(albuterol, USA)
Terbutaline (Bricanyl)(brethine, USA)
Bambuterol (Bambec)
Rimiterol (Pulmadil)
Fenoterol (Berotec)
Pirbuterol (Exirel)
Reproterol (Bronchodil)
Salmeterol (Serevent)
Tulobuterol (Brelomax; Respacal)

All the selective beta$_2$ agonists are potent bronchodilators. Salbutamol and terbutaline are the beta$_2$ agonists most frequently used in the UK. There are many formulations of salbutamol and terbutaline, including tablets, slow-release tablets, elixirs, aerosols and dry powder and solutions for injection and inhalation from a nebulizer. Inhalation is the route of choice because it is the most rapidly effective (1–2 minutes) and is associated with the fewest side-effects. Tremor is the only common side-effect after inhalation. The side-effects after oral administration include fine tremor (usually of the hands), nervous tension and headache. Tachycardia, peripheral vasodilation and hypokalaemia may occur after oral dosing but are commoner after intravenous injection. Tachycardia is most uncommon after aerosol inhalation. The duration of action of salbutamol and terbutaline after aerosol administration is approximately 4–6 hours. All but rimiterol and fenoterol are active after oral administration (Clark and Cochrane, 1984). Rimiterol has the shortest duration of action.

Historically, controversy over the use of sympathomimetics has centred upon the potential ergogenic value of the cardiovascular system and CNS side-effects that these drugs can evoke. Thus, alpha agonists, non-selective alpha/beta agonists and non-selective beta agonists have been banned. Ephedrine and related substances are classed as 'Sympathomimetic Amines' and belong in Class 1A (Stimulants) of the IOC doping classes. All but two, selective beta$_2$ agonists, are now classed within Doping Class 1A and are banned. **Only salbutamol and terbutaline are now permitted and then only by inhalation and following written notification to the relevant medical authority by the team physician** (IOC, 1994). The presence of a prohibited beta$_2$ agonist in a urine sample, either in or out of competition, may be reported by the laboratory. However, confusion may arise when sporting federations do not concur with the IOC. For example the use of salbutamol is banned by law by the French Cycling Federation and Ministry of Sport. This has led to four professional cyclists (including Miguel Indurain, five times winner of the Tour de France) testing positive in 1994. Indurain was quickly exonerated of misuse of salbutamol (which had been administered by inhaler to treat a pollen allergy) by cycling's ruling body, Union Cycliste Internationale, and by the IOC, in the person of Prince Alexandre de Merode (IOC Vice President and Chairman of the IOC Medical Commission). Clearly this is unacceptable and places the sportsperson in an invidious position.

The 1992 Olympics in Barcelona turned the spotlight on to a new controversy surrounding selective beta$_2$ agonists, namely the putative anabolic effects of beta$_2$ agonists, in general, and clenbuterol in particular. Subsequently, the classification of selective beta$_2$ agonists was changed dramatically. All beta$_2$ agonists, except salbutamol and terbutaline, were reclassified into Subgroup 2 (Other Anabolic Agents) of doping class C,

Anabolic Agents. This subgroup included only $beta_2$ agonists and specified clenbuterol as the example. Thus the IOC is unequivocal towards this drug. However, the justification for their decision is rather more equivocal.

Clenbuterol is a long-acting, $beta_2$ agonist which is licensed for the treatment of asthma in Germany, Italy and Spain. The drug is only available as an oral formulation. It is not licensed for human use in the UK. It is, however, licensed for veterinary use in horses and cattle (*Pharm. J.*, 1992). This dichotomy embodies the controversy concerning the anabolic, and hence ergogenic, potential of clenbuterol. Much of the evidence for anabolic activity is drawn from animal experiments. For example clenbuterol caused a 12% increase in muscle weight in rats (Yang and McElliott, 1989). The effect was selective for skeletal muscle and was the result of hypertrophy, not hyperplasia. It was blocked by the selective $beta_2$ receptor antagonist, ICI-118,551 (Choo, Horon, Little and Rothwell, 1992). The increase in muscle mass is not mediated by other anabolic hormones, e.g. growth hormone. The precise mechanism of increased protein accumulation is not understood. There is evidence that protein synthesis is increased and that protein degradation is decreased. Further evidence that clenbuterol affects skeletal muscle has been derived from denervation studies in which the drug prevented muscle atrophy and, what is more, induced hyperplasia. The German pharmaceutical company which manufactures clenbuterol is purported to claim not to have data from human studies on the effect of the drug upon skeletal muscle.

In addition to the potential for increasing skeletal muscle mass, $beta_2$ agonists have an incontrovertible effect upon lipid metabolism (Katzung, 1995). They increase lipolysis, decrease fat deposition and thereby increase lean body mass (Yang and McElliott, 1989). They also increase non-shivering thermogenesis via beta receptors in brown adipose tissue. The combination of increased muscle mass and decreased body fat leads to increased lean to fat ratio. This is a highly desirable characteristic for livestock and may underpin the anecdotal evidence of drug misuse by breeders.

The IOC banned the use of clenbuterol from July 1992. Two British weightlifters were withdrawn from the Olympic Games that year when they tested positive for clenbuterol. Two German athletes have also been banned for using the drug. There is anecdotal evidence that misuse of clenbuterol is epidemic amongst the sporting community. That the IOC acted so unequivocally to clarify the situation on clenbuterol suggests that the evidence for abuse of the drug is more than anecdotal, although, because of its nature, it might not be expected to be published in the scientific press.

2. Methyl xanthines
Both theophylline and aminophylline (the soluble ethylenediamine derivative of theophylline) are related to caffeine. They are classed as

additional bronchodilators and should be confined to Stages 3, 4 and 5 of the BTS guidelines (1993). They constitute the second line of broncho-dilator therapy. They must be given orally or intravenously, and the risk of side-effects is much greater than with selective beta$_2$ agonists. The dose should be adjusted to provide a therapeutic plasma theophylline concentration of 10–20 μg/ml. Although the absolute threshold varies between individuals, both the frequency and severity of side-effects increase with the plasma concentration. Thus 15 μg/ml is associated with nausea, vomiting, abdominal pains, headache, nervousness and muscle tremor. Plasma concentrations between 20 and 40 μg/ml can cause convulsions and ventricular arrhythmias, increasing in severity from tachycardia to fibrillation and ultimately cardiac arrest. Sustained-release tablets are now the formulation of choice because they have reduced the fluctuations in plasma concentrations of theophylline and hence have reduced the incidence of side-effects. Cardiovascular side-effects are associated more with theophylline, and CNS side-effects with caffeine. Caffeine is banned by the IOC if the urinary concentration exceeds 12 μg/ml.

The mode of action of methyl xanthines is contentious. The classical explanation is that they inhibit phosphodiesterase, the enzyme responsible for the inactivation of cAMP. However, the plasma concentration required to achieve this inhibition *in vivo* is a factor of 10 times the accepted upper limit of therapeutic plasma concentrations. Alternatively, there is evidence that methyl xanthines antagonize adenosine receptors. Theophylline and aminophylline also down-regulate the activity of pro-inflammatory cells. Whatever the mode of action, these drugs have a place in the treatment of both chronic and acute severe asthma.

3. Anticholinergic drugs
The PNS causes contraction of bronchial smooth muscle by the effect of acetylcholine upon muscarinic cholinergic receptors. Theoretically, therefore, anticholinergic drugs should be of benefit in the treatment of asthma. In practice, they have a greater bronchodilator effect in chronic bronchitics than in asthmatics. Inhaled ipratropium bromide, which is a quaternary derivative of atropine, is a useful alternative for individuals who cannot tolerate or respond to beta$_2$ agonists. It is classed as an additional bronchodilator and should be used in Stage 4 or 5 of the BTS guidelines (1993). It has a slow onset time (30–60 minutes), is active for 3–4 hours and hence should be taken four times per day. Oxitropium bromide, a derivative of ipratropium, has a longer duration of action and need only be taken twice daily. Neither drug will give rapid relief of symptoms. The side-effects of antagonism of the PNS are dry mouth, urinary retention and constipation. However, ipratropium bromide is poorly absorbed and is not associated with

significant side-effects when standard doses are administered by inhalation. The IOC permits the use of ipratropium bromide for the treatment of asthma.

Treatment of asthma is now directed at arresting and reversing the inflammatory process. The emphasis has shifted from the excessive and inappropriate use of beta$_2$ agonist bronchodilator therapy towards the early use of anti-inflammatory drugs. Beta$_2$ agonists merely relieve the symptoms of asthma without addressing the underlying inflammation. This has been likened to 'painting over rust'. Guidelines for the treatment of chronic asthma have been prepared in several countries, including Britain and the United States. They constitute a systematic approach to the treatment of increasing severity of symptoms. It must be remembered that the treatment of asthma can also be stepped down if the severity of the symptoms declines.

The following is a résumé of the guidelines published by the BTS in 1993.

Step 1
Occasional use of relief bronchodilators
Inhaled short-acting beta$_2$ agonists should be used as required. If they are needed more than once daily, then treatment should progress to Step 2.
N.B. patient compliance and inhaler technique should be assessed before progressing to the next stage in treatment.

Step 2
Regular inhaled anti-inflammatory drugs
Inhaled short-acting beta$_2$ agonists can be used as required, PLUS beclomethasone or budesonide (100–400 µg twice daily) by metered dose inhaler. A child may be prescribed SCG or nedocromil sodium. If this is not successful, then inhaled steroids should be substituted for the mast-cell stabilizer.

Step 3
High-dose inhaled steroids
Inhaled short-acting beta$_2$ agonists can be used as required, beclomethasone or budesonide (increased to 800–2000 µg daily) via a large volume spacer.
Alternatives: if the patient has unacceptable problems with high-dose inhaled steroids, the following drugs may be tried:

- long-acting inhaled beta$_2$ agonists (salmeterol);
- sustained-release theophylline;
- SCG or nedocromil sodium.

Step 4

High-dose inhaled steroids and regular bronchodilators

Inhaled short-acting beta$_2$ agonists can be used as required. Beclomethasone or budesonide (increased to 800–2000 μg daily) via a large volume spacer, PLUS a sequential therapeutic trial of one or more of the following:

- long-acting inhaled beta$_2$ agonists;
- sustained-release theophylline;
- inhaled ipratropium or oxitropium bromide;
- long-acting oral beta$_2$ agonists;
- SCG or nedocromil sodium.

Step 5

Addition of regular steroid tablets

Inhaled short-acting beta$_2$ agonists can be used as required, PLUS beclomethasone or budesonide (increased to 800–2000 μg daily) via a large volume spacer, PLUS one or more of the long-acting bronchodilators, PLUS regular prednisolone tablets in a single daily dose.

Stepping down

Treatment should be reviewed every 3 to 6 months. If the patient has been stable during that period, then it may be possible to introduce a slow, stepwise reduction in therapy.

Exercise-induced asthma

Exercise-induced asthma (EIA) can be defined as large changes in airway resistance induced by standardized exercise (Bundgaard, 1985). It is, perhaps, more appropriate to think of it as post-exercise bronchoconstriction, because the maximum decrease in peak expiratory flow rate (PEFR) and forced expiratory volume in the first second (FEV$_1$) normally occurs between 15 and 20 minutes after the exercise has been completed. The ventilatory changes in EIA are identical to those observed during a spontaneous asthma attack, i.e. decreased V$_t$ (tidal volume), PEFR, FEV$_1$, FVC (forced vital capacity) and increased residual volume (RV) leading to hyperventilation and dyspnoea. Between 50% and 70% of asthmatics experience bronchoconstriction after exercise. Non-asthmatics are not affected in this way.

Exercise of less than 1 minute duration actually increases FEV$_1$ in the asthmatic. After 1 minute the FEV$_1$ begins to decline, most dramatically once the exercise has been terminated. The response may consist of just an early phase or may also demonstrate a late phase. The severity of the bronchoconstriction is decreased by warm temperature and high humidity. Cooling and drying of the airways are thought to be responsible for EIA. The severity of the bronchoconstriction is directly related to the degree of hyperpnoea and hence to the duration and intensity of the workload. Warm-up can reduce EIA. Some asthmatics are refractory to EIA for up to 30 minutes after initial exercise and bronchoconstriction. Awareness of the potential benefits of warm-up and the refractory period can be incorporated into training sessions to maximize efficiency and to minimize bronchoconstriction. There is no diurnal variation in the response to exercise. The possibility of increased sensitivity during the pollen season is controversial (Bundgaard, 1985).

The management of EIA consists of both non-drug and drug interventions and is directed at two goals – optimal control of baseline symptoms and prevention of the induction of an asthmatic attack by exercise. Relief of symptoms of EIA should be considered as an indication that the first two goals have not been achieved satisfactorily.

Non-drug therapy

- Aerobic fitness. Fitness does not prevent EIA, as indicated by the number of Olympians who suffer from the syndrome. However, aerobic fitness does improve lung function, retards deterioration in lung function with age (in non-asthmatics) and enables asthmatics to exercise with less EIA. It also facilitates social interactions and improves self-esteem of asthmatics. There is no evidence to suggest that aerobic training is deleterious to asthmatics, provided that their treatment is optimal and that they have a satisfactory management plan which includes access to appropriate bronchodilator therapy, if required. The only contraindication for aerobic training in asthmatics would be if they demonstrated significant arterial desaturation upon exercise-testing during laboratory investigations.

- Minimize cooling and drying of the airways. This can be achieved in several ways. Firstly, if possible, select physical activities, such as walking and swimming, which are less likely to evoke bronchoconstriction. Secondly, utilize nasal breathing whenever possible. Thirdly, seek to avoid exercising in a cold, dry environment. If this is unavoidable, then a face mask may reduce cooling and drying of the airways.

- Warm-up. This can help to maximize the benefit of the training session and, if possible, should take cognizance of the refractory period that many asthmatics experience after an initial episode of EIA.

- Monitoring of PEFR. This can help the asthmatic to monitor the efficacy of baseline control. It will provide objective assessment of the current status of the asthmatic's airways. If bronchoconstriction is present prior to exercise, then either additional therapy is indicated or participation may be counselled against, depending upon the severity of the condition.

Drug therapy

1. Beta$_2$ agonists. These drugs are the most effective prophylactic treatment of EIA. Salbutamol and terbutaline are the only beta$_2$ agonists which are permitted by the IOC (September , 1994) and then only when administered by aerosol inhalation and accompanied by written notification to the IOC Medical Commission by the team doctor. Beta$_2$ agonists induce bronchodilation within 1 to 2 minutes and afford protection against EIA for approximately 2 to 4 hours (Morton and Fitch, 1992). Salmeterol is slower in onset but effective for up to 12 hours. It is indicated for the prevention of EIA (BNF, 1995; BTS, 1993). However, its use is not permitted by the IOC.
2. Mast-cell stabilizers. Neither SCG nor nedocromil sodium (a derivative of SCG) are as effective as beta$_2$ agonists in the prevention of EIA. They should be administered 10 to 15 minutes before the start of exercise and will provide up to 2 hours' protection against bronchoconstriction (Morton and Fitch, 1992). They are more likely to be effective in children than in adults. Even so, they are only completely effective in 45% of children. Their use is permitted by the IOC. It should be noted that SCG is available as a compound formulation with isoprenaline (BNF, 1995). Isoprenaline is banned by the IOC and hence the compound formulation should be avoided by sportspersons.
3. Methyl xanthines. Theophylline in plasma concentrations of 10–24 µg/ml afforded incomplete protection in a group of 12 child asthmatics (Bundgaard, 1985). In two other studies, theophylline relieved the symptoms of EIA but did not prevent EIA from occurring. The narrow therapeutic window of theophylline, coupled with the many factors that can elevate plasma concentrations and increase toxicity of the drug, mean that it is impracticable to administer a single dose as a prophylactic against EIA. The greater risk of cardiovascular side-effects from theophylline than from either inhaled beta$_2$ agonists or mast-cell stabilizers would relegate theophylline to the third line of therapy for EIA. Its role, albeit minor, in the prevention of EIA is in the establishment of better baseline control of symptoms as indicated in the BTS guidelines. Theophylline is not banned by the IOC.
4. Steroids. The time to onset of anti-inflammatory effects of steroids is 8 to 12 hours. Hence, single doses of inhaled steroids immediately prior to exercise do not afford protection against EIA. A 4-week trial of

inhaled betamethasone valerate produced a significant improvement in EIA, but this was probably related to better baseline control of asthma. Inhaled budesonide twice a day for 4 weeks produced a significant improvement in resting pulmonary function and in the benefit derived from pre-exercise terbutaline. The role of inhaled steroids in the treatment of EIA is now considered to be in the establishment of satisfactory baseline control of symptoms (BTS, 1993).

5. Anticholinergic drugs. These drugs are of minor importance in the treatment of EIA. Bronchodilation produced by inhalation of 0.5 mg ipratropium bromide was equal to that of a beta$_2$ agonist but was not effective against EIA (Bundgaard, 1985). Two studies have demonstrated a synergistic effect between SCG and ipratropium bromide in the treatment of EIA (Bundgaard, 1985). However, ipratropium bromide alone does not compare with beta$_2$ agonists in either the prevention or the reversal of EIA. The use of both ipratropium and its longer-acting derivative, oxitropium, is permitted by the IOC.

Cough and cold

Cough is a protective reflex that is initiated by either mechanical or chemical stimulation of the oral pharynx, larynx, trachea or bronchi. It is designed to remove mucus from the URT. Most commonly it is a symptom of a self-limiting URT infection which will normally resolve, without treatment, within 3 to 4 days. Antibiotics are of no value because the infection is normally viral and not bacterial. Less frequently, cough is a symptom of serious disease of the respiratory tract, but this is unlikely to be relevant to an individual who is participating in competitive sport.

The important therapeutic distinction is between productive and nonproductive coughs. A productive cough is often caused by a bacterial infection and may require antibiotic as well as antitussive therapy. A nonproductive cough is normally caused by a viral infection of the throat and often marks the onset of a 'cold'. Other causes of coughing include bronchoconstriction (in asthmatics), drainage of excess mucus from the nasopharynx (particularly when lying down) and tenacious mucus which cannot be moved adequately by the action of cilia on the respiratory epithelium.

Treatment of cough and cold

There are many preparations which can be bought over the counter (OTC) for the treatment of coughs and colds. Very often they contain more than one active ingredient, some of which are banned by the IOC, e.g. sympathomimetics and narcotic analgesics. Therefore, great care must be taken by the sportsperson when purchasing a cough or cold remedy for consumption during the competition season.

The major classes of antitussive drugs are:

- cough suppressants – narcotic analgesics and antihistamines;
- expectorants;
- demulcents;
- vasoconstrictors;
- bronchodilators.

1. Cough suppressants

Centrally acting cough suppressants reduce coughing by inhibiting the cough centre in the medulla oblongata in the brainstem. The three main drugs in this category are codeine, pholcodine and dextromethorphan. Codeine is a narcotic analgesic and related to morphine. As a group, these drugs can cause both physical and psychological dependence and hence are potentially drugs of abuse. Codeine also causes respiratory depression and constipation. What is more, there is no conclusive evidence that codeine can completely suppress a cough. However, although codeine belongs within Group B (Narcotic Analgesics) it is permitted for medical use (IOC, November, 1994). The use of other centrally acting cough suppressants (dihydrocodeine, diphenoxylate, pholcodine and dextromethorphan) is permitted (IOC, September, 1994). Pholcodine and dextromethorphan are preferable to codeine because they cause less respiratory depression and constipation. They are present in many OTC preparations. Sportspersons should choose carefully when selecting a cough suppressant.

2. Antihistamines

Antihistamines reduce coughing by two mechanisms. Firstly, they have a central suppressant action. Secondly, their anticholinergic action reduces the rate of mucus secretion. They are not banned by the IOC. Antihistamines are usually accompanied by a warning that they can cause drowsiness. They are present in many cough and cold remedies, especially those which are recommended for use at night.

3. Expectorants

These are meant to increase the volume and decrease the viscosity of respiratory mucus. They are emetics, i.e. they cause vomiting at high concentrations. At sub-emetic doses they are thought to irritate the gastric mucosa, which in turn stimulates secretion of respiratory mucus by a vagal reflex. There is little evidence to suggest that OTC expectorants are effective. Consequently, they are sometimes dismissed as little more than harmless placebos, but this is not the case. Expectorants, such as squill and ipecacuanha, can be cardiotoxic in patients with renal impairment. Therefore, they are only indicated when tenacious mucus cannot be expectorated. Thick tenacious mucus that cannot be cleared by coughing is normally a feature of bacterial infections of the lower respiratory tract, not of viral infections of the URT. The former require antibiotic therapy, in which case an expectorant may be prescribed by a doctor rather than sold over the counter by a pharmacist, though this is seldom done. An alternative approach is to decrease the viscosity of mucus with a mucolytic. Acetylcysteine, carbocisteine and methylcysteine are mucolytics which are permitted by the IOC. However, these are indicated for treatment of chronic bronchitics and more severe asthmatics and, therefore, are unlikely to be of wide application in sportspersons. Steam is an excellent expectorant and mucolytic. As such it is an acceptable alternative to those drugs mentioned above.

4. Demulcents

Demulcents substitute for the natural function of the mucus, i.e. a mechanical and chemical barrier which coats and protects the epithelium of the respiratory tract. Viral infections destroy epithelial cells which contribute to the production of mucus; hence there is less mucus to protect the inflamed mucosa. A dry, persistent cough exacerbates the removal of cells and should be prevented. Demulcents are very effective in preventing dry, non-productive coughs. Simple linctus, syrups and lozenges containing glycerin (glycerol), honey and lemon are widely available. Some lozenges also contain a local anaesthetic (benzocaine), which may be advantageous for a particularly troublesome cough, and an antibacterial agent, cetylpyridinium, which is of dubious merit. Note that demulcents are only effective in those areas that they can reach, i.e. the oral pharynx and larynx. However, they are often all that is needed to treat a dry, non-productive cough caused by a self-limiting viral infection and they are quite safe. Their use is permitted by the IOC. In that respect, they are preferable to centrally acting cough suppressants.

5. Vasoconstrictors

Selective alpha$_1$ agonists, phenlephrine, phenylpropanolamine (PPA), oxymetazoline and xylometazoline, will reduce nasal secretions by decreasing blood flow to the respiratory mucosa. These drugs are described as decongestants. However, they may also increase the viscosity of respiratory secretions and cause congestion in some individuals. They are most effective in preventing the runny nose (rhinnorrhoea) that accompanies the common cold (coryzal syndrome), and which makes the external nares and alae so sore.

Pseudoephedrine, norpseudoephedrine, phenylephrine and PPA are powerful, orally active vasoconstrictors. Because of their stimulant effects upon the CNS (headache and anxiety) and cardiovascular system (elevated blood pressure, tachycardia and arrhythmia) they are banned by the IOC under Class 1A, Stimulants. Moreover, since they cannot be targeted to the desired site of action, topical formulations, i.e. drops or sprays, are the preferred route of administration. Ephedrine, oxymetazoline and xylometazoline are available as topical decongestants in the UK. Ephedrine is banned by the IOC. Oxymetazoline and xylometazoline are permitted as topical decongestants. They are potent, long-acting vasoconstrictors that need only be applied twice daily. They are the drugs of choice for the treatment of rhinnorrhoea associated with the common cold. Topical decongestants which contain phenylephrine and other drugs (Table 3.3) are permitted by the IOC (September, 1994).

Table 3.3 Other drugs permitted for topical treatment of nasal disorders

Generic name	Drug class	Formulation
Beclomethasone	Glucocorticosteroid	Aerosol and atomizer
Betamethasone	Glucocorticosteroid	Drops
Budesonide	Glucocorticosteroid	Aerosol
Flunisolide	Glucocorticosteroid	Spray
Fluticasone	Glucocorticosteroid	Spray
Oxymetazoline	Sympathomimetic	Spray and drops
Xylometazoline	Sympathomimetic	Spray and drops
Ipratropium	Anticholinergic	Spray
Azelastine	Antihistamine	Spray
Sodium cromoglycate	Mast-cell stabilizer	Spray
Betamethasone and Neomycin	Glucocorticosteroid Antibacterial	Drops
Tramazoline and Dexamethasone and Neomycin	Antihistamine Glucocorticosteroid Antibacterial	Aerosol

6. Bronchodilators

Selective beta$_2$ agonists are not used in any cough or cold medicines. Instead either a non-selective sympathomimetic (ephedrine or pseudoephedrine) or a xanthine, e.g. caffeine or theophylline, is used as a bronchodilator (or possibly as a decongestant). Both non-selective beta agonists and caffeine (when the plasma concentration exceeds 12 μg/ml) are banned by the IOC. Bronchodilators are only appropriate for lower respiratory tract infections where there is bronchoconstriction or a wheeze. Bronchodilators are of no relevance to the treatment of a congested pharynx, larynx or nasal cavity. Preparations which include a bronchodilator cannot be recommended to the sportsperson.

Table 3.4 Some of the more common drugs contained in OTC cough and cold medicines

Class of drugs	Examples
Narcotic analgesics	Codeine Pholcodine Dextromethorphan
Non-narcotic analgesics	Acetylsalicylic acid (aspirin) Paracetamol
Antihistamines	Brompheniramine Carbinoxamine Chlorpheniramine Diphenhydramine Diphenylpyraline Doxylamine Pheniramine Promethazine Triprolidine
Sympathomimetics[1]	Ephedrine Pseudoephedrine Phenylephrine[2] Phenylpropanolamine (PPA) Oxymetazoline[2] Xylometazoline[2]
Xanthines	Caffeine[3] Theophylline
Expectorants	Ammonium citrate Sodium citrate Ipecacuanha Squill Guaiphenesin

[1] Banned by the IOC
[2] Permitted as topical decongestants
[3] Banned if urine concentration $> 12\,\mu g/ml$

Self-help

The following are recommendations for self-treatment of coughs and colds:

1. Hydration. This will prevent dehydration when there is copious secretion and will aid expectoration when a cough is non-productive.
2. Since a cough is designed to remove mucus, a productive cough should **never** be suppressed. A decongestant may be used if the secretions are watery and arise from the nasopharynx. A purulent secretion requires antibiotic therapy from a medical practitioner.
3. A cough should only be suppressed when it is dry and non-productive (often a prelude to a viral infection of the URT). However, demulcents are preferable to cough suppressants if the cause is an inflamed throat, because they have no side-effects and they are not banned by the IOC.
4. Many cough and cold remedies cannot be recommended because they contain irrational combinations of either cough suppressants and expectorants and antihistamines or decongestants and expectorants. Some compound preparations contain sub-therapeutic concentrations of the active ingredients. Many of the active constituents are banned by the IOC (Table 3.4). Therefore, always attempt to purchase a product with a single active constituent. Always check the list of active drugs in the pharmaceutical preparation against the list of banned drugs that is readily available. If in doubt about either the mode of action or the type of drug and whether it is likely to be banned, ask a pharmacist and then your coach. The major groups of drugs which are contained in OTC cough and cold medicines are summarized in Table 3.4.
5. Sportspersons should heed the following warning from the IOC (August, 1993): '**Thus no product for use in colds, flu or hay fever purchased by a competitor or given to him/her should be used without first checking with a doctor or pharmacist that the product does not contain a drug of the banned stimulant class**'.

3.4 ADRENERGIC ANTAGONISTS

3.4.1 BETA ANTAGONISTS (BETA BLOCKERS)

Beta antagonists block beta adrenoceptors and hence prevent adrenaline and noradrenaline from exerting those effects which are beta-receptor mediated. The significance of this group of drugs to the sportsperson is two-fold. Firstly, they are being prescribed increasingly for a wide variety of clinical conditions and people may be unaware of the effects that this will have upon their ability to perform exercise. Secondly, beta blockers are developing into a major group of drugs of abuse in sport, principally because of their ability to reduce the effects of anxiety.

Beta receptors are widely distributed throughout the tissues and organs of the body, e.g. heart, blood vessels, bronchi, eyes, liver, pancreas and gastrointestinal tract, adipose tissue, skeletal muscle and the brain

(Table 3.1). They can be subdivided into $beta_1$ and $beta_2$ receptors. $Beta_1$ receptors predominate in the heart. They also stimulate lipolysis in adipose tissue, thus increasing the plasma concentration of free fatty acids which can be metabolized by skeletal muscle. $Beta_2$ receptors cause bronchodilation, release insulin from the pancreas and stimulate glycogenolysis in liver and skeletal muscle. These last three effects all increase glucose availability to the exercising muscle. Hence, a $beta_2$ antagonist would be expected to decrease endurance capability. All beta blockers block $beta_1$ receptors. Those antagonists with a greater affinity for $beta_1$ as opposed to $beta_2$ receptors are described as cardioselective. Cardioselectivity is lost as the dose is increased, so the distinction may not be of great therapeutic significance (Hudson, 1985). Table 3.5 indicates the cardioselectivity of some common beta blockers.

Table 3.5   The cardioselectivity and lipid solubility of some commonly used beta blockers

Beta blocker	Cardioselectivity	Lipid solubility
Propranolol	−	+
Acebutolol	+/−	+
Oxprenolol	−	+
Metoprolol	+	+
Timolol	−	−
Pindolol	−	−
Sotalol	−	−
Betaxolol	+	−
Nadolol	−	−
Atenolol	+	−

Clinical uses of beta blockers

Beta blockers are used to treat a variety of conditions, including cardiac arrhythmias, glaucoma, hyperthyroidism, migraine and essential tremor. Most commonly, they are used to treat angina pectoris and hypertension.

Angina pectoris is a symptom of coronary artery disease. It is the pain associated with reduced oxygen availability to (i.e. ischaemia of) the myocardium. This means that the demand for oxygen from the myocardium is not matched by the supply of blood, i.e. coronary blood flow is inadequate. There are at least three causes of angina – effort, thrombo-embolism and vasospasm. The management of angina involves reduction of risk factors (e.g. obesity, cigarette smoking, lack of exercise, hyperlipidaemia and hypertension) and drug treatment.

Organic nitrates are the first-line treatment of angina. A significant proportion of patients cannot tolerate nitrates because they cause severe headaches. Beta blockers are the second choice for the treatment of angina of effort, but they are less effective in treating angina caused by vasospasm (Prinzmetal's syndrome). They are contraindicated in some patients because of their side-effects (see later). The third group of anti-anginal drugs, calcium channel blockers, are first-line therapy for Prinzmetal's angina. They are frequently used in combination with either nitrates or beta blockers to treat angina of effort when monotherapy is insufficient. They may also be used when either nitrates cannot be tolerated or when beta blockers are contraindicated. Unstable angina is associated with a high risk of heart attack (myocardial infarction). It is normally treated aggressively with nitrates, beta blockers, calcium channel blockers and aspirin, the latter in a dose of 75 mg per day which inhibits platelet aggregation and reduces the risk of thrombosis in the coronary arteries.

Hypertension is present when systemic arterial blood pressure is increased above an acceptable value following duplicate measurements on four or more separate occasions. The World Health Organization defines hypertension as systolic pressure greater than 160 mmHg and/or diastolic pressure greater than 90 mmHg. However, it is perhaps more appropriate to consider threshold levels for intervention in the context of the presence of absence of other risk factors (British Hypertension Society, 1993).

Anti-anginal and antihypertensive effects of beta blockers

Beta blockers affect both the heart and blood vessels. They reduce the work of the heart and hence its oxygen demand by reducing heart rate, myocardial contractility and peripheral resistance. A reduction in heart rate *per se* improves coronary blood flow because the latter occurs mainly during diastole which varies inversely with heart rate. The dose of beta blocker should be adjusted for each individual to obtain a resting heart rate of 50–60/minutes which should give a maximum rate of 100–120/minutes. The reductions in heart rate and myocardial contractility reduce cardiac output and hence arterial blood pressure. These anti-hypertensive effects of beta blockers are evident within 2 days to 2 weeks of regular treatment (Hudson, 1985). Subsequently, stroke volume may increase as peripheral resistance decreases and cardiac output at rest returns to pre-treatment values. However, blood pressure is still reduced because of the decrease in peripheral resistance. The decrease in peripheral resistance reduces the after-load against which the heart must pump. This in turn reduces the work of the heart and hence the oxygen requirement of the myocardium. The way in which beta blockers decrease peripheral resistance is controversial. Decreased renin release from the kidneys, noradrenaline release from post-ganglionic sympathetic nerve terminals and central SNS activity have been cited as possible explanations. However, some would maintain that beta blockers increase peripheral resistance (Walther and Tifft, 1985) by exposing alpha receptor-mediated vasoconstriction (Powles, 1981).

Beta blockers and exercise

Effects upon the cardiovascular and respiratory systems

Exercise in healthy individuals increases heart rate, myocardial contractility, stroke volume, cardiac output, oxygen consumption (VO_2) and artereo-venous oxygen (a-vO_2) difference. Antagonism of beta$_1$ receptors in the heart reduces heart rate and myocardial contractility at rest. This effect is absent or negligible in élite athletes with very low resting heart rates (Tesch, 1985). During sub-maximal exercise in healthy subjects, beta blockers decrease heart rate, systolic blood pressure and cardiac output, increase stroke volume and a-vO_2 difference, and have no significant effect upon diastolic blood pressure, ventilation and VO_2. Stroke volume is increased at both sub-maximal and maximal workloads. This effect is not related to cardioselectivity. The time taken by normotensive subjects to run 5000 m was increased by 33% by metoprolol. This was probably caused by reduction in maximal heart rate (Bengtsson, 1991).

Maximum cardiac output is decreased by beta blockers, but the decrease is less than the decrease in maximum heart rate because of the compensatory rise in stroke volume. Once again this effect is not related to cardioselectivity.

The majority of reports suggest that oxygen uptake at sub-maximal workloads is unaffected by beta blockade. However, VO_2 max. is reduced by beta blockade. A 30% reduction in heart rate causes a 10–15% reduction in VO_2 max. in patients and also in trained and untrained individuals. Such a decrease can be obtained after a single dose of propranolol or metoprolol (Tesch, 1985). The effects are dose related. The reported effects upon VO_2 max. vary between a decrease and no significant difference. This may be due to the control VO_2 max. of the subjects before beta blockade. Thus, beta blockade has little effect upon VO_2 max. in subjects whose control or unblocked VO_2 max. was <50 ml/kg/min but caused a significant reduction in VO_2 max. in individuals whose control VO_2 max. was >50 ml/kg/min. The decrease in VO_2 max. did not correlate well (r=0.42) with the decrease in heart rate for the group as a whole. However, when the subjects were divided into three subgroups on the basis of their unblocked VO_2 max., the correlation between the decrease in heart rate and that in VO_2 max. increased as the unblocked VO_2 max. increased (Wilmore *et al.*, 1985). The authors suggest that those subjects with an unblocked VO_2 max. of <50 ml/kg/min can compensate for a decrease in heart rate by increasing stroke volume and a-vO_2 difference. However, those subjects with a control VO_2 max. >50 ml/kg/min will be operating at maximum stroke volume and a-vO_2 difference and therefore cannot compensate adequately for the decrease in heart rate. There was no apparent significant difference between the effects of a cardio-selective beta blocker (atenolol) and those of the two non-selective blockers (propranolol and sotalol). Rather surprisingly, propranolol tended to produce a greater decrease in VO_2 max. than did atenolol (Wilmore et al., 1985).

Effects upon metabolism

Beta blockers do not affect muscle strength, power, speed of contraction or work capacity (Tesch, 1985). However, they do have profound effects upon metabolism and energy availability. Antagonism of beta$_2$ receptors reduces energy availability in skeletal muscle by three mechanisms. Firstly, it reduces the release of insulin from the beta cells in the Islets of Langerhans in the pancreas. Secondly, it reduces glycogenolysis in the liver which can lead to hypoglycaemia. Non-selective beta blockers cause a greater reduction in blood glucose levels at sub-maximal workloads than do selective beta$_1$ antagonists.Thirdly, it reduces glycogenolysis in skeletal muscle, so that less glucose is liberated from intramuscular glycogen stores. In addition, selective beta$_1$ antagonists reduce lipolysis in adipose tissue and hence the concentration of free fatty acids in the blood. These effects will be unimportant in explosive anaerobic events but will limit performance in endurance events. The ability to sustain sub-maximal work is reduced by beta blockers. The time to exhaustion on either a treadmill or a bicycle is reduced by beta blockade. Non-selective beta blockers (e.g. propranolol) inhibit lipolysis and glycogenolysis more than cardioselective beta blockers (e.g. metoprolol), so they have a greater inhibitory effect upon time to exhaustion. However, metoprolol (a cardio-selective beta blocker) inhibits lipolysis more than glycogenolysis, so that the muscle glycogen is reduced more rapidly in metoprolol-treated than in control subjects (Allen et al., 1984).

Effects upon psychomotor function

Non-selective beta blockers, e.g. propranolol, give effective relief of the physical symptoms of anxiety, e.g. palpitations, tremor, facial flushing and diarrhoea. The ability of a beta blocker to relieve the symptoms of anxiety increases with its lipophilicity which determines the rate at which it can cross the blood–brain barrier. Reduction in these physical symptoms *per se* reduces the state of anxiety. However, the more lipophilic beta blockers (Table 3.5) are also more likely to cause insomnia, nightmares and depression, which are the centrally mediated undesirable side-effects of beta blockers. Also, they preferentially inhibit lipolysis in adipose tissue. Essential tremor responds well to non-selective beta antagonists.

Side-effects of treatment with beta blockers

1. Bronchospasm. Blockade of beta$_2$ receptors may precipitate broncho-constriction in either asthmatics or chronic bronchitics. Consequently, beta blockers are contraindicated in asthmatics and chronic bronchitics.
2. Heart failure. Inhibition of sympathetic tone to the heart may precipitate cardiac failure in individuals with compromised cardiac function. The effects are enhanced by interaction with other cardiodepressant drugs, e.g. verapamil and lignocaine. Beta blockers are contraindicated in uncontrolled heart failure.
3. Heart block. Since these drugs are used to slow heart rate, they cannot be given to individuals who have an existing bradycardia due to a conduction defect, e.g. second or third degree heart block.
4. Cold extremities. Beta blockers reduce vasodilation and reveal alpha receptor-mediated vasoconstriction. This will aggravate peripheral vascular disease and may lead to intermittent claudication or to Raynaud's disease.
5. Destabilization of diabetes mellitus. Beta blockers can decrease glucose tolerance and reduce the response to hypoglycaemia in diabetics. This effect is more marked with cardioselective beta blockers. However, even these drugs are contraindicated for diabetics who suffer from frequent hypoglycaemic episodes. Beta blockers do not induce diabetes in normal subjects.
6. Fatigue is a common side-effect of the more lipophilic beta blockers. Atenolol, which is both cardioselective and only weakly lipophilic, is the beta blocker of choice in this case. A programme of exercise will often alleviate the symptoms of fatigue, whilst at the same time improving cardiovascular function. Moreover, the symptoms of fatigue tend to decrease with time as the body accommodates the effects of beta blockade.

Effects of beta blockade on the response to exercise of hypertensive and ischaemic heart disease (IHD) patients

Hypertensive subjects
Hypertensives have decreased cardiac output and stroke volume, together with increased heart rate and total peripheral resistance for the same intensity of workload as normotensive individuals. Beta blockers will impair performance of endurance exercise (30 minutes duration) in patients with asymptomatic, uncomplicated hypertension. Propranolol decreased the VO$_2$ max. response to an aerobic training programme in mild hypertensive males. Diltiazem, which is a calcium channel blocker that is indicated for the treatment of hypertension, did not have the same effect.

Thus, calcium channel blockade may be a more appropriate therapy for hypertensives who also wish to include exercise in the treatment of their disease. Neither propranolol nor diltiazem affected one-repetition maximal strength. These data are in accord with those from normotensive subjects in which neither propranolol nor atenolol affected isokinetic exercise. Thus, strength performance training will be unaffected by beta blockade prescribed for non-cardiac diseases, e.g. migraine, anxiety and glaucoma.

IHD subjects

Beta blockers will facilitate an initial increase in exercise capacity in IHD subjects because of the improvement in the availability of oxygen to the myocardium at rest. Any improvement in the symptoms of exercise-induced angina should be used to encourage the subject to undertake an exercise programme which will augment the improvement in cardiovascular status. The training effect will be limited by the inhibitory effects of the beta blocker upon maximal heart rate and muscle metabolism. However, long-term treatment with a selective beta$_1$ antagonist will have more of a favourable effect upon plasma lipids and less of an inhibitory effect upon exercise-induced changes in plasma lipids than will a nonselective blockade. Whether the cardioselective blocker should be more or less lipophilic remains the subject of conjecture (Tesch, 1985). Objective assessment of the interaction between exercise and beta blockade in IHD is difficult because of the criteria (changes in heart rate and VO$_2$ max.) that are normally used to assess responses to a training programme. Beta blockade, *per se*, reduces heart rate, and limitation of exercise testing by the onset of symptoms of angina introduces an element of subjectivity.

It should be remembered that beta blockade affects the physiological and biochemical responses to exercise, so that the warm-up and cooldown periods need to be increased accordingly. An increase in warm-up will permit a gradual increase in both muscle blood flow (thus reducing anaerobic metabolism) and lipolysis. A longer cool-down period will reduce the light-headedness and fainting that can result from post-exercise hypotension (Allen *et al.*, 1984).

Potential for abuse of beta blockers

The major area of potential abuse for beta blockers lies in those events in which motor skills can be affected by muscle tremor caused by anxiety. Beta blockers have been moved to Subgroup E of Group III, Classes of Drugs Subject to Certain Restrictions, i.e. they should be tested for in those sports where they are likely to enhance performance (e.g. archery, shooting, biathlon, modern pentathlon, bobsleigh, diving, luge and ski-jumping). Tests for beta blockers will also be performed at the request of the relevant international federation and at the discretion of the IOC Medical Commission. Other sports which control the use of beta blockers are fencing, figure-skating, equestrian sports, gymnastics, sailing and synchronized swimming.

Beta blockers cannot be recommended for individuals who wish to participate in those events in which sub-maximal and maximal oxygen utilization is of prime importance (Walther and Tifft, 1985). The IOC Medical Commission considers it unlikely that beta blockers will be abused in endurance events which require prolonged periods of high cardiac output and large stores of metabolic substrates, because they would have a markedly adverse effect upon performance. However, the IOC does retain the right to test where it deems it to be appropriate.

3.4.2 ALPHA ANTAGONISTS (ALPHA BLOCKERS)

These drugs are used in the treatment of hypertension and other vascular disorders. They produce their therapeutic effects by causing dilation of peripheral blood vessels following blockade of alpha adrenoceptors.

Alpha adrenoceptors are subdivided into $alpha_1$ and $alpha_2$ adrenoceptors. The $alpha_2$ adrenoceptors are located pre-synaptically, that is on the membrane of sympathetic nerve endings. Their physiological function is to control the amount of the neurotransmitter, noradrenaline, released from the nerve endings when the nerves are stimulated. Some of the released noradrenaline acts upon these pre-synaptic $alpha_2$ adrenoceptors, thereby inhibiting further release of noradrenaline. This is a negative feedback mechanism.

$Alpha_1$ adrenoceptors are found post-synaptically on the membranes of the smooth muscle, within the tissue being innervated by the sympathetic nerves. It is through these $alpha_1$ adrenoceptors that the neurotransmitter, noradrenaline, interacts to cause contraction of the smooth muscle. An important example of this is seen within the arterial blood vessels. Sympathetic nerve stimulation leads to noradrenaline release, which in turn acts on the $alpha_1$ adrenoceptors in the smooth muscle of the walls of the arterioles, resulting in vasoconstriction. This vasoconstriction, or narrowing of the arterioles, is responsible for maintaining normal blood pressure and is known as sympathetic tone.

Hypertension (elevated blood pressure) can result from an identifiable cause, removal of which abolishes the hypertension. However, the majority of cases of hypertension are of unknown origin and are referred to as 'essential hypertension'. Treatment of this condition is therefore symptomatic, in that the underlying cause cannot be treated as it is unknown. Consequently, patients suffering from essential hypertension are normally on drug therapy for life. This can present complications for hypertensives who are otherwise fit and well and who may therefore participate in a wide variety of sports.

There are several groups of drugs used to treat hypertensive patients which have widely differing modes of action. The most widely prescribed drugs are diuretics and beta blockers, because of their pharmacological effectiveness and their relatively low incidence of side-effects at the therapeutic dose levels used. Other groups of drugs include vasodilators, calcium antagonists, angiotensin-converting enzyme inhibitors and centrally acting drugs. The vasodilator group of drugs includes the alpha blockers.

In the past, alpha blockers, such as phentolamine, tolazoline and phenoxybenzamine, were used to treat hypertension but caused two major side-effects – postural hypotension, manifested by a tendency towards dizziness on standing up, and tachycardia or rapid heart rate. More recently, a second generation of alpha blockers has emerged which has a selective action on alpha$_1$ adrenoceptors. Prazosin and indoramin are members of this group of selective alpha$_1$ blockers in current therapeutic use.

The advantage of alpha$_1$ selectivity lies in the fact that alpha$_1$ adrenoceptors are occupied, thereby preventing the vasoconstrictor action of noradrenaline released from the sympathetic nerves. The resultant vasodilation leads to a decrease in blood pressure. With non-selective alpha blockers, the pre-synaptic alpha$_2$ adrenoceptors are also blocked; therefore the negative feedback mechanism is inhibited and a greater amount of noradrenaline is released from sympathetic nerve endings. In tissues where the post-synaptic receptors are of the alpha$_1$ type, this does not matter as these are protected by the alpha blocker. However, where the post-synaptic receptors are of the beta type, there is no protection against the increased noradrenaline released. This is the case in the heart, and accounts for the tachycardia associated with non-selective alpha blockers. Prazosin and indoramin have a reduced affinity for alpha$_2$ adrenoceptors, hence the incidence of tachycardia with these drugs is greatly diminished. The selective alpha blockers are also less likely to dilate venous blood vessels which carry the blood back to the heart. Venous return is, therefore, improved, and this helps to reduce the incidence of postural hypotension.

Alpha blockers are not drugs of abuse in sport, nor have there been any reports of their adverse effects in exercise performance. It is pertinent to note that patients who are hypertensive often experience no symptoms. All antihypertensive drugs, however, induce various degrees of side-effects. A patient may therefore end up with a poorer quality of life when treated with antihypertensive drugs than when their hypertension was untreated. It must be stressed, however, that untreated hypertension can lead to more serious diseases, such as a stroke, with a high risk of mortality. Long-term exercise has been proposed as an alternative to drug therapy for reducing blood pressure in hypertensives. Unfortunately, a study by Kenney and Zambaski (1984) provided equivocal evidence and led them to conclude that the effect of training on the chronic high blood pressure of hypertensives is still unclear.

3.5 REFERENCES

Allen, C.J., Craven, M.A., Rosenbloom, D. and Sutton, J.R. (1984) Beta blockade and exercise in normal subjects and patients with coronary artery disease. *Physician and Sports Medicine*, **12**, 51–63.

Alquist, R.P. (1948) Study of adrenotropic receptors. *Am. J. Physiol.*, **153**, 586–600.

Bengtsson, C. (1991) Effects of various antihypertensive drugs on the physical performance of a healthy person. *Scandinavian Journal of Medicine and Science in Sports*, **1**(1), 51–4.

British Hypertension Society (1993) Management guidelines in essential hypertension: report of the second working party of the British Hypertension Society. *British Medical Journal*, **306**, 983–7.

British National Formulary. Number 29 (March, 1995). British Medical Association and Royal Pharmaceutical Society of Great Britain.

British Thoracic Society (1993) Guidelines for the management of asthma: a summary. *British Medical Journal*, **306**, 776–82.

Bundgaard, A. (1985) Exercise and the asthmatic. *Sports Medicine*, **2**, 254–66.

Choo, J.J., Horon, M.A., Little, R.A. and Rothwell, N.J. (1992) Anabolic effects of clenbuterol and skeletal muscle are mediated by β_2-adrenoceptor activation. *American Journal of Physiology*, **263**, E50–56.

Clark, T.J.H. and Cochrane, G.M. (1984) *Bronchodilator Therapy: The Basis of Asthma and Chronic Obstructive Airway Disease Management*, UK, Auckland ADIS Press, pp. 17–46.

1992 editorial. Clenbuterol: muscle growth reported in animals but what effect in humans? *Pharmaceutical Journal*, 8 August, 169.

Eisenstadt, W.S., Nicholas, S.S., Velick, G. and Enright, T. (1984) Allergic reactions to exercise. *Physician and Sports Medicine*, **12**, 95–104.

Fitch, K.D. (1986) The use of anti-asthmatic drugs. Do they affect sports performance? *Sports Medicine*, **3**, 136–50.

Gordon, N.F. and Duncan, J.J. (1991) Effect of beta-blockers on exercise physiology: implications for exercise training. *Medicine and Science in Sports and Exercise*, **23**(6), 668–76.Hudson, S.A. (1985) Drug review: understanding β-blockers. *Pharmacy Update*, May, 74–7.

Hudson, S.A. (1985) Drug review: understanding beta-blockers. *Pharmacy Update*, May, 74–7.

IOC (1993) Doping Classes and Methods of the International Olympic Committee. IOC, Lausanne, August.

IOC (1994) Doping Classes and Methods of the International Olympic Committee. IOC, Lausanne, November.

Katzung, B.G. (1995) *Basic and Clinical Pharmacology*, 6th edn, Lange, Los Altos, Calif.

Kenny, W.K. and Zambaski, E.J. (1984) Physical activity in human hypertension. A mechanisms approach. *Sports Medicine*, **1**, 459–73.

Morton, A.R. and Fitch, K.D. (1992) Asthmatic drugs and competitive sport: an update. *Sports Medicine*, **14**(4), 228–42.

Powles, A.C.P. (1981) The effects of drugs on the cardiovascular response to exercise. *Medicine and Science in Sports and Exercise*, **13**, 252–8.

Tesch, P.A. (1985) Exercise performance and β-blockade. *Sports Medicine*, **2**, 389–412.

Walter, R.J. and Tifft, C.P. (1985) High blood pressure in the competitive athlete: guidelines and recommendations. *Physician and Sports Medicine*, **13**, 93–114.

Wilmore, J.H., Joyner, M.J., Freund, B.J. *et al.* (1985) Beta-blockade and response to exercise: influence of training. *Physician and Sports Medicine*, **13**, 61–9.

Yang, Y.T. and McElliott, M.A. (1989) Multiple Actions of β-adrenergic agonists on skeletal muscle and adipose tissue. *Biochem. J.*, **261**, 1–10.

Central nervous system stimulants

4

Alan George

Various drugs which stimulate the central nervous system (CNS) have been known for over 2000 years. A simple classification of these substances is complicated by their combination of central and systemic effects. Thus, though the compounds mainly stimulate CNS activity, many central stimulants have, in addition, direct effects on cardiovascular functions and on the sympathetic nervous system.

4.1 CNS NEUROPHYSIOLOGY

To understand the various mechanisms by which CNS stimulants produce their effects, it is necessary to understand the basic functioning of neurones in the CNS (Figure 4.1). The stimulant drug must pass from the circulation, across the blood–brain barrier and into the brain tissue spaces. Once in the brain it may: (a) increase neurotransmitter release on to receptors (amphetamine and ephedrine); (b) directly stimulate the post-synaptic receptors (ephedrine, caffeine); or (c) inhibit neurotransmitter re-uptake (cocaine and amphetamine).

CNS stimulants are thought to act mainly on the dopamine (DA), noradrenaline (NA) and 5-hydroxytryptamine (5HT) (serotonin) neurotransmitter systems. Caffeine is thought to affect adenosine neurotransmission.

4.2 AMPHETAMINES

Several structurally related drugs are known as 'amphetamines', includes dextroamphetamine, methamphetamine, phenmetrazine and methylphenidate. In this chapter the word amphetamine will refer to dextroamphetamine, the structure of which is shown in Figure 4.2.

Drugs in Sport, 2nd edn. Edited by David R. Mottram. Published in 1996 by E & FN Spon, London. ISBN 0 419 18890 8

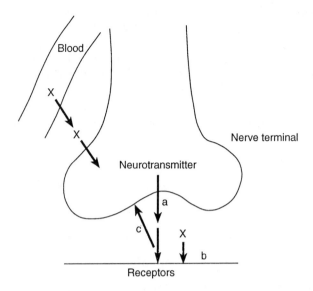

Figure 4.1 Sites of action of CNS stimulants (a) amphetamines; (b) caffeine; (c) amphetamine and cocaine.

Amphetamine is a phenyl isopropylamine (Figure 4.2) and was first synthesized in 1920. It was originally prescribed for the treatment of nasal congestion – inhalation of an amphetamine spray through the nose induced nasal vasoconstriction which resulted in decongestion. In 1935, amphetamine was first used to treat the neurological condition narcolepsy, and its use in the treatment of depression, anxiety and hyperactivity in children followed from this. Amphetamine was used widely during the Second World War to reduce fatigue and increase alertness, particularly amongst naval and airforce crew on patrol duties. Reference to this was made in 1974, in Ludovic Kennedy's account of the pursuit and sinking of the German battleship *Bismarck*. The rapid development of tolerance to amphetamine and the insidious occurrence of dependence have led to the drug being withdrawn from clinical use, except in certain controlled circumstances, in both Britain and the USA.

4.2.1 THE EFFECT OF AMPHETAMINES ON HUMAN MOOD AND PERFORMANCE

The desire to enhance mood or performance or both is usually the main reason for taking amphetamines. In their comprehensive review of amphetamines, Weiss and Laties (1962) agreed that amphetamine does produce an enhanced performance in many tasks and does not simply normalize fatigue responses. They examined various tasks, such as: (a) work output by subjects on a bicycle ergometer; (b) performance on arduous military exercises; and (c) performance during flying or driving missions. Apparent improvements in athletic performance in events as diverse as shot-put, swimming and running are produced by amphetamines as well as a reduction in reaction time and increased coordination and steadiness. These aspects will be discussed in detail later. Intellectual performance does not seem to be improved by amphetamines, unless the performance has been degraded by boredom and fatigue (Brookes, 1985).

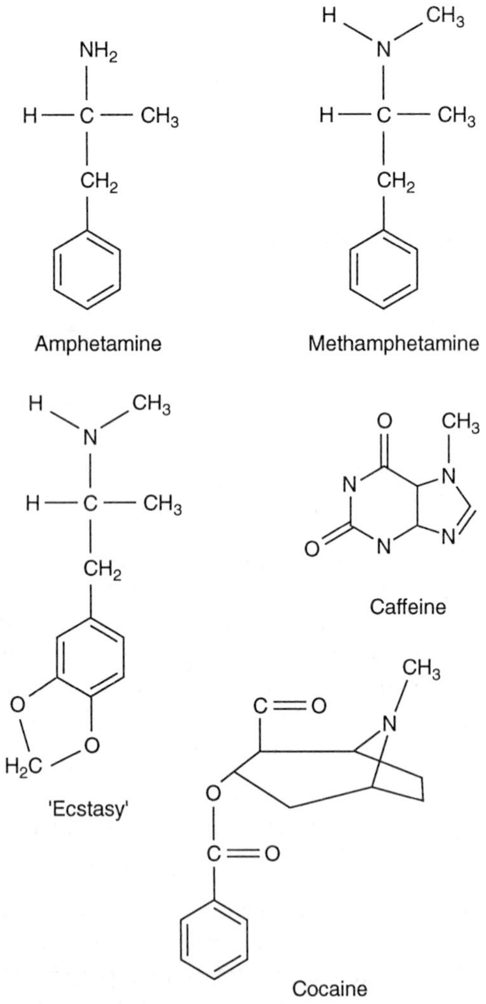

Figure 4.2 Some central stimulants.

In the short term, amphetamine increases the speed of learning of new tasks. The effects of amphetamine on judgement are uncertain and several conflicting studies have been published (Brookes, 1985). There is general agreement that amphetamines cause a mild distortion of time perception which may lead to misjudgement in planning manoeuvres or in manipulations, such as driving a car. Active avoidance learning is facilitated by amphetamine. Although there is considerable inter-individual variation in the effects of amphetamine on mood, the general effects are of positive mood enhancement. These positive effects include an increase in physical energy, mental aptitude, talkativeness, restlessness, excitement and good humour. Subjects taking amphetamine also report that they feel confident, efficient, ambitious and that their food intake is reduced.

Some 'negative' effects of amphetamine include anxiety, indifference, slowness in reasoning, irresponsible behaviour, irritability and restlessness, dry mouth, tremors, insomnia and, following withdrawal, depression. These effects of amphetamine on mood are dose-dependent and are thought to be produced by the stimulation of DA and NA receptors.

Tolerance and dependence

Tolerance develops rapidly to many of the effects of the amphetamines. Tolerance is said to be present when, over a period of time, increasing doses of a drug are required to maintain the same response. Brookes (1985) has reported several cases of subjects requiring as much as 1 g of amphetamine per day to produce the same effect on mood as a new taker of amphetamines who may require only 10–30 mg. There is much evidence to show that amphetamines induce drug dependence and the amphetamine-dependent person may become psychotic aggressive and antisocial. Withdrawal of amphetamines is associated with mental and physical depression.

4.2.2 THERAPEUTIC USE

The many varied uses of amphetamine following its original introduction are now largely discredited. It is interesting to compare the initial enthusiasm for amphetamine as the 'cure-all' for numerous mental problems with that for the use of cocaine some 50 years previously.

Until quite recently amphetamine was used to treat narcolepsy, but its use is now limited to the treatment of hyperactivity in children. A rare use of amphetamines is as a diagnostic aid in determining which patients are unsuitable for a particular anti-manic or anti-schizophrenic treatment.

Toxicity

The major side-effects of amphetamine administration (excluding those following withdrawal of the drug) include: (a) many of the negative effects described previously; (b) confusion, delirium, sweating, palpitations, dilation of the pupil and rapid breathing; and (c) hypertension, tachycardia, tremors and muscle and joint pain. Though amphetamines may initially stimulate libido, chronic amphetamine use often leads to a reduction in sex drive. Chronic amphetamine administration is also associated with myocardial pathology and with growth retardation in adolescents. Usually, the personality changes induced by chronic low doses of amphetamine are gradually reversed after the drug is stopped. However, high chronic doses may lead to a variety of persistent personality changes. Possibly the most serious of the severe personality disorders induced by amphetamine is the so-called amphetamine psychosis described by Connell in 1958. The frightening array of psychiatric symptoms he described in patients presenting with amphetamine psychosis include many commonly found in paranoid-type schizophrenics. An important distinction between amphetamine psychosis and schizophrenia is that amphetamine induces a preponderance of symptoms of paranoid and visual hallucinations.

4.2.3 THE MODE OF ACTION OF AMPHETAMINE

There are four mechanisms by which amphetamine may produce its effects. These are (1) release of neurotransmitter – DA, NA or 5HT – from their respective nerve terminals; (2) inhibition of monoamine oxidase activity; (3) inhibition of neurotransmitter re-uptake; and (4) direct action on neuro-transmitter receptors. Of these four possibilities, neurotransmitter release appears to be the most important (Brookes, 1985).

Amphetamine stimulates DA release by reversing the neuronal mem-brane uptake transporter (Seiden, Sabol and Ricaurte, 1993). It also inhibits the activity of the enzyme monoamine oxidase (Seiden, Sabol and Ricaurte, 1993). It also seems that several major behavioural changes induced by amphetamine are most closely mimicked by stimulation of central NA-releasing neurones. Thus, the amphetamine-induced locomo-tor activity and self-stimulation seen in animals and the increased alertness and elevation of mood produced in humans are closely related to increas-es in noradrenergic activity. Amphetamine is a potent anorectic and ele-vates plasma free fatty acid levels. Body temperature is also elevated. The cardiovascular, gastrointestinal and respiratory effects of amphetamine are sympathomimetic in nature. However, both animal and clinical experi-ments suggest that the effects of amphetamine are mediated by the release of at least two neurotransmitters, NA and DA, and that, in the rat, the development of tolerance to amphetamine involves the release of 5HT. However, the stereotyped behaviour induced in the rat by amphetamine administration appears to depend on DA release. The euphoriant action of amphetamine can be abolished by the DA receptor antagonist, pimozide. There is some evidence to suggest that the positive behavioural effects of amphetamine may be mediated by DA, whilst the effect of amphetamine on food intake may be mediated by NA. However, Silverstone and Goodall (1985) produced conflicting evidence of this.

Pharmacokinetics

Amphetamines are readily absorbed, mainly from the small intestine, and the peak plasma concentration occurs in 1–2 hours following administration. Absorption is usually complete in 2.5–4 hours and is accelerated by food intake.

The metabolism of amphetamines has been difficult to investigate because of the wide variation between species in the metabolic effects of amphetamines. The principal amphetamine metabolites are p-hydroxy-ephedrine and p-hydroxyamphetamine. Both these metabolites have similar pharmacological effects to the parent amphetamine. Amphetamine is lost from the blood by renal filtration. Some secretion of amphetamine into the urine also occurs. Amphetamine excretion is enhanced by an acid urine, and treatments which increase the acidity of urine enhance amphetamine loss – a reaction which is useful in the treatment of amphetamine overdose.

4.2.4 THE EFFECTS OF AMPHETAMINE IN SPORT

In the USA, the increasing use of amphetamines in all sports led the American Medical Association to initiate research projects to test the effects of amphetamine on sports performance and the incidence of side-effects associated with the drug. One of these studies (Smith and Beecher, 1959) reported that 14–21 mg/kg body weight of amphetamine sulphate when administered 2–3 hours prior to running, swimming or weight throwing, improved performance in 75% of the cases investigated. This was a double-blind study in which 14 out of 15 swimmers and 19 out of 26 runners showed a statistically significant improvement in performance after amphetamine administration. However, the improvements demonstrated were quite small (usually 1%). This study also demonstrated that the performance of athletes in throwing events was improved by an average of 4% following amphetamine administration. Criticism of the study soon followed because the athletes were sometimes allowed to time themselves, there was little control for weather conditions, a wide range of distances (600 yards to 12 miles) was used to test the athletes and a minor dosage of amphetamine was administered. Chandler and Blair (1980) reported that amphetamine improved athletic performance in terms of acceleration, knee extension strength and time to exhaustion, but that it had no effect on sprinting speed.

Haldi and Wynn (1959) reported that 5 mg of amphetamine 90 minutes before a 100 yard swim had no effect on the time of the swim. A more sophisticated double-blind investigation of amphetamine was carried out by Golding and Barnard (1963) using a treadmill. They studied the effect of amphetamine on treadmill running in trained and untrained subjects. Each subject undertook an initial run, followed 12 minutes later by a second 'fatigued' run. Thus, the effects of amphetamine on initial performance and fatigue could be examined in the same subject. Their subjects showed that amphetamine had no effect on performance during the initial and fatigued runs in either the trained or the untrained athletes. During the fatigued runs, amphetamine retarded the recovery rates for heart rate and blood pressure. Only one of the subjects was able to tell that he was receiving amphetamine.

Many of the studies on the effects of amphetamine on athletic performance have been carried out on cyclists. One reason for this is that there are numerous examples of fatalities arising from the use of amphetamines by cyclists, notably the incidence of death from heatstroke. Wyndham *et al.* (1971) carried out a wide-ranging placebo-controlled biochemical and physiological investigation on two champion cyclists exercising on a bicycle ergometer. Whilst working at rates between 12 000 and 16 000 ft/lb/min there was no difference between amphetamine and placebo in terms of sub-maximal or maximal oxygen uptake, heart rate or minute ventilation; however, there were significant increases in blood lactate levels with amphetamine compared to placebo. The authors concluded that amphetamines have no effect on the ability to do aerobic work, but they significantly increased the cyclists' ability to tolerate higher levels of anaerobic metabolism. The dangers inherent in these results are that an athlete taking amphetamine might be better able to ignore the usual internal signals of over-exertion and heat stress, which may therefore explain the incidence of heatstroke and cardiac problems in cyclists who take amphetamines during long-distance cycling events.

Since amphetamine was last reviewed in this book (George, 1988) there have been no significant new findings relating to the ergogenic effects of amphetamine. This has been attributed to a decline (in the USA) in the abuse of amphetamine by athletes and by the general public, following increased controls on its prescription and availability (Wadler and Hainline, 1989). Several reviewers, including Conlee (1991), have remarked on the considerable inconsistency of amphetamine effects in humans, particularly with regard to ergogenicity. A poorly explored feature of amphetamine action is its effect on fatigue. Most studies have concentrated on the central aspects of fatigue whilst neglecting peripheral contributions. However, the few studies of amphetamine effects on muscle glycogen stores before and during exercise have been contradictory (Conlee, 1991).

Since no significant improvement in performance is associated with amphetamine use, why does it continue to be taken? The answer could be an effect on mental attitude in terms of improved mood, greater confidence and optimism, and increased alertness. It should also be remembered that, like anabolic steroids, amphetamine could be abused for different reasons by different athletes. Thus, baseball and football players may use them to increase alertness and concentration; runners or swimmers to increase energy and endurance (Smith and Perry, 1992).

An interesting insight into the differential abuse of amphetamine in an American football team has been provided by Mandell, Stewart and Russo (1981). They reported that amphetamine dosage would be adjusted according to the players' position in the team. The lowest doses, 5–15 mg per man per game, were given to those players, such as wide receivers, whose concentration needed to be heightened whilst maintaining near normal perception. The high doses, 10–60 mg per man per game (linebackers) and 30–150 mg per man per game (defensive linemen), went to those players in whom aggression was paramount.

It is also possible that amphetamine might increase preparedness and make the athlete more keyed up for his event. To examine this possibility, the effects of amphetamine sulphate were compared with the tranquillizer, meprobamate, and with placebo control in 126 male medical students. The results showed that none of the students was able to tell which drug he was taking, and, also, there was no correlation between either subjective feelings of increased alertness in those taking amphetamine or lethargy in subjects on meprobamate with any change in reaction time or manipulative skills (Golding, 1981).

Several studies thus indicate that the effect of amphetamine on the psychological state of athletes is almost certainly self-induced and occurs as a result of the athlete expecting to perform better and be more alert.

Side-effects of amphetamine in relation to sport

Some side-effects of amphetamine are particularly important in athletes, and have often only been revealed in individuals undertaking extremely arduous training or sporting schedules.

One of the most widely publicized side-effects of amphetamine, from which a number of fatalities have occurred, is heatstroke. This has been most prominent in cyclists, owing to the intensity of their exercise, the endurance required and the high ambient temperatures at which the exercise often occurs. Amphetamine causes a redistribution of blood flow away from the skin, thus limiting the cooling of the blood. As a result of this, two cyclists (Jenson and Simpson), who had both been taking amphetamine, died of heatstroke and cardiac arrest respectively during gruelling road races. The former occurred in the intense summer heat of Rome, the latter whilst climbing the infamous Mont Ventoux during the 1967 Tour de France.

The ability of amphetamines to obscure painful injuries has enabled many American footballers to play on and exacerbate injuries which would normally have resulted in their withdrawal from play.

The side-effects of amphetamine on behaviour are also important in sport. Mandell (1979) has reviewed amphetamine abuse amongst American footballers and found extensive abuse, as much as 60–70 mg average dose per man per game. In this sport, amphetamine was administered apparently to promote aggression and weaken fatigue in the footballers. However, there are several accounts quoted by Golding (1981) in which the euphoriant effects of such doses have rendered the takers unaware of the errors and misjudgements they were making on the pitch.

Why take amphetamines?

Why take amphetamines when the chance of increased injury, dependence, heatstroke and cardiac arrest is enhanced by these drugs, and the actual improvement in performance, if it does occur, is so small – in the order of 1 or 2%? The simple answer to this was proposed by Laties and Weiss (1981) who examined the improvements in world records in athletic events over the past 100 years. As an example, the 1500 m world record has improved by only 15% since 1880, and, on average, in the past 50 years it has improved by only 1% in every 7 years. They concluded, therefore, that a top athlete who could consistently maintain a 1% improvement in performance would be at an advantage over competitors. This advantage they termed 'the amphetamine margin'.

4.2.5 CONCLUSION

The prescription and administration of amphetamines are strictly controlled by law in most developed countries. They produce powerful stimulating effects on the CNS, which include euphoria, excitation and increased aggression and alertness. These effects are achieved at the expense of judgement and self-criticism. Amphetamine administration may be followed by severe bouts of depression and dependence. Increases in athletic performance induced by amphetamine are very small and several studies have failed to show that amphetamine produces any physical advantage. Some evidence suggests that amphetamine may increase confidence before and during an event, and laboratory studies have shown that it may also reduce fatigue in isometric muscle contraction.

The induction of dependence and the increased susceptibility to heatstroke and cardiac abnormalities seem to suggest that amphetamine taking is of little value as a performance-enhancing drug.

4.2.6 ECSTASY

This is an amphetamine derivative and was synthesized as early as 1914, being used initially as an appetite suppressant. It has been a Class A illegal substance since 1977 in the UK and a controlled drug in the USA since 1985. Ecstasy has amphetamine-like stimulant properties and is associated with increased stamina and endurance. Its abuse is most commonly associated with social activities, such as dancing. However, it is described here as a prelude to its **possible** misuse by athletes.

Ecstasy produces its effects by stimulating the release of the neurotransmitter, 5HT (serotonin), from 5HT-releasing neurones in the CNS, and can induce the destruction of these neurones. Its most serious physical side-effects are hyperpyrexia, which is the most common cause of death, and seizures. It is addictive.

4.2.7 OTHER SYMPATHOMIMETICS: EPHEDRINE AND PHENYLPROPANOLAMINE

The drugs in this group are structurally related to amphetamine (Figure 4.2). Both drugs exert their effect indirectly on neurones of the sympathetic and central nervous systems, by displacing NA and possibly other monoamine transmitters from neuronal storage sites. Both drugs also exert direct effects on alpha and beta receptors and are weak inhibitors of monoamine uptake. They are also resistant to oxidation by monoamine oxidase.

Both phenylpropanolamine and ephedrine are reported to be five times less potent than amphetamine. The CNS effects of phenylpropanolamine and ephedrine are much less than those of amphetamine. For example a 75 mg/ 70 kg body weight dose of ephedrine is required before it will cross the blood–brain barrier. This may explain why both drugs produce much less depletion of brain monoamines than amphetamine (Wadler and Hainline, 1989).

The effects of phenylpropanolamine and ephedrine are produced within 40 minutes after administration and can last up to 3 hours, with therapeutic effects being associated with plasma levels of between 60 and 200 mg/ml (Wadler and Hainline, 1989).

Uses

Both phenylpropanolamine and ephedrine are sold in pharmacies in the UK and USA as 'cold cures' (see Chapter 3).

Adverse effects

At the usual therapeutic doses quoted previously, the most common side-effects are tachycardia, hypertension, headache and dizziness.

Phenylpropanolamine appears to produce serious hypertensive side-effects at doses sometimes as low as 25 mg (Wadler and Hainline, 1989). Both drugs may cause anorexia, insomnia, irritability and nervousness at low to medium doses, whereas high doses are associated with mania and a psychosis similar to that occasionally seen with amphetamine .

Abuse in sport

Abuse of ephedrine and phenylpropanolamine by athletes is nebulous, since many of those detected as having taken them have claimed they were using the drugs as 'cold cures'. The first and only comprehensive study of the possible ergogenic effects of these drugs was carried out by Sidney and Lefcoe (1977). They examined the effect of 25 mg of ephedrine v. placebo in a double-blind crossover study using three separate athletic trials during a 3-week period. In this comprehensive experiment, 10 variables were measured, including strength, endurance, reaction time, anaerobic capacity and speed of recovery from effort. The results showed that though exercise heart rate and resting pulse pressure increased and post-exercise recovery rate slowed, none of the physical performance measures improved. It was also interesting that no subjective improvements in performance were noted. There is evidence that ephedrine and phenylpropanolamine may become abused as anorexic agents by gymnasts (Wadler and Hainline, 1989).

Adverse effects in athletes

The adverse effects observed in athletes are similar to those seen in the general population. However, a number of investigators have warned of possible interactions between phenylpropanolamine and ephedrine and non-steroidal anti-inflammatory agents (NSAIDS). The pharmacology of these anti-inflammatory drugs is described in Chapter 5, and it will be seen that they inhibit the production of endogenous vasodilators, the prostaglandins. Since many athletes may take these anti-inflammatory drugs, an interaction leading to a larger than expected rise in blood pressure may occur when NSAIDS and phenylpropanolamine and ephedrine are taken together. Another possible dangerous interaction may occur with phenylpropanolamine and ephedrine taken with caffeine.

Can abuse be justified?

The prescription of ephedrine- and phenylpropanolamine-like drugs has been criticized (Wadler and Hainline, 1989). In the 1972 Olympics, US swimmer, De Mont, was disqualified because of the presence of ephedrine in his urine, which he admitted originated from a medicine. At

Seoul, in 1988, the eventual 100 m silver medallist, Linford Christie, narrowly escaped disqualification when small traces of 'a cold-cure substance' were found in his urine. It has been argued that since caffeine is not completely proscribed but is limited to a urine concentration of 12 mcg/ml, a similar rule should apply to ephedrine and phenylpropanolamine once dose/response relationships have been established (Wadler and Hainline, 1989). However, it has also been suggested that phenylpropanolamine and ephedrine may indicate more serious abuse of substances like amphetamine, and their presence may be a sign of weaning-off from, or a mask for, the more powerful drug.

4.3 COCAINE

Cocaine first became available commercially in the 1880s. It was an ingredient of the famous Vin Mariani, beloved by Pope Leo XIII, which was named 'the wine for athletes'.

Sigmund Freud took the drug to try and cure his own depression, and suggested it as a 'cure-all' for others. He exclaimed, 'I took for the first time 0.05 g of cocaine and a few moments later I experienced a sudden exhilaration and a feeling of ease'.

The drug fell out of medical use by the 1920s and social use 10 years later, only to reappear in the 1960s as a major drug of abuse.

4.3.1 PHARMACOLOGY

Cocaine affects the brain in a complex way. The most obvious initial effects are a decrease in fatigue, an increase in motor activity and an increase in talkativeness, coupled with a general feeling of euphoria and well-being. These mood changes soon subside and are replaced by a dysphoria (mood lowering). Cocaine is possibly the most addictive agent known.

The mechanism by which cocaine produces these effects is not known fully. Animal studies show that cocaine is a powerful 'reinforcer' and rewarding agent. It stimulates elements of the brain's pleasure and reward 'centres' which are distributed throughout the limbic system of the brain and include the DA-rich mesocortical and mesolimbic systems. Much of the reinforcing and rewarding behaviour induced by cocaine in animals, i.e. rats who will repeatedly administer cocaine to themselves in preference to food, can be reduced by DA receptor antagonists. The evidence for the action of cocaine on these systems has been reviewed recently by Fibiger, Phillips and Brown (1992).

Further evidence for the involvement of cocaine with DA-releasing neurones comes from studies at the molecular level, reviewed by Kuhar (1992). He has shown that cocaine inhibits the re-uptake of DA into the nerve terminals of DA-releasing neurones. This leads to a potentiation of the action of DA at post-synaptic receptor sites. However, though DA receptor antagonists appear to block the actions of cocaine in rats, in humans they appear to block cocaine craving but not the euphoria (Kuhar, 1992). Some investigators have linked the dysphoria and craving following a cocaine dose with an increase in post-synaptic receptor numbers (Wadler and Hainline, 1989). There is some evidence that the different actions of cocaine may be mediated by separate DA receptor sub-types, principally D_2 and D_4. Tricyclic antidepressants which antagonize these post-administration effects are thought to do so by inducing receptor subsensitivity.

Metabolism

Cocaine is mainly metabolized by plasma and liver cholinesterases to benzoyl ecgonine and ecgonine methyl ester which are excreted in the urine.

Pharmacokinetics

Cocaine may be administered by injection, orally, intranasally or by inhalation. Oral administration produces peak effects at variable times with behavioural changes lasting up to 1 hour. The most popular route is via nasal 'snorting', which produces peak effects from 5 to 15 minutes lasting for an hour. Inhalation of 'free-base'cocaine produces peak effects in less than 1 minute, but also a short-lived physiological effect measured in minutes. Inhalation results in the most intense cravings (Wadler and Hainline, 1989).

Adverse effects

Cocaine is highly addictive (more so than amphetamine) and the abuser may experience acute psychotic symptoms and undertake irrational actions, in addition to the well-known adverse effects of euphoria. Chronic symptoms include a paranoid psychosis similar to that induced by amphetamine, coupled with spells of delirium and confusion. Other CNS side-effects include epileptogenesis – stimulation of epileptic seizures. This adverse effect is particularly dangerous, since animal studies have revealed that the epileptogenic effect increases with frequency of cocaine abuse, a process known as reverse tolerance (Smith and Perry, 1992). This is important when the powerful reinforcing properties of the drug are considered. The epileptogenic effect can be produced even by repeated small doses of the drug (Wadler and Hainline, 1989).

Cocaine abuse is strongly associated with cerebrovascular accidents (strokes) arising either from the rupture or spasm of cerebral blood vessels. Some of these incidents may be due to pre-existing vascular pathologies, but there are several cases where no predisposing cause has been found at autopsy (Wadler and Hainline, 1989). Cocaine is also responsible for a number of cardiovascular side-effects which are discussed later. Smith and Perry (1992) have suggested that the increase in cardiovascular and cerebrovascular side-effects seen in recent years is due to the rise in abuse of 'crack' cocaine which is rapidly absorbed and produces a concentrated effect on cerebral and cardiac arterioles. A detailed account of cocaine side-effects is given by Wadler and Hainline (1989).

4.3.2 EFFECTS IN ATHLETES

Cocaine was used by South American natives for centuries to increase efficiency, vigour and physical endurance. In 1884, Freud tested the effects of 0.1 g of cocaine hydrochloride, taken intranasally, on hand-grip strength and on reaction time. He noted that the positive effect of cocaine was greatest when he was fatigued (Freud, 1885, quoted by Conlee, 1991).

In 1930, Theil and Essing reported that 0.1 g of cocaine administered to subjects before exercising on a cycle ergometer improved work efficiency, as determined by VO_2 measurements per unit work, and that exercise could be maintained for longer. The results were attributed to reduced CNS perception of fatigue. A second study, using the same cocaine dose, revealed no increase in work efficiency but a more rapid increase in recovery after exercise (Conlee, 1991). In his review of pre-1983 studies of the effects of cocaine on exercise, Conlee (1991) concluded that they were all contradictory and were usually poorly controlled and carried out. Many of the studies reviewed since 1983 have been in animals, because of ethical considerations, and have involved measurements undertaken in rats trained to run on treadmills connected to ergometers.

Early studies demonstrated that cocaine had no beneficial effect on running times within a dose range of 0.1–20.0 mg/kg body weight, and at doses above 12.5 mg/kg the cocaine actually reduced running time. At all doses used, cocaine significantly increased glycogen degradation whilst increasing plasma lactate concentration without producing consistent changes in plasma catecholamine levels. In 1991, Conlee and co-workers demonstrated in rats exercising voluntarily that cocaine increases glycogen metabolism and enhances the exercise-induced sympathetic responses. None of these studies have explained how cocaine reduces endurance performance. Conlee (1991) has suggested three possible mechanisms to explain cocaine's action which could operate in parallel: (1) cocaine releases catecholamines which increase glycogenolysis and lactate production leading to early fatigue; (2) cocaine may induce skeletal muscle vasoconstriction, reducing oxygen delivery, oxidative metabolism, strength and reaction time, and stimulating glycogen breakdown; and (3) cocaine may have a direct effect on muscle glycogen breakdown. Indirect evidence suggests that mechanism (2) is less likely since cocaine-induced reduction of myocardial blood flow is not associated with increased myocardial glycogen breakdown.

These experiments in animals may explain the detrimental effects of cocaine, but do not explain the continued use of the drug and the claims made for it. It may be that cocaine's positive ergogenic effect is manifested only on activities of short duration requiring a burst of high intensity energy output and activities associated with the drug's central stimulatory effect rather than its action on peripheral metabolism. It has been suggested that it is precisely for these central heightened arousal and increased alertness effects, achieved principally at 'low' doses, that cocaine is used in sport (Wadler and Hainline, 1989).

A 1984 study quoted by Wadler and Hainline (1989) stated that 17% of 2039 US National Collegiate Athletic Association (NCAA) athletes admitted to using cocaine in the year preceding the study. Two years later 50% of the respondents in a survey of US National Football League players revealed that they felt cocaine was 'the number one drug of abuse in the NFL'. It is not clear from these surveys whether the cocaine was abused for social or athletic reasons.

Side-effects in athletes

In the previous edition of this book, a paper detailing the deaths of two athletes from cocaine abuse was described (George, 1988). These sudden deaths of a basketball player and a US footballer from cocaine-induced coronary occlusion provided the most dramatic evidence of the potential adverse side-effects of cocaine abuse in athletes. Cantwell and Rose (1981) describe the recovery of a 21-year-old cocaine- and amphetamine-abusing athlete from a coronary occlusion. These cases were followed by the cocaine-related deaths of basketball players, Bias and Rogers, in 1986 (Wadler and Hainline, 1989). These authors have also described the reported experiences of several US baseball players who testify to the mood-enhancing but often performance-inhibiting effects of cocaine. Significantly, baseball players complained of the deleterious central effects of cocaine, i.e. they were most liable to misjudge pitching and hitting. They also reported time disorientation in basketball players. Recently, the New York Yankees' pitcher, Steve Howe, was arraigned on charges of cocaine abuse, but escaped a lifetime ban from baseball. The apparent leniency of US Baseball League administrators towards drug transgression has been criticized (Hoffer, 1992).

There have also been reports of athletes combining cocaine abuse with other drugs, such as alcohol and anabolic steroids. According to Welder and Melchert (1993), heavy alcohol consumption combined with cocaine abuse enhances cocaine's cardiotoxicity, possibly by the production of a unique metabolite, 'cocaethylene'. This may well have been the ultimate cause of death of the Canadian ice-hockey player, John Kordic, who abused cocaine, alcohol and anabolic steroids. His downfall has been chronicled in detail (Scher, 1992), and included frequent fights on the pitch with opponents, team-mates and officials. In the UK, the Arsenal footballer, Paul Merson, admitted to 'recreational' cocaine and alcohol abuse in the autumn of 1994.

4.3.3 CONCLUSION

I concluded earlier (George, 1988) that 'whatever sporting advantage might be gained by cocaine abuse is far outweighed by the serious cardio-vascular consequences'. It is quite possible that it is the occasional short-term abuse in sport which is the major problem, and athletes think that such an abuse pattern will prevent their experiencing harmful side-effects. However, as with anabolic steroids the cardiotoxic damage is probably insidious, with any current cardiac damage causing problems in later life. Another aspect is that much of the cocaine abuse in sport may be social, with young, naive individuals, suddenly with massive salaries, able to fund an experimental abuse that leads to addiction.

4.4 CAFFEINE

The three psychoactive drugs most commonly used are alcohol, nicotine and caffeine and all are self-administered! It has been suggested that caffeine has been in use as a stimulant since the Stone Age! Caffeine is a member of the methyl xanthine group of compounds (Figure 4.2) which also includes theophylline and theobromine. Caffeine occurs naturally in coca, coffee beans and tea leaves. The amount of caffeine obtained from each source depends on the method of extraction and the particle size of the extracts. Caffeine is added to soft drinks, such as many types of colas, and is also present in a number of 'over-the-counter' medicines (Table 4.1).

4.4.1 PHARMACOLOGY

Caffeine usually exerts an effect on the CNS in doses ranging from 85 to 200 mg and, in this dose range, it produces a reduction in drowsiness and fatigue, an elevation in mood, improved alertness and productivity, increasing capacity for sustained intellectual effort and a rapid and clearer flow of thought. This dose range of caffeine also causes diuresis, a relaxation of smooth muscle, activation of gastric acid secretion and an increase in heart rate, blood pressure and blood vessel diameter. A caffeine dose in excess of 250 mg is considered to be high and may cause headaches, instability and nervousness. The American Psychiatric Association considers caffeine intoxication as occurring at doses greater than 250 mg.

Table 4.1 Caffeine content of some beverages, drinks and medicines

	Caffeine content (mg)
Coffee (per 5 oz cup)	
Percolated	64–124
Instant	40–108
Filter	110–150
Decaffeinated	2–5
Tea (per 5 oz cup)	
1 minute brew	9–33
5 minute brew	25–50
Soft drinks (per 12 oz serving)	
Pepsi Cola	38.4
Coca Cola	46
Proprietary medicines	
Anadin tablet	15
Cephos tablet	10
Coldrex cold treatment tablet	25
Phensic tablet	50

The pharmacokinetics of caffeine has recently been comprehensively reviewed by Sawynok and Yaksh (1993). They concluded that caffeine absorption after oral administration is almost 100% and that caffeine can appear in the blood as little as 5 minutes after ingestion. An important point is that though peak plasma concentrations usually occur 30–60 minutes after oral administration, the range can be as wide as 15–120 minutes because of individual variations in gastric emptying. Using an oral dose of 175 mg, it can be shown that almost 90% of the caffeine dose can be absorbed from the stomach, giving rise to plasma concentrations of 5–10 µg/ml. In 17 subjects who consumed coffee and tea, with an average daily consumption of 6.8 mg/kg per day of caffeine, mean 24 h plasma levels of 4.4 µg/ml were observed. The range of concentrations during the 24 h sampling period was 1.2–9.7 µg/ml (Lelo et al., 1986). This information has important consequences for athletes who drink caffeine-containing beverages regularly and who might take additional pure caffeine, as the plasma levels of the two ingestions will be additive. They should also be aware that caffeine is absorbed more slowly from soft drinks, such as Coca Cola, than from tea or coffee. Caffeine is rapidly distributed through all tissues from the plasma and moves into the brain rapidly by simple diffusion. The plasma half-life, that is the time for a given concentration in the plasma to reduce by half, varies from 3 to 5 hours (Sawynok and Yaksh, 1993).

Five important features governing caffeine disposition relevant to athletes have been discussed by Sawynok and Yaksh (1993). These are age, genetics, exercise, smoking and drugs. Several studies have shown that age has very little effect on caffeine metabolism, but there can be marked genetic variabilities in the ability to metabolize it. Moderate exercise appears to increase peak plasma concentrations of caffeine. Smoking increases caffeine removal from the plasma, by increasing the rate at which it is metabolized. Drugs as varied as oral contraceptives and alcohol reduce caffeine metabolism, thus raising its plasma levels.

Many athletes are convinced that caffeine improves their performance, whilst many a student (and this author) have improved their mental concentration by taking drinks containing caffeine. These uses aside, it must be remembered that caffeine consumption (as coffee) has been associated with a number of systemic disorders, which include hypertension, myocardial infarction, peptic ulcer and cancers of the gastrointestinal tract and urinary tract.

4.4.2 THE EFFECTS OF CAFFEINE

Caffeine causes:

- increased gastric acid and pepsin secretion, plus increased secretion into the small intestine;
- increased heart rate, stroke volume, cardiac output and blood pressure at rest;
- tachycardia;
- increased lipolysis;
- increased contractility of skeletal muscles;
- increased oxygen consumption and metabolic rate;
- increased diuresis;
- increased anti-nociceptive action of NSAIDS, and it exerts a mild anti-nociceptive action itself.

Mechanism of action

Caffeine is a powerful inhibitor of the cyclic nucleotide phosphodiesterase group of enzymes, of which there are five distinct types. These enzymes inactivate the so-called intracellular 'second messengers', such as cyclic AMP which acts as one of the links between receptor stimulation and cellular response. When these cellular enzymes are inhibited, the action of intracellular messengers, such as cyclic AMP, is increased. Many researchers have doubted that this is the main mechanism of action of caffeine, since the intracellular concentration of caffeine (0.1–1 mM) required to achieve significant enzyme inhibition could not be produced by the blood concentrations provided by normal caffeine dosing (Sawynok and Yaksh, 1993). However, phosphodiesterase inhibition as a mechanism of action should not be entirely dismissed. Caffeine also inhibits 5'-nucleotides which convert AMP to adenosine, but this is not thought to be of consequence in the mechanism of action of caffeine.

It is now widely accepted that the majority of the pharmacological effects of caffeine are mediated by antagonism of adenosine receptors, though some of the cardiac and renal actions may be brought about by inhibition of phosphodiesterases. In 1983, Daly, Butts-Lamb and Padgett showed that the central stimulatory activity of caffeine is correlated with its ability to bind to the adenosine receptors. There are currently three known types of adenosine receptor (A_1, A_2 and A_3), and the relative importance of these in relation to caffeine action is unclear. Most recently, *in vitro* experiments have demonstrated that caffeine can influence Ca^{2+} movements in muscle and nerve cells (Dodd, Herb and Powes, 1993).

Central effects

Caffeine is widely accepted as a mild stimulant, though clinical tests often reveal a wide variability in its action. Caffeine increases vigilance and attention and prevents the decrement in performance and information processing that occurs during fatigue or where boring repetitive jobs are being carried out (Weiss and Laties, 1962). Compared to controls, subjects taking caffeine report improved alertness, reaction times and attention span. The common finding of most placebo-controlled studies carried out in the last 30 years is that caffeine produces the most consistent improvements in tests where fatigue or a stressful workload are part of the research protocol (Sawynok and Yaksh, 1993). Investigations into the effects of caffeine on numerical reasoning, verbal fluency, short-term memory or digital skill have produced conflicting results. This may be explained by the effect of differences in personality on the action of caffeine; that is extroverts may react differently to introverts. The impulsiveness of subjects may also influence their response to caffeine, as may their normal pattern of caffeine consumption.

Many subjects report an increased feeling of well-being, indicated by improvements in mood, vigour and euphoria. However, some researchers have shown that the response to caffeine is dependent on expectations and that, in controlled trials, subjects are able to detect caffeine from placebo (Sawynok and Yaksh, 1993). The most favourable improvements in mood seem to occur when doses of 100–200 mg are taken. When the dose exceeds 400 mg the major response seems to be dysphoria (lowering of mood) and increased anxiety (Sawynok and Yaksh, 1993). It has been suggested that caffeine may act as a reinforcing agent, in that caffeine abstinence for up to 24 hours following chronic caffeine consumption leads to a withdrawal state characterized by irritability, insomnia, muscle twitching and headaches. Avoidance of this negative state could therefore act as a reinforcement of caffeine administration.

Caffeine has been shown to be anxiogenic in a number of studies (Sawynok and Yaksh, 1993), and this has led to the description of a clinical syndrome, caffeinism, by Greden (1974).

Adverse reactions

When coffee drinking became fashionable in Great Britain during the seventeenth century, the effects of caffeine were immediately noticed and there were suggestions that it should be banned.

The average intake of caffeine in the USA is 206 mg per person per day, and 10% of the population consume greater than 1000 mg per day (Conlee, 1991). The major side-effects have been described and categorized as acute, severe and chronic by Wadler and Hainline (1989). Mild effects include nervousness, irritability, insomnia and gastrointestinal distress. Severe effects, including peptic ulcer, delirium, coma, seizures and supraventricular and ventricular arrhythmias are associated with doses greater than 200 mg/kg. Chronic effects mainly involve raised serum cholesterol levels. A particular cluster of side-effects, involving anxiety, mood changes, sleep disruption, psychophysiological changes and withdrawal symptoms, has been recognized as caffeinism and is described by Greden (1974). The *Diagnostic and Statistical Manual of Mental Disorders* (1989) of the American Psychiatric Association describes caffeine intoxication as a condition simulating an anxiety attack, in which the person experiences nausea, insomnia, restlessness and jitteriness.

4.4.3 EFFECTS IN ATHLETES

In 1965, Bellet, Kershbaum and Aspe described the elevation of blood fatty acids that occurred with caffeine ingestion. They concluded that caffeine improved endurance by enhancing fat utilization, thus sparing glycogen stores. Using nine competitive cyclists, Costill, Dalsky and Fink (1978) studied the effects of caffeine on their general metabolism. Each cyclist exercised to exhaustion on a cycle ergometer at 50% of their aerobic capacity, after ingesting either decaffeinated or normal coffee (containing

330 mg caffeine). The caffeine takers managed to exercise for 19.5% longer than the control group and had significantly higher levels of plasma fatty acids and blood glycerol. In the caffeine group, the respiratory quotient was reduced, possibly indicating a shift from carbohydrate to fat utilization. It was suggested that increased lipolysis postponed exhaustion by slowing the rate of glycogen utilization in liver and skeletal muscle.

Ivy, Costill and Fink (1979) found that caffeine increased work production in athletes by 7.4% compared to control conditions and, in the same study, fat oxidation was elevated by 31% during the last 70 minutes of the trial. Essig, Costill and Von Handel (1980) measured the effect of caffeine on insulin secretion and glycogen utilization in seven untrained male cyclists. Compared to controls, the caffeine group had a 51% increase in lipid oxidation. Muscle biopsies showed a 39% reduction in glycogen utilization. They concluded that caffeine ingestion can increase oxidation of fatty acids and glycerol in muscle. In contrast, Perkins and Williams (1975) could find no effect with 4, 7 or 10 mg of caffeine per kg body weight in 14 male students exercising to exhaustion. They found no significant difference between control and caffeine-taking groups in exercise time to exhaustion, even though there was a caffeine-induced increase in fatty acid level.

The results of the pioneering studies of the putative ergogenicity of caffeine led me to summarize in the previous edition of this book that 'caffeine has a positive ergogenic effect on large muscles and on short-term exercise which requires both strength and power' (George, 1988). Since then a number of studies have been carried out in both animals and humans, some of which support and some of which refute this statement. In addition, some reviewers have doubted whether caffeine is a true ergogenic aid. In his 1991 review, Conlee listed six crucial factors which he claimed accounted for the variability in the effect of caffeine on athletic performance. These were dose, type of exercise, intensity of exercise, pre-exercising feedings, previous caffeine use and training status. He also identified from his literature survey optimal conditions for the ergogenic effect of caffeine, which are: use of untrained, caffeine-abstaining subjects, caffeine doses of 6–10 mg/kg, abstinence from high carbohydrate diets and an experimental protocol involving prolonged activities at 70–85% VO_2max.

Some of the questions raised by Conlee (1991) had also been addressed previously by Powers and Dodd (1985) who reviewed the evidence for caffeine ergogenicity prior to 1985 and, in particular, noted discrepancies between the positive effect of caffeine during graded exercise but its lack of effect on VO_2max. Research evidence has been further complicated by the increasing number of animal studies, particularly those involving isolated muscle preparations. A detailed analysis of the conflicting results produced by these various studies has been made by Dodd, Herb and Powers (1993). They examined all the studies of caffeine on exercise performance since 1985 and found that they could be divided into three major groups, i.e. short-term high intensity exercise, graded incremental exercise and prolonged endurance exercise, each group containing both human and animal studies.

High intensity, graded incremental and prolonged endurance exercise

During short-term, high intensity exercise, caffeine has been shown to enhance muscle force production in isolated muscle preparation whilst most human studies demonstrate no effect. Caffeine appears to increase peak muscular tension and decrease the time required to achieve peak tension, and this is associated with increased release of Ca^{2+} from the sarcoplasmic reticulum. However, in this situation, the muscle Ca^{2+} was also depleted more rapidly, resulting in earlier fatigue. Studies in humans, however, have shown that caffeine does not increase force, electromyograph EMG activity or muscular power during either hand-grip exercise or short maximal bouts of cycle exercise. Dodd, Herb and Powers (1993) have concluded that the major source of discrepancy between human and *in vitro* animal studies is the dosage of caffeine used. They have calculated that most *in vitro* studies utilize caffeine doses of 200–3500 μmol/L, whilst human studies have used caffeine doses below 10 mg/kg. In the blood, even assuming the caffeine remained unbound to plasma proteins, the concentration of caffeine would be 60–100 μmol/L. If allowance is made for 15–17% binding of caffeine to plasma proteins, then the amount of caffeine available for cellular action is some 100 μmol **less** than the lowest dosage used in *in vitro* studies. Conversely, to produce a positive ergogenic effect in humans of the same order as that achieved in *in vitro* experiments, it would require caffeine doses which would produce urinary caffeine concentrations well in excess of the International Olympic Committee (IOC) limits of 12 mcg/ml urine. It is surprising that so few caffeine studies have involved determinations of blood caffeine levels following administration and during exercise.

More recently, the effects of caffeine on graded incremental exercise have been investigated. Two studies, both of which administered caffeine 10–15 mg/kg to moderately fit, caffeine-naive subjects, 1–3 hours before exercise testing, demonstrated an improved performance during graded incremental exercise (McNaughton, 1987 and Flinn *et al.*, 1990). Performance improvement was identified as an increase in time to exhaustion and a reduced lactate threshold. The significance of the results is that they were obtained using high doses of caffeine, and it is unclear whether they were influenced by any caffeine intolerance of the subjects. However, in 1991, Dodd and co-workers produced evidence to show that the caffeine tolerance within a subject has no effect on performance during exercise of moderate intensity and duration. From these findings it was concluded that the results of the original studies were associated with the high dosage of caffeine used (Dodd, Herb and Powers, 1993).

The other major area of exercise research involving caffeine concerns prolonged endurance exercise, the subject of the much quoted early research of Costill, Dalsky and Fink (1978). In the past four years the initial findings have been disputed. Conlee (1991) has stated that the evidence supporting the positive ergogenic effect of caffeine during prolonged exercise is inconclusive. In contrast, Dodd, Herb and Powers (1993) have reviewed the studies of caffeine and prolonged exercise since 1978 and have produced a detailed re-analysis of the series of tests.

There was a considerable variability in the experimental design used. For example some studies used caffeine-naive, and others caffeine-habit-uated subjects, and dietary control was employed in some subjects but not in others. With the exception of one study that involved a 21 km ski run, all the studies quoted involved cycle ergometer or treadmill measurements. From these Dodd, Herb and Powers (1993) concluded that moderate to high doses of caffeine are ergogenic during prolonged moderate intensity exercise in both caffeine-naive and caffeine-habituated subjects. It was argued in their review that the positive ergogenic effect of caffeine on endurance exercise is apparent only when studies of high intensity exercise are omitted from the analysis. Thus, in their table of endurance studies, two of which used continuous low intensity exercise (50–60% of VO_2max.) for 2–8 hours followed by exercise to exhaustion at 90% of VO_2max., there was no evidence of an ergogenic effect of caffeine.

The biochemical and physiological basis of the ergogenic effect of caffeine during endurance exercise is unclear. The possible explanations cited by Ivy, Costill and Fink (1979) and Essig, Costill and Von Handel (1980) have been added to by Conlee (1991) and now include: (1) a stimulatory effect on the CNS; (2) enhanced release of catecholamines; (3) free fatty acid mobilization from adipose tissue, leading to increased β oxidation in muscle and the sparing of glycogen; (4) indirect inhibition of muscle glycogenolysis, thus sparing muscle glycogen; and (5) increased use of muscle triglycerides also leading to muscle glycogen sparing.

In studies where caffeine effects on glycogen depletion have been investigated simultaneously with prolonged exercise (Essig, Costill and Von Handel, 1980; Erickson, Schwarzkopf and McKenzie, 1987 and Spriet *et al.*, 1992), all show that caffeine brings about glycogen sparing, thus confirming the original hypothesis of Bellet, Kershbaum and Aspe (1965) quoted earlier. Research by Essig, Costill and Von Handel (1980) suggesting that fat metabolism, fuelled by increased lipolysis, is enhanced following caffeine ingestion has not been unequivocally supported by recent research.

Dodd, Herb and Powers (1993) quote the results of seven experiments, five of which demonstrated increased plasma free fatty acid levels during exercise following caffeine ingestion, which, however, was not accompanied in any study by a rise in the respiratory quotient. Thus caffeine may well antagonize adenosine-mediated inhibition of lipolysis, but the consequent increased availability of free fatty acids does not appear to influence energy production. The anomalous results obtained with caffeine on free fatty acids and the respiratory quotient may be explained by the observation that caffeine ingestion raises plasma catecholamine levels. This may lead to a pre-exercise increase in free fatty acid utilization which masks any effect of caffeine during the exercise period (Conlee, 1991). However, French *et al.* (1991) showed that caffeine ingestion immediately prior to exercise to exhaustion improved the distance that was run by six trained athletes. In this experiment, blood lactate was raised only at the end of the study and blood triglycerides were elevated by caffeine only after 45 minutes' exercise.

The future of caffeine as an ergogenic aid seems unpredictable. Only one exercise category, long-term endurance exercise (75–80% $VO_2max.$) seems to be positively enhanced by caffeine, and even this modest improvement may not be attainable within the IOC limit of 12 mcg/ml urine. It would be of interest to know what is the exact mechanism of caffeine's ergogenic action.

4.5 THE FUTURE

As a percentage of the total positive doping tests in the UK, abuse of central stimulants is declining. In 1988–89, the UK Sports Council reported that stimulants accounted for 29 (45%) of the total positive tests in Britain, but by 1992–93 this had fallen to 18 (30%). A similar trend has been observed in the USA and has been explained by more stringent legislation (USA) and the impact of drug testing (USA and UK). However, another interpretation of the US findings is the increasing impact of cocaine which appears to be less of a problem in British sport. One answer to the problem of stimulant abuse, which may also help to detect the onset of abuse in the young, is the introduction of out-of-competition testing, particularly during training sessions and summer schools. In response to the Paul Merson case, in 1994, Arsenal Football Club decided to test all their first team squad for drug abuse. The next decade may see a further decline in abuse of traditional stimulants in favour of designer drugs, such as Ecstasy, or their derivatives. This may present abusers with fewer unpredictable central side-effects. The possibility of doping with negative ergogenic drugs, as suggested for anabolic steroids in Chapter 7, should not be ignored.

Future research might be devoted to understanding the underlying psychological processes that influence the abuse of central stimulants by athletes. Begel (1992) has reviewed the psychodynamic factors influencing the development of the athlete and the maintenance of his/her performance. It may be that athletes particularly resort to central stimulants when coaches fail to identify or help to rectify problems in the athletes' approach and technique, or fail to counsel them adequately when their performance drops. It would also be interesting to know, as Begel has concluded, what particular personalities are associated with central stimulant abuse in sportspersons, and whether psychiatric disorders contribute to abuse of stimulants by them.

4.6 REFERENCES

American Psychiatric Association (1989) *Diagnostic and Statistical Manual of Mental Disorders. Third Edition Revised*, (DSM 3R), American Psychiatric Press, Washington, DC.

Begel, D. (1992) An overview of sport psychiatry. *Am. J. Psychiat.*, **149**, 606–14.

Bellet, S., Kershbaum, A. and Aspe, J. (1965) The effect of caffeine on free fatty acids. *Arch. Intern. Med.*, **116**, 750–52.

Brookes, L.G. (1985) *Central Nervous System Stimulants in Psychopharmacology: Recent Advances and Future Prospects*, (ed. S.D. Iverson), Oxford University Press, Oxford, pp. 264–77.

Cantwell, J.D. and Rose, F.D. (1981) Cocaine and cardiovascular events. *Physician and Sports Medicine*, **14**, 77–82.

Chandler, J.V. and Blair, S.N. (1980) The effect of amphetamines on selected physiological components related to athletic success. *Med. Sci. Sports Exerc.*, **12**, 65–9.

Conlee, R.K. (1991) Amphetamine, caffeine and cocaine, in *Perspectives in Exercise Science and Sports Medicine*, 4, (ed. D.R. Lamb and M.H. Williams), Brown and Benchmark, New York, pp. 285–328.

Conlee, R.K., Han, D.H., Kelly, K.P. and Barnett, D.W. (1991) Effects of cocaine on plasma catecholamine and muscle glycogen concentrations during exercise in the rat. *J. Appl. Physiol.*, **70**, 1323–7.

Connell, P.H. (1958) *Amphetamine Psychosis*. Chapman and Hall, London.

Costill, D.L., Dalsky, G.P. and Fink, W.J. (1978) Effects of caffeine ingestion on metabolism and exercise performance. *Med. Sci. Sports*, **10**, 155–8.

Daly, J.W., Butts-Lamb, P. and Padgett, W. (1983) Sub-classes of adenosine receptors in the central nervous system interaction with caffeine and related methyl xanthines. *Cell. Mol. Neurobiol.*, **3**, 69–80.

Dodd, S.L., Herb, R.A. and Powers, S.K. (1993) Caffeine and exercise performance – an update. *Sports. Med.*, **15**, 14–23.

Erickson, M.A., Schwarzkopf, R.J. and McKenzie, R.D. (1987) Effects of caffeine, fructose, and glucose ingestion on muscle glycogen utilisation during exercise. *Mod. Sci. in Sport Exerc.*, **19**, 579–83.

Essig, D., Costill, D.L. and Von Handel, P.J. (1980) Effects of caffeine ingestion on utilisation of muscle glycogen and lipid during leg ergometer cycling. *Int. J. Sports Med.*, **1**, 86–90.

Fibiger, H.C., Phillips, A.G. and Brown, E.E. (1992) The neurobiology of cocaine-induced reinforcement, in *Cocaine: Scientific and Social Dimensions*, Ciba

Foundation Symposium 166, (ed. G.E.W. Wolstenholme), John Wiley, Chichester, pp. 96–124.

Flinn, S., Gregory, J., McNaughton, L.R. *et al.* (1990) Caffeine ingestion prior to incremental cycling to exhaustion in recreational cyclists. *Int. J. Sports Med.*, **11**, 188–93.

French, C., McNaughton, L., Davies, P. and Tristram, S. (1991) Caffeine ingestion during exercise to exhaustion in élite distance runners. *J. Sport Med. Phys. Fitness*, **31**, 425–32.

George, A.J. (1988) CNS stimulants, in *Drugs in Sport*, (ed. D.R. Mottram), E. and F.N. Spon, London.

Golding, L.A. (1981) Drugs and hormones, in *Ergogenic Aids and Muscular Performance*, (ed. W.P. Morgan), Academic Press, London, pp. 368–97.

Golding, L.A. and Barnard, J.P. (1963) The effect of d-amphetamine sulphate on physical performance. *J. Sports Med.*, **3**, 221–4.

Greden, J.F. (1974) Anxiety or caffeinism: a diagnostic dilemma. *Am. J. Psychiat.*, **131**, 1089–92.

Haldi, J. and Wynn, W. (1959) Action of drugs on efficiency of swimmers. *Res. Quarterly*, **31**, 449–553.

Hoffer, R. (1992) A career of living dangerously. *Sports Illustrated*, **76**, 38–41.

Ivy, J.L., Costill, D.L. and Fink, W.J. (1979) Influence of caffeine and carbohydrate feedings on endurance performance. *Med. Sci. Sports*, **11**, 6–11.

Kennedy, L. (1974) *Pursuit. The Chase and Sinking of the Bismarck*, Collins, London.

Kuhar, M.J. (1992) Molecular pharmacology of cocaine: a dopamine hypothesis and its implications, in *Cocaine: Scientific and Social Dimensions*, Ciba Foundation Symposium 166, (ed. G.E.W. Wolstenholme), John Wiley, Chichester, pp. 81–95.

Laties, V.G. and Weiss, B. (1981) The amphetamine margin in sports. *Fed. Proc.*, **40**, 2689–92.

Lelo, A., Miners, J.O., Robson, R. and Birkett, D.J. (1986) Assessment of caffeine exposure: caffeine content of beverages, caffeine intake and plasma concentrations of methylxanthines. *Clin. Pharmac. Ther.*, **39**, 54–9.

Mandell, A.J. (1979) The Sunday syndrome: a unique pattern of amphetamine abuse indigenous to American professional football. *Clin. Toxicol.*, **15**, 225–32.

Mandell, A.J., Stewart, K.D. and Russo, P.V. (1981) The Sunday syndrome from kinetics to altered consciousness. *Fed. Proc.*, **40**, 2693–6.

McNaughton, L. (1987) Two levels of caffeine ingestion on blood lactate and free fatty acid response during incremental exercise. *Res. Quart. Exerc. Sport*, **58**, 255–9.

Perkins, R. and Williams, M.H. (1975) Effects of caffeine upon maximal muscular endurance of females. *Med. Sci. Sports*, **7**, 221–4.

Pierson, W.R., Rasch, P.J. and Brubaker, M.L. (1961) *Med. Sport*, **1**, 61–6.

Powers, S.K. and Dodd, S. (1985) Caffeine and endurance performance. *Sports Med.*, **2**, 165–74.

Sawynok, J. and Yaksh, T.L. (1993) Caffeine as an analgesic adjuvant. A review of pharmacology and mechanisms of action. *Pharmac. Revs.*, **45**, 43–85.

Scher, J. (1992) Death of a goon. *Sports Illustrated*, **76**, 112–16.

Seiden, L.S., Sabol, K.E. and Ricaurte, G.A. (1993) Amphetamine: effects on catecholamine systems and behaviour. *Ann. Rev. Pharmac. Tox.*, **32**, 639–77.

Sidney, K.H. and Lefcoe, W.M. (1977) The effects of ephedrine on the physiological and psychological responses to submaximal and maximal exercises in man. *Med. Sci. Sports*, **9**, 95–9.

Silverstone, T. and Goodall, E. (1985) How amphetamine works, in *Psychopharmacology. Recent Advances, Future Prospects*, (ed. S.D. Iversen), Oxford University Press, Oxford, pp. 315–25.

Smith, D.A. and Perry, P.J. (1992) The efficacy of ergogenic agents in athletic competition. Part II: other performance-enhancing agents. *Annal. Pharmacother.*, **26**, 653–9.

Smith, G.M. and Beecher, H.G. (1959) Amphetamine sulphate and athletic performance. *J. Am. Med. Assoc.*, **170**, 542–51.

Sports Council Doping Control Unit (1993) *Report on the Sports Council's Doping Control Service*, UK Sports Council, London.

Spriet, L., MacLean, D., Dyck, D. *et al.* (1992) Effects of caffeine on muscle glycogenolysis and acetyl group metabolism during prolonged exercise in humans. *Am. J. Physiol.*, **262**, 891–8.

Theil, D. and Essing, B. (1930) Cocaine und muskelarbeit I. Der einfluss auf leistung und gastoffwechsel. *Arbeitsphysiologie*, **3**, 287–97.

Wadler, G.A. and Hainline, B. (1989) *Drugs and the Athlete*, F.A. Davies Company, Philadelphia.

Weiss, B. and Laties, V.G. (1962) Enhancement of human performance by caffeine and the amphetamines. *Pharmac. Rev.*, **14**, 1–36.

Welder, A.A. and Melchert, R.B. (1993) Cardiotoxic effects of cocaine and anabolic-androgenic steroids in the athlete. *J. Pharmac. Tox. Method.*, **29**, 61–8.

Wyndham, G.H., Rogers, G.G., Benade, A.J.S. and Strydan, N.B. (1971) Physiological effects of the amphetamines during exercise. *S. Afr. Med. J.*, **45**, 247–52.

Drug treatment of inflammation in sports injuries

5

Peter Elliott

5.1 SUMMARY

Following a brief introduction putting sports injury in perspective, the nature of the inflammatory response is described. The role of chemical mediators of inflammation and the contribution of leucocytes to the inflammation is detailed.

The treatment of sporting injuries is then discussed, with particular reference to the use of aerosol sprays, oral and topical aspirin-like drugs, proteolytic enzymes and anti-inflammatory glucocorticoids. The place of each therapy is discussed and possible mechanisms of action of the drugs outlined.

5.2 INTRODUCTION

All sports have developed from the natural capabilities of the human mind and body, and so, when partaken at a modest level, few sports involve great risk of physical injury. This situation changes, however, when sporting pursuits are undertaken at higher competitive levels. As it becomes necessary to push the body further, in an effort to achieve greater performance, a point may well be reached where the stresses and strains exerted on the structural framework of the body may exceed that which the body is capable of withstanding, resulting in connective tissues being torn or joints being dislocated. Many sports carry their own peculiar additional risks of injury to the body; the boxer may suffer repeated blows to the face causing extensive bruising and laceration and the footballer may receive kicks to the legs resulting in bruising or even bone fracture.

Any traumatic injury to a competitor will result in a reduced level of performance capability and may require abstention from sport for a period of recuperation. As well as the pain and personal discomfort

Drugs in Sport, 2nd edn. Edited by David R. Mottram. Published in 1996 by E & FN Spon, London. ISBN 0 419 18890 8

associated with injury, the person's performance is likely to deteriorate during a period of inactivity, and an extended training period will subsequently be required to regain peak fitness.

In a sport where a career may be of limited duration and where there is a short season of competition, the result of even minor trauma may be devastating. To the keen amateur, years of training may be wasted by an inability to participate competitively in a once in a lifetime event. To the top international professional, a day on the bench may represent the loss of vast sums of money to the individual or club. Whatever the injury, one of its undoubted features will be the occurrence of an inflammatory reaction at the damaged site.

5.3 THE INFLAMMATORY RESPONSE

Inflammation (a word derived from the Latin *inflammare*, meaning to set on fire) is a term widely employed to describe the pathological process which occurs at the site of tissue damage. A precise definition of the condition is difficult, but a useful description is that it is a process which enables the body's defensive and regenerative resources to be channelled into tissues which have suffered damage or are contaminated with abnormal material (such as invading micro-organisms). It is a process which aims to limit the damaging effects of any contaminating material, to cleanse and remove any foreign particles and damaged tissue debris and allow healing processes to restore the tissues to some kind of normality. Inflammation is a process which is fundamentally important for survival. Protection against noxious stimuli and the repair of damaged tissue are essential processes.

Inflammation is a phenomenon well known to ancient civilizations. The classical description of inflammation was undoubtedly given by Celsus in the first century AD. In his *De re medicina*, he states that 'the signs of inflammation are four, redness and swelling with heat and pain'. To these four signs was added a fifth, loss of function, by Virchow (1858), the founder of modern cellular pathology. Loss of function is a consequence of the swelling and pain associated with inflammation and is clearly an indication that affected tissues require rest for rapid rehabilitation.

Prior to the twentieth century the principal tool employed to study the processes of inflammation was the microscope. Defence mechanisms typical of those seen in mammals were found in many simple organisms, and it was maintained that the primary movement of the inflammatory reaction was the direction of protoplasm to digest any noxious agent. This activity can be seen in many different phyla of the animal kingdom. In protozoans, phagocytic (that is engulfing) activity is exerted by the organisms as a whole, but in more complex animals this function is attributed to specialized cells. The phagocytic cells of multicellular organisms are able to move to the site of the noxious agent by amoeboid movement (a directed flowing movement of the cytoplasm). This movement is greatly enhanced in, but not restricted to, those organisms having a vascular system for transport of these cells to the affected area.

Nineteenth century physiologists recognized the importance of the circulation and proposed that it was the vascular system itself that was responsible for inflammation. Undoubtedly, the vascular system is of fundamental importance in the inflammatory process of mammals, but it is well to remember that defensive reactions can occur in simple organisms which do not possess a vascular system. The reaction of such organisms to noxious stimuli, however, will not be accompanied by all the classical signs of inflammation. Without a vascular system there can be no redness or heat, and indeed, with the exception of mammalia and avia which are warm-blooded, inflammation of the tissues in animal species will not be accompanied by heat at the affected site.

However inflammation may be defined, it is a dynamic process, and this process may, on occasions, be capable of causing more harm to the organism than the initiating noxious stimulus itself would. The necrotic lesions produced on dogs at the feeding site of a tick, for example, are brought about by the dog's defence system; they are not caused directly by the tick. The necrosis can be virtually eliminated by the prior destruction of polymorphonuclear leucocytes (blood cells which have a phagocytic role in the defence system). Similarly, some immunologically induced reactions to seemingly harmless agents result in tissue damage out of all proportion to the threat from the sensitizing agent, and there is no obvious reason why the inflammatory reactions which occur in diseases such as rheumatic fever or rheumatoid arthritis benefit organisms. Clearly not all inflammation can be useful. The combined effect of the components of the body's defensive mechanism may often be excessive.

Whilst there are many and varied kinds of inflammation, it is possible to consider that the basic components of the inflammatory reaction are due to the combined effects of changes in the microcirculation, alteration of permeability of the blood vessel walls, migration of leucocytes and phagocytosis.

5.3.1 CHANGES IN THE MICROCIRCULATION DURING THE INFLAMMATORY RESPONSE

The immediate reaction of skin to a burn or irritant is to become reddened. This reddening will persist for a variable time depending on the severity of the stimulus. The redness is due to an increased volume of blood flowing through the inflamed area. Consequently, the temperature of the inflamed skin rises and approaches that of the deep body temperature. This effect on the microcirculation is seen clearly if a firm line is drawn with a blunt point over the surface of the forearm. As Lewis (1927) demonstrated, a red line appears in exactly the position that the stimulus is applied. This dull red area is then surrounded by a bright red halo and a weal begins to form, firstly at the red line and then spreading outwards. Lewis confirmed earlier suggestions that many different types of injury could induce inflammation, including heat, cold, electric shock, radiation and chemical irritants, as well as mechanical injury.

Detailed studies of vascular changes occurring during inflammation have been made by many physiologists who have observed vascular changes in sheets of living connective tissue arranged on microscope stages. Using this technique, it is possible to observe mild inflammatory reactions over long periods of time. In this way it has been demonstrated that the whole capillary bed at the damaged site becomes suffused with blood at an increased pressure. Capillaries dilate and many closed ones open up. The venules dilate and there is an increased flow of blood in the draining veins. This rapid flow gradually slows in the central capillaries and venules even though the vessels are still dilated. This slowing may gradually spread to the peripheral areas of the lesion and the flow may even stop completely. Despite this stasis the capillary pressure remains high, probably due to a resistance to outflow. The pressure in the small veins may be increased by a rise in pressure of the interstitial fluid due to oedema. Two of the cardinal signs of inflammation, heat and redness, are caused by this increase in blood flow to the affected area.

Another of the principal signs, swelling, is also the consequence of a change in the vascular system. In this case it is a change in the permeability of the blood vessel wall to protein. Normally the fluid found outside the blood system, in the tissues, is composed of water with some low molecular weight solutes, such as sodium chloride. The protein content of this fluid is very low, whilst the protein content of blood is relatively high. This state of affairs is maintained by virtue of the fact that the blood vessel wall is permeable only to water and salts. Proteins cannot normally move from the blood vessel through the vessel wall into the surrounding tissues.

Water is forced out of small blood vessels at the arteriolar end of capillary beds due to the internal pressure which is generated by the pumping action of the heart on the blood enclosed in the vascular system. The colloid osmotic pressure exerted by the protein present in the blood counterbalances this force, causing water to be drawn back into the blood system. Without the presence of the plasma protein, blood volume would very rapidly diminish due to the net movement of water from the blood to the tissues.

At the inflammatory site, the balance of forces is altered. The permeability of small blood vessels changes to allow plasma protein to leak out of the vessel into the surrounding tissue, and this change in distribution of protein is followed by a net passage of water from the blood into the tissues, giving rise to the oedema which may ultimately be seen as a swelling. Electron microscopic examination of blood vessels, to which vasoactive substances have been applied, reveal the production of gaps $0.1\,\mu m$ to $0.4\,\mu m$ in diameter between adjacent endothelial cells. These gaps are temporary and there is no apparent damage caused to the endothelium of the leaking vessel.

Another consequence of oedema formation is the development of pain. Pain is, at least in part, due to the increased pressure on sensory nerves caused by the accumulation of the oedematous fluid. The common experience of relief that occurs instantly after the rupture of a painful boil lends support to this idea. There is, however, some evidence that pain may also be due to the release of pain-inducing chemicals at the site of the reaction. The cardinal signs of inflammation can thus be accounted for by the various changes that occur to the vasculature of the affected area. Vasodilation results in the increased redness and temperature of the affected area, whilst the change to the protein permeability of blood vessels results in the development of swelling and pain.

Even though each inflammatory reaction is unique, very similar reactions can be induced by widely differing stimuli. This has led to the idea that some intermediary control system exists to link the stimulus and the effect. The most popular idea is that the inflammatory insult causes the release of chemicals within the body which then trigger the inflammatory reactions. This mediator concept was exemplified by Lewis (1927), who proposed that the local vasodilation and increased vascular permeability observed in the triple response could be mediated by a substance, liberated by the tissue, which he termed 'H-substance'. The search for chemical mediators of inflammation has been particularly directed towards finding substances capable of increasing vascular permeability, largely because this parameter may be quantified quite easily. It should be remembered, however, that mediators of increased vascular permeability may not necessarily be responsible for mediation of other aspects of the inflammatory reaction. The time course of vasodilation differs markedly from increased vascular permeability in many types of inflammatory reactions induced by chemical irritants. In general, investigations of permeability change mediation centre on endogenous substances which exhibit high permeability-increasing potency and can be demonstrated in normal or inflamed tissues. A number of such substances have been investigated to determine their possible role in the inflammatory response.

Histamine

One of the first substances to be examined as a potential mediator of inflammation was histamine. Histamine is formed by the decarboxylation of the amino acid, histidine, and is a normal constituent of most tissues. The most abundant source of histamine in the body is to be found in the mast cells where it is stored in granules in association with the anti-coagulant substance, heparin. Mast cells are found in high levels in the lungs, gastrointestinal system and skin. When released from the mast cell, or when injected, histamine produces vasodilation and an increase in blood vessel permeability to protein. At high concentration histamine can also induce pain, and so this particular locally acting hormone has the properties that could contribute to all four cardinal signs of inflammation.

Histamine has been found to be released following chemical, thermal, ionizing irradiation and immunological challenge. The contribution of histamine to most inflammatory reactions is limited, however, to the very early phase, and, in most cases, after the first few hours antihistamine drugs have no anti-inflammatory activity. The most notable exception is in the case of immunological reactions where histamine activity may persist throughout the duration of a type 1 hypersensitivity reaction (Figure 5.1), such as hay fever or urticaria, where antihistamine drugs represent an effective therapeutic approach.

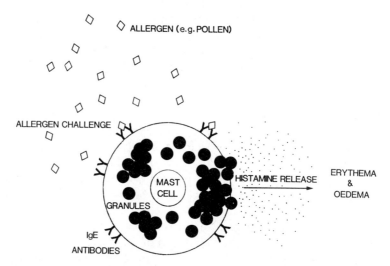

Figure 5.1 Histamine release in allergic reactions.

Kinins

The body can generate a number of highly active polypeptide hormones which exert local actions on the tissues in a variety of circumstances. A characteristic feature of these substances is that they are intensely vaso-active. One particular group of these polypeptides is known as the kinins, and the best known of these is bradykinin, a polypeptide of nine amino acid residues. Kinins can be released in all body fluids by the action of an enzyme, kallikrein, on a globulin protein. In glandular tissue, kinins may be responsible for the functional vasodilation that occurs during periods of glandular activity. During exercise, bradykinin may be released in response to increasing activity that occurs in active muscles and cause vasodilation of the tissues and promote sweating. It is possible that kinins may contribute to ischaemic pain where the vasodilation has proved inadequate. Kinins are also generated, however, where tissue damage occurs, and may promote both vasodilation and an increase in blood vessel permeability. They are extremely potent in these respects but are very labile, having a half-life in blood of only a few seconds. Despite the difficulties that exist in handling the material, some evidence has been produced that kinins do contribute to inflammatory reactions, but, as with histamine, this may well be restricted to the fairly early stages of an acute reaction.

A substance capable of inhibiting kallikrein has been detected in a number of bovine tissues. This substance, aprotinin, is available commercially and has been tried in the treatment of acute pancreatitis; here it owes its possible usefulness to inhibition of kinin release and to blocking the activity of pancreatic protease. It has been shown to be active as an anti-inflammatory agent in experimental animals, but clinical trials in human inflammatory diseases have failed to provide convincing evidence of efficacy. It would seem, therefore, that whilst kinins may contribute to the early development of an inflammatory reaction, their inhibition would not seem to be an important target for drug treatment in musculoskeletal injuries.

Arachidonic acid metabolites

With respect to the chemical mediation of inflammatory reactions, the most interesting areas that are currently being studied are the various products of arachidonic acid metabolism. Every cell in the body has the capacity to generate some products from arachidonic acid, which is a 20-carbon straight-chain polyunsaturated fatty acid. This substance is usually found only at very low levels in the free form, but an abundant supply is normally available in a bound form, principally as cell membrane phospholipid. Following hormone activity or perturbation of the cell, the phospholipids are split by the action of enzymes, such as phospholipase A_2, releasing arachidonic acid. Once made available, arachidonic acid is metabolized in a way that is characteristic for the particular cell. This metabolism is generally rapid, since it is the availability of arachidonic acid that is the rate-limiting factor. Two enzyme systems are available for this metabolism: a cyclo-oxygenase and a lipoxygenase. None of the biologically active products of these enzymes have long half-lives in the body and they are not generally stored. They tend to exert their activities locally, and it has become apparent that many of them exhibit opposing properties, giving rise to the idea that they are involved in the local modulation of physiological processes.

The first class of these products to be discovered was the prostaglandins, so named because it was thought that they were secreted by the prostate gland, although it was subsequently found that the principal source of these substances found in seminal fluid was the seminal vesicles. Prostaglandins are formed by the action of the cyclo-oxygenase on arachidonic acid. This enzyme causes the oxygenation and internal cyclization of the fatty acid to give an unstable cyclic endoperoxide, PGG_2. This unstable 15-hydroperoxy compound rapidly reduces to the 15-hydroxy derivative, PGH_2, this change being accompanied by the release of a free radical into the medium. (It is worthy of mention here that free radicals are extremely damaging to biological tissues and may be responsible for some of the tissue destruction that occurs in the course of inflammatory reactions. Free radicals are also generated by cells during phagocytosis.) The second stage of synthesis involves another enzyme which is tissue-specific and results in the conversion of the cyclic endoperoxide to either PGE_2, PGF_{2a}, PGI or to a thromboxane, depending on the tissue (Figure 5.2).

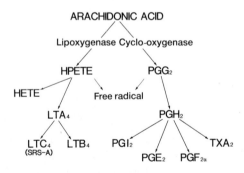

Figure 5.2 Some biologically active metabolites of arachidonic acid.

Tremendous interest has been shown in these highly biologically active substances since the discovery of their presence in exudates. A number of properties exhibited by prostaglandins are compatible with the idea that these locally acting hormones are mediators of the inflammatory response. Firstly, they can cause profound vasodilation at very low concentrations, and the erythema that they induce is very long lasting, persisting even after the prostaglandins have been broken down. Prostaglandins by themselves do not greatly affect vascular permeability, nor do they evoke a pain response at physiological concentrations. Prostaglandins do, however, radically enhance the vascular permeability-increasing and pain-provoking activity of other substances, such as histamine and bradykinin. These properties, coupled with the fact that raised prostaglandin levels are readily detectable in a number of inflammatory conditions, make them ideal candidates for the role of mediators of inflammation.

5.3.2 LEUCOCYTES IN INFLAMMATION

Some types of inflammatory reaction, such as acute allergic responses, are restricted to changes in the microcirculation alone. More chronic conditions of the type common to sports injuries, however, involve another major physiological change – the influx of leucocytes.

Normal tissues contain few extra vascular polymorphs, but in an inflammatory reaction these cells may pass from the microcirculation into the damaged tissue site. Following an injury, blood polymorphs stick momentarily to the endothelium; they roll along the inside surface of the vessel wall, adhering briefly until they re-enter the circulation. After a few minutes, more and more cells adhere and, eventually, these are not dislodged by the blood flow. In this way the endothelium comes to be lined. This process is called margination. Other leucocytes, platelets and red cells may also stick. The marginated polymorphs leave the intra-vascular site by 'emigrating', or diapedesis. A pseudopodium insinuates itself between the endothelial cells, and the bulk of the polymorph, including the nucleus, passes between the endothelial cells and comes to lie outside the endothelial cell but within the basement membrane. The manner in which the cell passes through the basement membrane is not known. That these cells make an important contribution to the inflammatory process has been demonstrated by the reduced inflammatory response that occurs in experimental animals when their polymorphonuclear leucocytes have been depleted. To achieve this reduction, the number of both circulating polymorphs and polymorphs which enter the circulation (presumably from the bone marrow) following an inflammatory stimulus must be reduced to very low levels.

Polymorphonuclear leucocytes are the first circulating cells to accumulate in large numbers in an injured area. These cells are phago-cytic and play a protective role by ingesting and subsequently digesting invading micro-organisms or tissue debris in the affected area. Polymorphs do not survive for more than a few hours outside blood vessels, and when they die they release their contents, which include a wide range of catabolic enzymes, into the surrounding area. These highly destructive enzymes may be responsible for additional damage occurring to the tissues.

As well as the emigration of polymorphonuclear cells from the blood, there is also a movement of mononuclear cells. Monocytes begin to move into the affected site at the same time as the polymorphs, but they are slower and are therefore generally outnumbered by polymorphonuclear cells at the start of a reaction. Mononuclear cells are, however, much more enduring than the polymorphs and, in many reactions, begin to pre-dominate after a day or so. Outside of the circulation monocytes go through a maturation phase, becoming macrophages which, as the name implies, are large phagocytic cells. These cells can undergo cell division that also contributes to the large number of mononuclear cells which accumulate at the inflamed site. In the same way that changes in the microcirculation are brought about by chemical mediation, the influx of leucocytes is also subject to chemical control. The simplest explanation of the phenomenon of cell migration is that a chemical stimulus originating from the damaged site is recognized by leucocytes, which respond by moving along a concentration gradient of the chemical towards the highest concentration in a process called chemotaxis. There are a number of chemotactic substances known to be released from inflammatory sites and, whilst cells may respond in a minor way to the mediators which affect changes in the vasculature, the most potent agents have little effect on the microcirculation.

Chemotaxis

Arachidonic acid can be metabolized by a lipoxygenase system to generate a range of hydroxyeicosatetraenoic acids, one of which is 5,12-dihydroxyeicosatetraenoic acid or leucotriene $B_4(LTB_4)$. LTB_4 is a potent chemotactic agent for polymorphonuclear leucoytes and mononuclear cells. LTB_4 also stimulates the general activity of leucocytes, as well as inducing more rapid movement and the release of degradative enzymes into the area. Thus, when arachidonic acid is released from cell mem-branes, the resultant prostaglandins and leucotrienes produced may, between them, mediate the development of all the major processes involved in an inflammatory response.

Another important source of chemotactic agents is the complement system. This is a complex system of plasma proteins which can be activated by a variety of stimuli, including antigen–antibody interaction and endotoxin release to produce a powerful cytolytic, membrane-attack unit. In the course of this activation a number of fragments of the com-plement components, which are powerfully chemotactic, are released into the area. These include components $C3_a$ and $C5_a$, which are also potent histamine releasers, and the aggregate C567 fraction. The complement system represents about 10% of plasma protein and has been implicated in a variety of inflammatory reactions. Other chemotactic material can be released from the breakdown of the structural protein, collagen, and from the breakdown of the blood clotting protein, fibrin.

Leucocyte contribution to inflammatory reaction

The contributions of the leucocytes to the inflammatory reactions are various. The presence of cells capable of phagocytosis at an injured site is an advantage. The removal of damaged tissues and any foreign material, such as micro-organisms, is of obvious importance. The local increase in leucocyte numbers at the site of inflammation at least warrants the hypothesis that there is a general increase in the concentration of proteolytic enzymes, because the lysosomes of the leucocytes contain cathepsins and hydrolases and the mast cells are rich in proteolytic enzymes. Release of these enzymes may be an important factor in the maintenance of inflammation by the production of altered tissue proteins and by the non-specific activation of thrombin, kinin-forming and plasmin systems. Polymorphs also provide a source of enzymes with more specific activities for maintaining the inflammatory reaction. The release of kininogenases from polymorphs has been reported, and the presence of a specific collagenase in human polymorphs has been noted. In some experimental models of inflammation, the phase in which prostaglandins are released corresponds in time to the migration of leucocytes into the inflamed area, and it has been proposed that the main source of prostaglandins at the inflammatory site is the polymorph.

The initial reaction to most types of injury is an acute inflammatory response exhibiting the prominent feature of increased vascular permeability. This reaction will normally resolve in time, and, if actual tissue necrosis is slight, no identifiable trace of the reaction will be left. In a more severe situation, repair is effected by the synthesis of connective tissue to form a scar.

Chronic inflammation

In some circumstances, however, inflammation may persist. This chronic reaction may be caused by the presence of some foreign material which is not easily removed from the inflammatory site. It has been found that the resolution of an inflammatory lesion is invariably associated with the disappearance of the inflammation-inducing irritant, but persistent inflammation may not necessarily be caused by any detectable irritant, for example, the aetiology of rheumatoid arthritis is uncertain.

The characteristic feature of chronic inflammation is the presence of white cells at the site of reaction. Some acute inflammatory reactions, such as the dextran-induced paw oedema in the rat, may proceed without migration of white cells into the extravascular spaces of the paw, but chronic inflammation is invariably associated with large numbers of extra-vascular white cells. Chronic inflammation is characterized by concurrent tissue destruction and resultant inflammation. The death of invading polymorphs at an inflamed site, with the resultant release of all the cellular enzymes, can give rise to a suppurative lesion. A suppurative lesion may continue at the site of some foreign material, but the necrotic area may become surrounded by a deposition of fibrous material and white cells to give rise to an **abscess**. A separation of degenerative and synthetic processes, as in the case of an abscess, is not always seen, the two processes often occurring simultaneously at the same site. Such a chronic inflammatory mass is called a **granuloma**.

Chronic inflammation can occur, however, without passing through an acute or suppurative phase, by the gradual development directly into the chronic state. Histological examination of chronic inflammatory lesions reveals the presence of a variety of different types of white cell. In rheumatoid synovial fluids, large numbers of white cells, principally polymorphs, can be found. These have extremely short half-lives of the order of only 3–4 hours, and the variety of damaging agents which can be released from these cells has already been outlined. Polymorphs are also actively phagocytic, but this function may not be important in chronic inflammatory situations since their short lifespan will frequently result in the release of any ingested material on the death of the cell. The predominant variety of polymorph is the neutrophil, but eosinophilic polymorphs, which share many of the properties of the neutrophil, also occur in inflammatory foci, possibly as a marker of general polymorph involvement, although in certain reactions the eosinophilic polymorph may predominate.

Most chronic inflammatory reactions are characterized by the presence of large numbers of mononuclear cells. Those mononuclear cells in a chronic inflammatory state may be derived either by emigration or division, and the persistence of these cells may be due to their great longevity. Macrophages, like polymorphs, are phagocytic, and this would seem to be an important function, the removal of foreign material and tissue debris being necessary for resolution of a reaction.

Within an area of chronic inflammation, macrophages may be transformed into two other cell types: epithelioid cells and foreign body giant cells. Epithelioid cells are a common feature of granulomatous inflammation and can be transformed into epithelial cells by natural maturation, if they live long enough and do not have undigested phagocytozed material within the cell. Giant cells are multinucleate and have been shown to be produced by cell fusion, although this fusion may be followed by nuclear division without cytoplasmic fission. These cells are found in large numbers around foreign bodies which are too large for macrophages to engulf. Other cells present in chronic inflammatory reactions are fibroblasts, which probably are derived from local connective tissue fibroblasts and are responsible for collagen deposition, and lymphocytes and plasma cells, responsible for the production of antibodies which facilitate the elimination of micro-organisms.

The contribution that any of the factors examined here may make in the inflammatory sequel to a sporting injury cannot be specified, but undoubtedly there will be an increased influx of blood, giving rise to the characteristic heat and redness; a movement of plasma protein and associated water into the tissue, caused by the swelling and pain and due, perhaps, to pressure on the nerve endings caused by the swelling or to the effect of released chemical mediators of pain; and finally, and perhaps most importantly to the sportsman, there will be a loss of function − Virchow's (1858) fifth cardinal sign. The persistence of the problem depends on many factors, but certainly the influx of leucocytes and the release of their enzyme-rich content will compound the damage already caused and tend to prolong the duration of the reaction. Given that no further aggravation occurs and that there are no complications, resolution should occur within days or weeks and, at worst, months. A pertinent question to ask at this point is whether the inflammation that follows a traumatic injury is necessary. Clearly, the body automatically takes the safest course of action when injured and directs its defensive systems to the area to make sure that no microbial invasion occurs and that all the necessary resources are made available to repair the damage. It is evident, however, that the body has a tendency to over-react. The response in many cases may be more serious than the stimulus.

5.4 TREATMENT OF SPORTING INJURIES

A number of treatments are available to deal with sporting injuries by the reduction of pain and inflammation. It is clear, however, that great care must be taken in judging the severity of an injury. Pain is the cue that intimates the severity of a problem. There are many drugs which can reduce our appreciation of pain, but a reduction of pain sensation may lead to the induction of further damage to an injury due to the failure to respond to the natural inclination to rest. Clear evidence of the dangers of masking pain sensation can be seen amongst those who suffer peripheral mutilation common amongst people with impaired sensory nerve activity, such as that which occurs in untreated lepers.

A common sight these days is the arrival on the field of play of the trainer who reaches into a bag for the aerosol can with which to spray some area of the prostrated player needing attention. The injured player stands gingerly and, cautiously at first, runs on. The trainer collects up the bag with the 'magic' spray and walks off. These aerosol sprays contain volatile compounds which evaporate on the skin surface causing rapid chilling of the area. The practice of cooling an injured area, whether by volatile spray, cold compress, ice-packs, etc. applied rapidly, may well reduce the immediate response to minor trauma by inhibiting the active processes which are involved in the initiation of an inflammatory reaction. Problems have arisen because of the abuse of these solvent-based products for 'sniffing'.

Other non-specific topical applications which are used successfully for the treatment of injured tissues include liniments. These preparations are rubefacients and act by counter-irritation. This is a phenomenon where mild or moderate pain can be relieved by irritating the skin. Counter-irritation is effective in providing relief from painful lesions of muscles, tendons and joints. There is, however, little evidence that the topical application of preparations containing adrenaline or aspirin is of value in the relief of pain.

5.4.1 MODES OF ACTION OF ANTI-INFLAMMATORY DRUGS

Although the treatment of inflammation with anti-inflammatory agents was practised by Hippocrates, who recommended the chewing of willow bark for a variety of ailments, the use of such measures was largely for-saken during subsequent centuries. It was not until 1876 when a physician named MacLagan, who was unimpressed with the treatments – including such measures as blood letting – that were available for rheumatic fever (a condition characterized by extensive inflammatory lesions), revolutionized the treatment of this condition by the re-introduction of an extract of willow bark called salicin. A synthetic analogue of this glycoside was soon produced and, in 1899, a German pharmaceutical company, Bayer, introduced a more palatable derivative, acetylsalicylic acid, under the trade name, Aspirine. Almost 100 years later we still have aspirin readily available as a simple, cheap and effective remedy for a wide variety of ailments. It has been the subject of innumerable clinical trials in many diverse areas of medicine, ranging from the treatment of food intolerance to the prevention of heart attacks. Without doubt, though, the bulk of the tens of thousands of tons of aspirin consumed each year is taken for the alleviation of pain, inflammation and fever.

Since the introduction of aspirin, many other drugs with similar therapeutic profiles have been developed and there are now about 20 aspirin-like drugs available for clinical use in the UK, although only aspirin and ibuprofen are available for general purchase. These aspirin-like drugs all have proven anti-inflammatory activity in the treatment of chronic inflammatory conditions, such as rheumatoid arthritis. Countless clinical trials have demonstrated the efficacy of these agents in alleviating both objective and subjective symptoms of inflammatory disease. Whilst some of these agents are more popular than others, there is no clear indication that any one of these drugs is more effective than any other. Indeed it is difficult to find convincing proof that any of the new drugs in this class is more effective than aspirin. The assessment of activity of this type of drug is, however, fraught with difficulties. It is not easy to find large numbers of patients with similar disease states who are prepared to be subjected to the withdrawal of active drugs in order to act as controls in such trials, and it is not easy to quantify a reduction in inflammation.

Testing anti-inflammatory agents

Given that these difficulties exist, when testing drugs on common chronic conditions it can be perceived that the difficulties involved in testing anti-inflammatory agents in acute sporting injuries, which may affect any part of the body, are considerably greater. Since a chronically inflamed joint in a patient with rheumatoid arthritis may remain in a similar condition for weeks on end, the effect of introduction and withdrawal of an effective anti-inflammatory agent on the level of inflammation of that joint should be seen fairly easily. Following a traumatic sporting injury, however, it is probable that the inflamed part will progressively heal over a fairly limited period without intervention. How, then, can one measure the efficacy of an anti-inflammatory drug superimposed on a naturally regressing inflammatory condition? The simple answer is: with great difficulty!

The majority of clinical trials published on the efficacy of aspirin-like drugs in sports injury are organized into two groups of injured subjects, given different members of this group of drugs. Usually no significant difference is established between the two drugs under test. Whilst these drugs are clearly effective in the treatment of chronic disease, evidence that they do have a role to play in acute traumatic injury treatment is much more limited. To establish firmly that drugs like aspirin can effectively treat a sports injury, a number of criteria would have to be met. Firstly, suitable injuries, preferably all of a certain type, would be needed in reasonable numbers. Secondly, some measure of effectiveness would be required which would have clear meaning, and, thirdly, a comparison would have to be made with a group of similar patients receiving no drug treatment, that is a control group. Because many individuals are responsive to suggestion, this control group would have to be given what appears to be the same treatment as the test group, but with the active drug missing. In other words, one group would be given tablets of the drug whilst the other group would be given identical-looking tablets but with no drug in them, so-called placebos.

With regard to the first two criteria, perhaps a good place to look for a plentiful supply of similar sports injuries would be in a club where members are involved in the same sport with, therefore, the same injury tendencies. A measurement of the period of time following injury until the injured person is fit for competition or full training again could serve as the key to assess effectiveness. If this time is reduced in the drug-treated group then it could be concluded that the drug was a success. With regard to the third criterion, however, there is a substantial ethical and moral problem. If the drug works, or even if it is thought to work, it is difficult to justify the withholding of that treatment for the purpose of a trial since this action might prolong unnecessarily the period of absence from the sport, which in many professional clubs would be an unacceptable action.

Aspirin-like anti-inflammatory drugs

Despite the relative paucity of convincing trials which demonstrate the effectiveness of these anti-inflammatory drugs, their use in the treatment of sports injuries is very widespread. The commencement of a course of aspirin-like drugs immediately after the injury occurs appears to be an effective way to reduce the recovery time. The most commonly used drugs in this class are aspirin, diclofenac, ibuprofen, indomethacin, naproxen and piroxicam. The use of these drugs, though widespread, remains largely empirical as there is no universally accepted explanation of how they reduce inflammation. Indeed, our understanding of the processes involved in soft-tissue injury is far from complete.

Several suggestions have been made, however, to explain the anti-inflammatory activity of the aspirin-like drugs. Considerable attention has been focused on the possible interaction of these drugs with various factors involved in the inflammatory process.

Many early attempts to explain the anti-inflammatory activity of these drugs considered their ability to interfere with proteolytic enzymes. These enzymes are involved both in the early stages of inflammation and in the later stages when the process is well established. An inhibition of proteolytic enzyme activity either at the start of the reaction, preventing the activation of the complement kinin, fibrin or plasmin systems, or during the later, autocatalytic stage of inflammation, could be the mechanism of action. Certainly, many anti-inflammatory drugs have been shown to have some measure of anti-protease activity, but the general correlation between enzyme inhibition and anti-inflammatory activity is not impressive. Aspirin derivatives are known to inhibit a large number of enzyme systems, but inhibition is generally seen only at drug concentrations which exceed the normal therapeutic level. Another explanation closely related to this idea is that the anti-inflammatory drugs reduce inflammation by preventing the release of enzymes from lysosomes during the more established phase of the reaction. Again, whilst there is some experimental evidence available to support this idea, overall it is not a convincing explanation.

Anti-inflammatory drugs and prostaglandins

With an improved understanding of the mediation of inflammation came the idea that the action of anti-inflammatory drugs might be due to an interference with the activities of one or more of the proposed chemical mediators of inflammation. It was not, however, until 1971 that any major headway was made in this area of our understanding. In a series of three papers published in *Nature*, John Vane (1971) and his colleagues (Ferreira, Moncada and Vane, 1971; Smith and Willis, 1971) outlined a hypothesis that the action of the aspirin-like drugs could be attributed to their ability to suppress the synthesis of prostaglandins. Virtually all the non-steroidal anti-inflammatory drugs have been shown to inhibit the synthesis of prostaglandins, and they generally exhibit this property at concentrations which are low enough to be achieved with normal therapeutic doses of the drugs. The predictable consequences of the inhibition of prostaglandin synthesis on an inflammatory process, based on the known pro-inflammatory activities of the prostaglandins, easily lead us to the conclusion that this property of the non-steroidal anti-inflammatory drugs provides an explanation for their mechanisms of action. A reduction in the level of prostaglandins at an inflammatory site should result in a reduction of the symptoms of heat and redness, since prostaglandins would normally promote an increased blood flow to the area by virtue of their ability to cause profound erythema. A reduction in the pain associated with the reaction could also be anticipated, since, in the absence of prostaglandins, there would be no state of hyperalgesia. In other words, the tissue would not exhibit a greater sensitivity to painful stimuli than normal. Oedema would also be reduced in severity as the permeability-increasing effect of chemical agents on blood vessel walls would not be subject to the normal exaggerating action of the prostaglandins. Thus we can see that the reduction in synthesis of the prostaglandins that can be demonstrated when using the non-steroidal anti-inflammatory drugs could account for the reduction of all the cardinal signs of inflammation.

As additional support for this idea of a single, common mechanism of action for the non-steroidal anti-inflammatory drugs, other properties exhibited by this group of drugs can also be explained by an inhibition of prostaglandin synthesis. For example, as well as being analgesic, anti-inflammatory drugs are invariably antipyretic agents as well; that is they have the ability to reduce elevated body temperature. During fever, prostaglandins are detectable in increased quantities in the cerebrospinal fluid which fills the cavities of the brain, and it has been shown in animals that the injection of prostaglandins into the anterior hypothalamus evokes a pyrexic response. The inhibition of prostaglandin synthesis, therefore, offers an explanation for this property of these drugs, in addition to their anti-inflammatory action.

Antiplatelet activity of anti-inflammatory drugs

Another property which is common to most of these agents is that they inhibit platelet aggregation. To repair damaged blood vessels, platelets come together to form a plug to fill the gap and prevent bleeding. This activity is in part mediated via the synthesis of thromboxanes by the platelets. Drugs such as aspirin, which inhibits the cyclo-oxygenase enzyme, will prevent the synthesis not only of prostaglandins but of thromboxanes as well, preventing normal platelet function. In some circumstances, notably when there is already some impairment to normal platelet function, this activity of these drugs may represent a hazard. There is, however, much interest in the potential use of this antiplatelet activity to prevent the development of thrombosis. Small blood clot fragments may lodge in the vascular beds of the brain or heart, and it is possible that a very small regular dose of aspirin may protect a subject from a stroke or a heart attack.

Another common feature of these agents is their tendency to cause gastric irritation, and this, too, can be explained by a mechanism of prostaglandin synthesis inhibition. Prostaglandins normally limit the amount of hydrochloric acid secreted by the parietal cells in the main gastric glands, probably by an action on the enzyme adenylate cyclase. In addition, prostaglandins may promote the functional vasodilation necessary for the parietal cells in their secretory mode. If the levels of prostaglandins in the stomach are reduced then a greater amount of acid will be secreted, and this acid will be produced by cells which have been forced into this synthetic activity without the usual increased provision of oxygen. This situation may thus result in a gastritis in which some mucosal tissue may be damaged by the ischaemia which can result from the increased metabolic activity occurring without increased blood flow.

We therefore have a mechanism of action for the non-steroidal anti-inflammatory drugs which can be invoked to explain not only their anti-inflammatory activity but also their antipyretic and antiplatelet activities, and even serves to explain their most common side-effect. This brief account of mechanism would be less than complete, however, if it did not at least indicate one or two of the many observations that have been reported which do not easily fit within this explanation. Firstly, as was made clear in Vane's (1971) original paper, sodium salicylate is of the order of 100 times less effective as an inhibitor of prostaglandin synthesis than is acetylsalicylic acid (aspirin) whereas they are of similar anti-inflammatory activity. Secondly, in experiments in which inflammation has been induced in animals rendered incapable of generating prostaglandins by being fed diets deficient in polyunsaturated fatty acids (e.g. arachidonic acid), aspirin has been shown to be as effective as it is in normal animals (Bonta *et al.*, 1977).

As a final example of the type of observation that is not compatible with this theory, it has been shown that even small sub-anti-inflammatory doses of aspirin render the inflamed synovial tissue of arthritic joints incapable of producing prostaglandins for several days (Crook *et al.*, 1976). Clearly, if this is the mechanism of action of aspirin, an explanation is required as to why regular high doses of the drug are needed to achieve an anti-inflammatory action, when two or three tablets, two or three times a week would seem to be all that is necessary to induce effective inhibition of prostaglandin synthesis.

The relationship between prostaglandin synthesis and the aspirin-like drugs is, thus, confused. On the one hand, we have a convincing and attractive hypothesis which explains the many and varied activities, and even side-effects, of this group of drugs by one simple and elegant mechanism. On the other hand, we have evidence that not all anti-inflammatory drugs are good inhibitors of prostaglandin synthesis, that aspirin can exert an anti-inflammatory effect in the absence of any prostaglandin synthesis and that it is too good at inhibiting prostaglandin synthesis in rheumatic patients to explain why such large amounts of the drug are needed in clinical practice.

5.4.2 ORAL NON-STEROIDAL ANTI-INFLAMMATORY DRUGS IN SPORTS INJURY

Whatever the mechanism by which these drugs exert their effect, their use in the treatment of chronic inflammatory disease is well established and their efficacy beyond question. Similarly, in the treatment of acute traumatic injury, their use has become commonplace and, although far too many clinical trials have failed to furnish proof of their efficacy, clear evidence that these drugs are of benefit in sports injury has been produced. These drugs represent a simple and safe means of reducing the response to an injury and speeding the return of an injured sport participant to competitive fitness. Whilst many trials compare the use of two different anti-inflammatory drugs, frequently no significant difference between the two drugs is found, and where differences are reported they are not consistent. It would, therefore, be difficult to indicate a rank order of efficacy for these drugs. Instead, it is proposed to describe the use of some of the commonly selected members of this group of drugs in sports injuries. Sprains (rupture of ligaments, which may be partial), strains (partial tearing of muscles) and bruises are all examples of painful sports injuries. Commonly, they may warrant the use of pain-killing (analgesic) drugs, such as paracetamol (acetaminophen, USA), or even in severe cases a narcotic analgesic compound, such as dihydrocodeine. Since, however, these conditions are generally associated with an inflammatory component, the use of an analgesic drug with anti-inflammatory activity would seem to be a more logical choice.

About 20 different non-steroidal anti-inflammatory drugs are available which could be used to treat sports injuries, and some details are given here of a small selection of them (Figure 5.3).

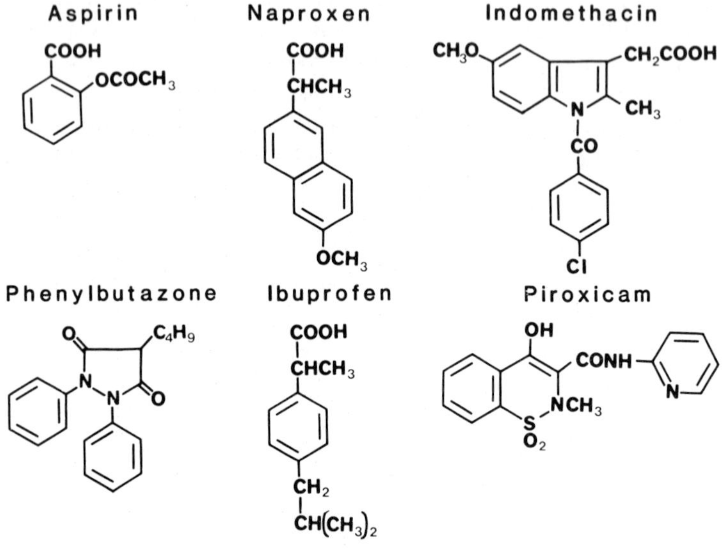

Figure 5.3　Some examples of commonly used non-steroidal anti-inflammatory drugs.

Aspirin

Aspirin (acetylsalicylic acid) is a very effective analgesic drug at a dose of 2–3 g per day. At higher doses, that is in excess of 4 g per day, aspirin will reduce the swelling of an inflamed joint, a property not shown at the lower, analgesic level. Whilst anti-inflammatory activity is seen only at higher doses, it is inadvisable to exceed the normal recommended doses without qualified medical supervision. Despite the antiquity of this preparation, unequivocal evidence that any of the newer challengers offers an all-round superior performance is lacking. The general availability and low cost of aspirin make it an ideal candidate for self-treatment following sports injury.

Aspirin is, however, not without toxicity, although the risks involved with the use of the drug are probably generally overstated. Given that the injured athlete is an otherwise normal, healthy adult, the major problem liable to be encountered following the use of aspirin (or indeed, for that matter, any of the non-steroidal anti-inflammatory drugs) is gastric irritation which may be experienced as a form of dyspepsia. Attempts to reduce this problem by modifying the tablets in a variety of ways have not been particularly successful, as it is now generally recognized that the effect of these drugs on the stomach is due not so much to the unabsorbed drug in contact with the gastric mucosa as to the drug in the circulation. It is generally believed that the most effective way to minimize this problem is to avoid the use of these drugs when the stomach is empty. If the drugs are taken following a meal, then any increased acid production that ensues can be utilized in the digestive process rather than being free to attack the lining of the stomach itself.

In a study comparing aspirin with naproxen in patients with sports injuries, no significant differences were detected between the two drugs, although the dose of aspirin used (2 g per day) was arguably on the low side for an anti-inflammatory action (Anderson and Gotzsche, 1984). What this study did demonstrate, however, was that significantly better results were obtained when the interval between injury and the start of treatment was shorter. This effect is widely appreciated now and is exactly what would be predicted from experimental inflammation studies in animals. In laboratory tests of the type used to screen for anti-inflammatory activity of potential new drugs for the treatment of arthritis, it can be clearly shown that aspirin-like drugs can profoundly reduce the development of an inflammatory response to an irritant. The effect of these drugs on the inflammatory response to the same irritant after it is established is marginal.

Clearly, if it is deemed necessary to use an anti-inflammatory drug to treat a sports injury it should be given as early as possible after the damage is sustained.

Naproxen

Naproxen has become one of the mainstays of treatment for chronic inflammatory conditions. Its efficacy and safety record are excellent and it is one of the most frequently prescribed drugs for the treatment of arthritis. Since its introduction in the early 1970s, naproxen has been the subject of a large number of trials in the treatment of soft-tissue injuries and, whilst many of these compare naproxen to another non-steroidal anti-inflammatory drug and find no difference in activity, several trials have shown naproxen to be better than the other drug in some respects, and naproxen has been shown to be superior to placebo. In view of the popularity of this drug and the generally good reports of its efficacy in the literature, naproxen must rank high amongst the most suitable drugs for the treatment of sporting injuries. The drug is given at a dose of 0.75–1.25 g per day in three or four divided doses. Initially, a high loading dose of 500 mg may be given to aid the rapid attainment of suitable plasma levels of the drug (750 μg/ml). The drug may be taken at meal times to help combat any gastric discomfort felt, although in the presence of food the drug is absorbed more slowly. More rapid absorption occurs with the use of naproxen sodium.

Ibuprofen

Ibuprofen is another non-steroidal anti-inflammatory drug with a similar structure to naproxen. It is the oldest propionic acid derivative anti-inflammatory agent in use, and considerable experience has, therefore, been obtained with it. This drug is also one of the few drugs of this class available without prescription. It has a reputation for being well tolerated, that is it is widely felt that this particular anti-inflammatory agent does not induce the same degree of dyspepsia as many of its rivals. It is possible, however, that much of this reputation is based on early experiences with the drug when it was used at relatively low dose levels. To improve the often disappointing activity of ibuprofen the doses used have been increased and, whilst the drug is still generally well tolerated, it is certainly not without gastric irritant activity at these higher levels.

Trials using ibuprofen at doses as low as 1200 mg per day have been shown to reduce pain and recovery time of soft-tissue sports injuries. Hutson (1986) found no significant differences between the activity of ibuprofen given at doses of 1800 mg or 2400 mg daily amongst 46 patients with sporting injuries to the knee. The ibuprofen-treated groups showed increased joint mobility and weight-bearing capability when compared to a placebo-treated group, again demonstrating the usefulness of anti-inflammatory drug therapy in sporting injuries. In this trial, only one subject reported moderate gastric upset, and this was a patient in the high-dose group. The normal recommended dose range for ibuprofen for musculoskeletal disorders is 1.2–1.8 g daily in three to four divided doses, preferably after food. This may be increased if necessary to 2.4 g daily. Whilst the maximum recommended dose for the drug is now 2400 mg daily, higher levels have been used on some occasions.

Indomethacin

Indomethacin has been used for treating inflammatory conditions since the mid-1960s and remains a very frequently prescribed drug. Whilst being an effective anti-inflammatory drug it does suffer, apart from the gastric irritant activity somewhat typical of this type of drug, from a number of central nervous system side-effects such as headaches, dizziness and light-headedness. Generally, indomethacin is found to be of similar efficacy to other non-steroidal anti-inflammatory drugs, such as naproxen, in the treatment of soft-tissue sports injuries.

As might be expected, the drop-out rate due to side-effects of this drug is generally higher than for other members of this group of drugs, with normal therapeutic doses of indomethacin (50–200 mg daily). As many as half the patients experience some untoward symptoms, and many of these will have to withdraw from using the drug. The drug is normally initiated as 25 mg, two or three times daily and gradually increased if necessary. It is possible that at this low starting dose toxicity is less of a problem. Edwards *et al.* (1984) found it necessary to withdraw only one patient from a group of 53 who were receiving 75 mg indomethacin daily for acute soft-tissue sports injuries.

Indomethacin is also available in 100 mg suppositories for night-time use and these may be of benefit in some individuals. It should be remembered that the combined rectal and oral doses should not amount to more than 200 mg in a 24-hour period.

Piroxicam

Piroxicam is an example of one of the newer anti-inflammatory agents to become generally available. It is often difficult to assess the place of a particular drug in a field of therapy until considerable experience has been obtained with it. Initial results suggest that piroxicam is comparable to indomethacin or naproxen in treating acute musculoskeletal injuries, but that it is better tolerated than aspirin or indomethacin. One particular advantage of piroxicam is that it has a long half-life which permits its use as a single daily dose, usually of 20 mg. Some concern has been expressed about the gastrotoxicity of piroxicam. It is now generally accepted that it is similar or only marginally more toxic in this respect than other similar compounds. It may be more troublesome in the elderly, however.

In a large study of acute sports injuries in Norway, the authors concluded that piroxicam, 40 mg daily for the first 2 days and 20 mg daily for a further 5 days, resulted in significant improvements in mobility and reductions in pain when compared to placebo (Lereim and Gabor, 1988). This treatment gave a marginally superior response when compared to naproxen, 500 mg twice daily, and both drugs were well tolerated.

Diclofenac

Diclofenac is another relatively new drug of this class which has been used in the treatment of sporting injury. In a trial involving subjects with severe sprained ankles, diclofenac, 50 mg three times daily, was shown to be superior to both placebo and piroxicam, 20 mg daily (Bahamonde and Saavedra, 1990). Both drugs were well tolerated. One particular advantage of this drug is that it is available in a slow-release form which is administered once daily, although this may be less of an advantage in the acute situation.

Phenylbutazone

Phenylbutazone was introduced into clinical medicine in 1949 to take its place alongside the salicylates for the treatment of arthritic conditions. It is a powerful anti-inflammatory drug and is capable of treating acute exacerbations of rheumatoid arthritis and severe ankylosing spondylitis (an inflammatory condition of the spine). Compared to the many, newer anti-inflammatory agents now available it is subject to a large number of toxic side-effects, some of which have led to fatal outcomes. Whilst many physicians believe this to be an extraordinarily useful anti-inflammatory agent, others have argued that it is too dangerous to use. The most serious side-effects are undoubtedly the retention of fluid, which in predisposed individuals may precipitate cardiac failure, and the interference with normal blood cell production, most commonly resulting in aplastic anaemia and agranulocytosis which can occur within the first few days of treatment. Its use, therefore, in trivial, self-limiting musculoskeletal disorders is difficult to justify. In the UK, phenylbutazone is now only indicated for the treatment of ankylosing spondylitis in hospital situations and its closely related congener, oxyphenbutazone, has been withdrawn completely.

In the past phenylbutazone has been somewhat abused, particularly in the United States. A report by Marshall (1979) indicates that in the National Football League, for example, an average of 24–40 unit doses of phenylbutazone was used per player per season. The treatment of sports injuries is not, however, a licensed indication for Butazolidin (phenylbutazone) in the United States.

Whatever the role of phenylbutazone in injuries in sportsmen and sportswomen, there is no doubt that this drug is used considerably in the field of equestrian sports. In show jumping, the horses' feet are subjected to constant concussion. By the age of 10 many show jumping horses will have suffered pathological changes in their feet, but in many cases will be at their peak. Similarly, three-day event horses are subject to considerable physical stress, with strain of a tendon or the suspensory ligament being common injuries. Even without jumping-related competition, the regular galloping activity, as in flat racing or polo, may result in substantial changes in bones, joints and ligaments of a horse and, when pushed too hard or for too long, lameness may develop due to the pain and inflammation of the particular injury. The time-honoured remedy for reducing the pain and inflammation of these injuries in horses is to administer an anti-inflammatory drug, the most frequently used example being phenylbutazone.

Horses generally tolerate phenylbutazone very well and may be treated with the drug to improve their comfort. Whilst there are many indications for the use of phenylbutazone in horses, dilemmas do arise as to whether their use may mask an injury and lead to a complete breakdown of an affected limb. The governing bodies of equestrian sports generally recognize the usefulness of this drug but exclude the use of the drug on, or immediately before, competition days in order that no unfair advantage may be gained by improving performance and also to protect unfit horses from being used competitively.

5.4.3 TOPICAL NON-STEROIDAL ANTI-INFLAMMATORY DRUGS IN SPORTS INJURY

Several pharmaceutical companies have introduced topical preparations of non-steroidal anti-inflammatory drugs for the relief of musculoskeletal pain. Topical preparations of benzydamine, piroxicam, ibuprofen, keto-profen, felbinac (the active metabolite of fenbufen) and diclofenac are currently available in the UK. The concept of applying a non-steroidal anti-inflammatory drug locally in an effort to maximize the level of the drug at the site of injury whilst minimizing the systemic level of the drug is an interesting one. It is possible that this technique may achieve a good therapeutic effect without the troublesome gastrointestinal side-effects sometimes encountered with systemic therapy.

There is good evidence that these preparations afford good penetration of the drug through the skin and that high levels of the active drug are achieved in the underlying tissues. Clinical trials with these preparations generally demonstrate that active drug formulations are more effective than placebo, but the differences are generally slight. In a double-blind study, in which patients suffering bilateral inflammatory knee joint effusions were treated with diclofenac gel to one knee and a placebo gel to the other, Radermacher *et al.* (1991) found that there were small reductions in swelling in both knees, and no significant difference between the drug-treated and placebo-treated knees could be detected.

It has been suggested that the massage of an affected area with a gel or cream may in itself be beneficial, irrespective of the presence of a non-steroidal anti-inflammatory drug. A significant point which should be considered here is whether these compounds actually exert their anti-inflammatory action at the inflamed site or elsewhere. If, for example, the reality of the situation is that the drugs reduce inflammation by interacting in some way with components in the bloodstream, then the concept of local application would be flawed. The statement found in the British National Formulary (1995) that these preparations 'may provide some slight relief of pain in musculoskeletal conditions' would seem to be a reasonable conclusion to this section.

5.4.4 PROTEOLYTIC ENZYMES AS ANTI-INFLAMMATORY AGENTS

Several reports have been published suggesting that proteolytic enzyme preparations are useful for the treatment of soft-tissue sports injuries. Hyaluronidase, which splits the glucosaminidic bonds of hyaluronic acid, reduces the viscosity of the cellular cement. Local injections of this enzyme have been shown to reduce healing time of sprained ankles. Chymotrypsin preparations, which are available in tablet form, have also been found to be useful in sporting injuries. Whilst these enzymes are obviously vulnerable to gastrointestinal breakdown, there is evidence that some active enzyme is absorbed. A number of clinical trials have been conducted amongst professional players of association football and, whilst not all have shown favourable results, some trials have found significant reduction in recovering time to match fitness, particularly where haematomata or sprains were the major feature of the injury. In one notable trial, where an enzyme preparation was compared with placebo in a London club, the physicians monitoring the trial were so impressed by the apparent efficacy of the enzyme that the trial was abandoned, since it was considered unjustifiable to withhold the enzyme from the placebo group (Boyne and Medhurst, 1967). This was deemed especially so since the club was in the running for major honours in that season!

Here, though, we have an enigma. On the one hand, we have apparently convincing reports that proteolytic enzyme preparations aid recovery from sports injury. On the other hand, we are faced with the fact that the bulk of these reports are over 20 years old. If these preparations could significantly reduce recovery time and return players to match fitness in perhaps only 70% of the usual time it takes, why are they not in use? Perhaps the optimistic initial reports have not been subsequently reproducible, or perhaps toxicity has limited their use; it is true that, occasionally, serious hypersensitivity reactions do occur. Whilst not now used for treating mechanically induced trauma, these preparations are regularly used in a variety of post-surgical situations to reduce oedema.

5.4.5 ANTI-INFLAMMATORY STEROIDS

Without question the most powerful anti-inflammatory agents known to man are the glucocorticoids. These are drugs which are based on the chemical structure of adrenal corticosteroids. In 1949 Hench and his colleagues demonstrated the beneficial effects of high doses of cortisone in patients with rheumatoid arthritis. Considerable interest was generated in this hormone as a potential cure for inflammatory disorders, but it rapidly became apparent that this substance was not curative and that it had no lasting effect on the disease process. More potent activity was found in hydrocortisone (cortisol), the predominant glucocorticoid secreted in man. The anti-inflammatory activity of these steroid hormones appears to be secondary to their glucocorticoid function as, despite the severe metabolic derangement which accompanies adrenal gland insufficiency (Addison's disease), there is no general precipitation of inflammatory reactions. Many attempts have been made to increase the anti-inflammatory activity of these steroids. A large number of anti-inflammatory steroids are now available, many of which are an order of magnitude more potent than cortisol, but all have significant glucocorticoid activity which renders their long-term use liable to affect the general metabolic activity of the body in much the same way as occurs in conditions of hyperactive secretion of the adrenal cortex (Cushing's syndrome). It is therefore important that a distinction is made between the long-term use of anti-inflammatory steroids and their use in acute situations.

The long-term use of these drugs may lead to a number of side-effects, some of which may be particularly unfortunate for an athlete. Osteoporosis is frequently encountered during corticosteroid therapy. This serious weakening of the skeletal structure affects principally those bones with the most trabecular structure, such as the ribs and vertebrae, and vertebral compression fractures are a frequent complication of steroid therapy. Long-term use of a drug, which may weaken the bone structure of an individual whose activities may subject that structure to greater than normal stress, should not be contemplated lightly.

Perhaps a more significant problem, however, is the catabolic effect of glucocorticoids on skeletal muscle. Weakness of muscles in the arms and legs can occur soon after treatment is started, even with quite modest doses of these anti-inflammatory drugs. Experiments with rats have shown that very significant reductions in muscle weight can occur within 7 days of treatment (Bullock *et al.*, 1971). Interestingly, the effect is restricted to skeletal muscle, with cardiac muscle being noticeably spared. If long-term systemic steroid treatment is initiated, it must be realized that as well as the anti-inflammatory effect which will be achieved, the administered drug will largely take over the glucocorticoid role of the natural adrenal hormone. Due to negative feedback mechanisms operating in both the hypothalamus and the anterior pituitary, the release of adrenocorticotrophic hormone (ACTH) is inhibited and so the adrenal cortex is not stimulated to produce its own glucocorticoids normally. Over a period of time the adrenal cortex regresses to a state such that if the drug treatment is stopped suddenly the adrenal gland can no longer respond to the demands placed on it and fails to produce sufficient quantities of glucocorticoid. It is important, therefore, that following long-term treatment with a steroid, the drug is only gradually withdrawn by a progressive lowering of the daily dose.

Steroids are double-edged weapons in the armoury of anti-inflammatory therapy. They are powerful anti-inflammatory drugs, but they are, unfortunately, subject to a great many side-effects. The direct application of these drugs to an affected site, such that a high concentration of the steroid is achieved locally but without the attainment of significant systemic levels, offers the possibility of gaining the maximum usefulness of steroids with minimal toxicity. Direct application of steroids to the skin is not an entirely satisfactory method as, although they are generally well absorbed, large proportions of the active drug will be transported away by the blood and, therefore, accumulation in affected muscle or connective tissue is limited. Additionally, topical application of steroids tends to cause thinning of the skin and a slowing down of wound healing. The local injection of a corticosteroid preparation does offer considerable advantages in the treatment of an inflammatory condition restricted to a small area of the body. Early attempts to inject steroids locally were not particularly successful as these highly soluble drugs were rapidly redistributed from the site. The development of less soluble esters of hydrocortisone and prednisolone to give fairly insoluble microcrystalline preparations, which are injected as suspensions, has markedly improved the successfulness of this particular technique. A single dose of an insoluble steroid preparation will provide relief for several days or even several weeks. If necessary these local injections can be repeated to extend the period of effectiveness. Great care must be taken when injections of steroids are given that aseptic precautions are taken to minimize the risk of the introduction of infective agents. This is especially the case where injections have to be administered intra-articularly to improve mobility and restrict damage of an affected joint. In the case of intra-articular injection, the use of a long-acting preparation, such as triamcinolone hexacetonide, is indicated so that repeated injections are less necessary or, at least, less frequent (Figure 5.4).

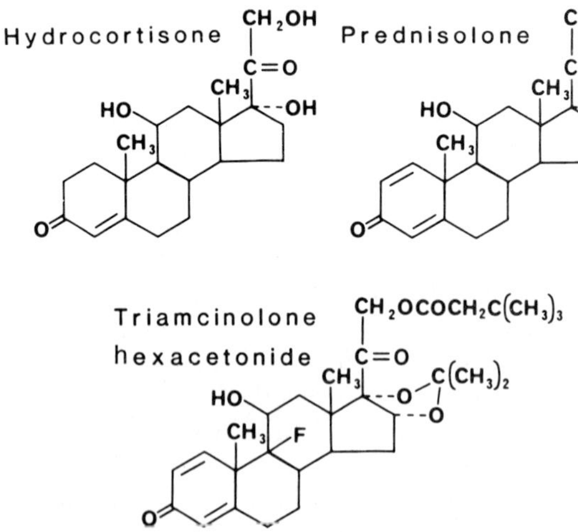

Figure 5.4 Some examples of anti-inflammatory steroids.

Local injections of steroids are also valuable for the treatment of soft-tissue injuries. They may be injected into the interior of a bursa (the fibrous sac, filled with synovial fluid, which may be found between muscles or between a tendon and bone and which facilitates frictionless movement between the surfaces that it separates); they may also be injected into a tendon sheath to reduce the inflammation of an affected tendon or infiltrated around the area of an inflamed ligament. Tendonitis of the elbow (tennis elbow) is a classical example of the type of injury which responds well to local corticosteroid injection. The injection of steroids into soft tissues is not without risk, however, particularly when stress-bearing tissues are involved. The repeated injection of steroids into load-bearing tendons carries the risk of tendon rupture.

Steroids do have the property of delaying the wound-healing process and so particular care should be taken in their use when extensive new tissue has to be produced to repair damage, as is the case, for example, where collision on the sports field has led to an open wound. In this instance, the use of steroids to reduce inflammation may not be appropriate.

The means by which these steroids exert their anti-inflammatory effects is not clear. It is probable that they have a number of activities, all of which contribute to their anti-inflammatory effects. They have been shown to reduce the output of chemical mediators of inflammation and to inhibit the effects of mediators on the vascular endothelium, resulting in a reduction of oedema formation. They have also been shown to have a number of inhibitory actions on the responsiveness of white blood cells. They are, for example, particularly effective in reducing the activity of thymocytes, which are involved with delayed hypersensitivity reactions. Whatever their mechanism of action, and despite the potential hazards of long-term, high-dose therapy, glucocorticoids are profoundly effective in the reduction of inflammatory reactions and their place in the treatment of sporting injuries is assured.

The use of corticosteroids is subject to stringent regulation by the International Olympic Committee (IOC). Topical application for ear, eye or skin problems is allowed, but general systemic application is banned. Local or intra-articular injection or inhalation (for respiratory problems, such as asthma or hay fever) is permissable. However, written notification, using an official Medical Notification Form which was introduced by the IOC in September 1994, must be given to the relevant authority.

5.5 REFERENCES

Anderson, L.A. and Gotzsche, P.C. (1984) Naproxen and aspirin in acute musculoskeletal disorders: a double-blind, parallel study in patients with sports injuries. *Pharmacotherapeutica*, 3, 531.

Bahamonde, L.A. and Saavedra, C. (1990) Comparison of the analgesic and anti-inflammatory effects of diclofenac potassium versus piroxicam versus placebo in ankle sprain patients. *J. Int. Med. Res.*, **18**, 104.

Bonta, I.L., Bult, H., Vincent, J.E. and Ziglstra, F.J. (1977) Acute anti-inflammatory effects of aspirin and dexamethasone in rats deprived of endogenous prostaglandin precursors. *J. Pharm. Pharmacol.*, **29**, 1.

Boyne, P.S. and Medhurst, H. (1967) Oral anti-inflammatory enzyme therapy in injuries in professional footballers. *Practitioner*, **198**, 543.

British National Formulary (1995) Number 29. Joint publication of BMA and RPSGB, March, London.

Bullock, G.J., Carter, E.E., Elliott, P. *et al.* (1971) Relative changes in the function of muscle ribosomes and mitochondria during the early phase of steroid-induced catabolism. *Biochem. J.*, **127**, 881.

Crook, D., Collins, A.J., Bacon, P.A. and Chan, R. (1976) Prostaglandin synthetase activity from human rheumatoid synovial microsomes. *Ann. Rheum. Dis.*, **35**, 327.

Edwards, V., Wilson, A.A., Harwood, H.F. *et al.* (1984) A multicentre comparison of piroxicam and indomethacin in acute soft tissue sports injuries. *J. Int. Med. Res.*, **12**, 46.

Ferreira, S.H., Moncada, S. and Vane, J.R. (1971) Indomethacin and aspirin abolish prostaglandin release from the spleen. *Nature, New Biol.*, **231**, 232.

Hench, P.S., Kendall, E.C., Slocumb, C.H. and Polley, H.F. (1949) The effect of a hormone of the adrenal cortex (17-hydroxy-11-dehydrocorticosterone: compound E) and of pituitary adrenocorticotropic hormone on rheumatoid arthritis. *Proc. Staff Meet., Mayo Clinic*, **24**, 181.

Hutson, M.A. (1986) A double-blind study comparing ibuprofen 1800 mg or 2400 mg daily and placebo in sports injuries. *J. Int. Med. Res.*, **4**, 142.

Lereim, P. and Gabor, I. (1988) Piroxicam and naproxen in acute sports injuries. *Am J. Med.*, **84**, (Suppl. 5A), 45.

Lewis, T. (1927) *The Blood Vessels of the Human Skin and their Responses*, Shaw and Sons, London.

MacLagan, T. (1876) The treatment of acute rheumatism by salacin. *Lancet*, **1**, 342.

Marshall, E. (1979) Drugging of football players curbed by central monitoring plan, NFL claims. *Science*, **203**, 626.

Radermacher, J., Jentsch, D., Scholl, M.A. *et al.* (1991) Diclofenac concentrations in synovial fluid and plasma after cutaneous application in inflammatory and degenerative joint disease. *Br. J. Clin. Pharmac.*, **31**, 537.

Smith, J.B. and Willis, A.L. (1971) Aspirin selectively inhibits prostaglandin production in human platelets. *Nature, New Biol.*, **231**, 235.

Vane, J.R. (1971) Inhibition of prostaglandin synthesis as a mechanism of action for aspirin-like drugs. *Nature, New Biol.*, **231**, 232.

Virchow, R. (1858) *Cellular Pathology*.

5.6 FURTHER READING

Campbell, W.B. (1990) Lipid derived autocoids: eicosanoids and platelet activating factor, in Goodman and Gilman's *The Pharmacological Basis of Therapeutics*, (8th edn), (eds A.G. Gilman, T.W. Rall, A.S. Neis and P. Taylor) Pergamon, Oxford.

Haynes, R.C. (1990) Adrenocorticotropic hormone: adrenocortical steroids and their synthetic analogs; inhibitors of the synthesis and actions of adreno-corticol steroid, in Goodman and Gilman's *The Pharmacological Basis of Therapeutics*, (8th edn), (eds A.G. Gilman, T.W. Rall, A.S. Neis and P. Taylor, Pergamon, Oxford.

Insel, P.A. (1990) Analgesic-antipyretics and anti-inflammatory agents: drugs employed in the treatment of rheumatoid arthritis and gout, in Goodman and Gilman's *The Pharmacological Basis of Therapeutics*, (8th edn), (eds A.G. Gilman, T.W. Rall, A.S. Neis and P. Taylor), Pergamon, Oxford.

Ryan, G.B. and Majno, G. (1977) *Inflammation*, Upjohn Company, Kalamazoo, Michigan.

Alcohol, anti-anxiety drugs and sport

6

Thomas Reilly

6.1 INTRODUCTION

Throughout civilization and up to the present day human ingenuity has found various ways of coping with the stresses that life brings. Sometimes these entail a form of escapism into a drug-induced illusory world to eschew temporary troubles. A resort to alcohol, for example, can bring a transient euphoric uplift from pressing matters of the day. These strategies are perhaps truer today than they were in Dionysian cultures, exceptions being certain countries where alcohol is taboo for religious reasons. Indeed, it is generally believed that stress-induced illness is a phenomenon of contemporary urban civilization. The widespread prescription of tranquillizers and the high incidence of alcohol addiction support this view. Their impact on fitness and well-being has received scant attention.

Amongst athletes, participation in sports brings its own unique form of stress, usually before the more important contests. Though a certain amount of pre-competition anxiety is inevitable, the anxiety response varies enormously between individuals, with some coping extremely poorly. Many find their own solutions to attenuate anxiety levels, albeit sometimes with exogenous aids. Anxiety may adversely affect performance, especially in activities highly demanding of mental concentration and steadiness of limbs. This has prompted the use of anti-anxiety drugs, although some are not permitted in many sports.

In this chapter the relationship between anxiety and sport performance is first explored. The next section concentrates on alcohol, its metabolism in the body and its effect on the central nervous system. The interactions between alcohol and health are then considered. Its impact on physiological responses to exercise and the uses in sport are examined next. The

Drugs in Sport, 2nd edn. Edited by David R. Mottram. Published in 1996 by E & FN Spon, London. ISBN 0 419 18890 8

main 'minor' tranquillizers, the benzodiazepines, are discussed before, finally, the uses and abuses of other anti-anxiety drugs are described.

6.2 ANXIETY AND PERFORMANCE

The psychological reaction to impending sports competition is variously referred to as anxiety, arousal, stress or activation. Though these concepts are not synonymous, their relationships to performance have sufficient similarities to lump them together for the present purposes. Anxiety denotes worry or emotional tension, arousal denotes a continuum from sleep to high excitement, stress implies an agent that induces strain in the organism and activation refers to the metabolic state in the 'flight or fight' reaction. Irrespective of which concept is adopted, the effects of the biological responses on performance are generally assumed to fit an inverted-U curve. A moderate level of 'anxiety' about the forthcoming activity is deemed desirable to induce the right levels of motivation for action. The simpler the task the higher will be the level of anxiety that can be tolerated before performance efficiency begins to fall (Figure 6.1).

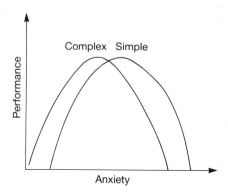

Figure 6.1 The relationship between level of anxiety and performance efficiency for simple and complex tasks.

Although the inverted-U model is somewhat simplistic, it does illustrate that over-anxiety has a detrimental effect on the physical and psychomotor elements that comprise sports performance. In such instances anxiety-reducing strategies will have an ergogenic effect. The athlete or mentor may have to choose between mental relaxation techniques or drugs to alleviate anxiety.

There are various indices which the behavioural scientist employs in measuring anxiety in field conditions, such as sport, especially pre-competition. These include hand tremor, restlessness or other subjective estimates of 'tension', paper and pencil tests and so on. Linked to these are physiological indices which demonstrate increased sympathetic tone. These include muscular tension as measured by electromyography, galvanic skin response or skin conductance and elevated concentrations of stress hormones or their metabolites in blood or in urine. These may be important to consider if the mechanisms by which the ergogenic or adverse effects of anxiety-reducing drugs operate are to be understood.

High levels of anxiety generally militate against performance and so favour attempts to reduce anxiety. Anxiety level depends very much on the nature of the sport as well as on the individual concerned. Generally, high anxiety is associated with brief and high-risk activities. A league table of anxiety responses pre-start (Figure 6.2), as reflected in the emotional tachycardia, shows motor-racing, ski-jumping and downhill skiing to be top of the list. Activities like parachuting and high acceleration rides in leisure parks induce strong anxiety reactions. In these cases heart rates have been found to correlate highly with adrenaline levels in blood and in urine (Reilly *et al.*, 1985). American football is lowest in the table, possibly because of the practice of meditation and relaxation techniques and the long duration of such games.

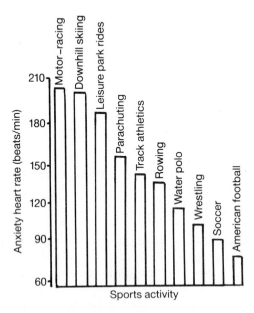

Figure 6.2 Pre-activity heart rate for various sports and recreations.

Professional athletes regularly subjected to situations of high psychological stress tend to adapt. At this élite level highly anxious personalities are rare. The anxiety reaction of professional soccer players, for example, is highly reproducible although there are noticeable trends. Heart rates in the dressing-room tend to be higher when playing at home rather than away, because players are subject to more critical scrutiny by a home audience. Anxiety is highest in goalkeepers, for whose mistakes the team is usually punished severely. Players returning to the team after a spell of injury or making an initial appearance in the premier team show higher heart rates than their normal pre-match values. It is hardly surprising to find that goalkeepers are the most vulnerable members of the team to stress-related illnesses such as stomach ulcers.

Avoiding over-anxiety may be important in game players for reasons of safety. Anxiety has been found to correlate with joint and muscle injuries in soccer, the more anxious players tending to get injured most often. This supports the notion of injury proneness: the mechanism is probably lack of commitment or hesitancy in critical events (such as tackling) that might promote injury (Sanderson, 1981). Some soccer players are in the habit of taking a nip of whisky immediately prior to going on to the pitch, the communal bottle being euphemistically referred to as 'team spirit'. The inhibiting effects of alcohol are exploited by tournament rugby players, who are not averse to drinking beer in between rounds of 'rugby sevens' competitions for example.

Obviously there is a thin line to tread between, on the one hand, reducing anxiety to enhance well-being and mental states prior to competing in sport and, on the other hand, impairing performance because of a disruption in motor coordination accompanying the treatment. The outcome depends on the concentrations of the drug, the timing of ingestion and the individual susceptibility to it. There are also possibilities of tolerance to the drug with chronic use or of drug dependence developing. Residual effects may carry over to the following day, affecting training or subsequent competitive performance. These aspects are now considered in the context of alcohol in sports and exercise.

6.3 ALCOHOL

6.3.1 METABOLISM OF ALCOHOL

The alcohols are a group of chemicals, most of which are toxic. The most common is ethanol or ethyl alcohol which is obtained by the fermentation of sugar. It is non-toxic, except in large and chronic doses, and has been enjoyed as a beverage for many centuries.

Ethyl alcohol is both a drug and a food, accounting for about 100 kcal (420 kJ) of energy per adult of the UK population each day. Its energy value per unit weight (kcal/g), the Atwater factor, is 7 compared with a value of 9 for fat, but this is higher than the value of 4 for both carbohydrate and protein. Wine contains about 12% alcohol, and so a litre bottle will contain about 120 g with a calorific content of 840 kcal (3516 kJ). The value of alcohol as a food stuff is limited, as it is metabolized mainly in the liver and at a fixed rate of about 100 mg/kg body weight/hour. For a 70 kg individual this amounts to 7 g of alcohol hourly. The energy is not available to active skeletal muscle and consequently it is not possible to exercise oneself to sobriety. Beer contains some electrolytes but its subsequent diuretic effect makes it less than the ideal agent of rehydration after hard physical training.

Alcohol is a polar substance which is freely miscible in water. This is due to the fact that alcohol molecules are held together by the same sort of intermolecular forces as water, namely hydrogen bonds. The alcohol molecule is also soluble in fat, it is small and has a weak charge. (As the lipophilic alkyl group becomes larger and the hydrophilic group smaller, the alcohol molecules associate preferentially with other alcohol, hydrocarbon or lipid molecules rather than water.) It easily penetrates biological membranes and can be absorbed unaltered from the stomach and more quickly from the small intestine. The rate of absorption is influenced by the amount of food in the stomach, whether there are gas molecules in the drink and the concentration of alcohol in the drink. Absorption is quickest if alcohol is drunk on an empty stomach, if gas molecules are present in the drink and the alcohol content is high. Intense mental concentration, lowered body temperature or physical exertion tend to slow the rate of absorption.

From the gastrointestinal tract the alcohol is transported to the liver by means of the hepatic circulation. The activity of the enzyme alcohol dehydrogenase, present chiefly in the liver, governs the disappearance of alcohol from the body. In the liver, alcohol dehydrogenase converts the alcohol to acetaldehyde; it is then converted to acetic acid or acetate by aldehyde dehydrogenase. About 75% of the alcohol taken up by the blood is released as acetate into the circulation. The acetate is then oxidized to carbon dioxide and water within the Krebs (or citric acid) cycle. An alternative metabolic route for acetate is its activation to acetyl co-enzyme A and further reactions to form fatty acids, ketone bodies, amino acids and steroids.

Ethyl alcohol is distributed throughout the body by means of the circulatory system and enters all the body water pools and tissues, including the central nervous system. Its distribution amongst the body fluids and tissues depends on several factors, such as blood flow, mass and permeability of the tissue. Organs such as the brain, lungs, liver and kidneys reach equilibrium quickly, whilst skeletal muscle with its relatively poorer blood supply attains its peak alcohol concentration more slowly. Initially, alcohol moves rapidly from blood into the tissues. When absorption is complete, arterial alcohol concentration falls and alcohol diffuses from the tissues into the capillary bed. This means that alcohol concentrations remain high in the peripheral venous blood due to the slower rates of metabolism and excretion.

The metabolism of alcohol in the liver is unaffected by its concentration in the blood. Some alcohol is eliminated in the breath, but this is usually less than 5% of the total amount metabolized. This route is utilized in assessing safe levels for driving, forming the basis of the breathalyser tests. Small amounts of alcohol are excreted in urine and also in sweat if exercise is performed whilst drunk. Higher excretion rates through the lungs, urine and sweat are produced at high environmental temperatures and at high blood alcohol levels.

With a single drink the blood alcohol level usually peaks about 45 minutes after ingestion. This is the point where any influence on performance will be most evident. Effect on performance will generally be greater on the ascending limb than for a corresponding value on the descending limb of the blood alcohol curve; the rate of change and the direction of change of the blood alcohol concentration are more crucial factors than is the length of time alcohol is in the bloodstream. The peak is delayed about 15 minutes if strenuous exercise precedes the ingestion. This may be due to the reduction in blood flow to the gut that accompanies exercise, the increased blood flow to skeletal muscle and the needs of the thermoregulatory system post-exercise.

Besides the exogenous ethanol in body fluids, trace amounts of ethanol are synthesized endogenously. This endogenous ethanol is thought to arise both from bacterial fermentation in the gut and from the action of alcohol dehydrogenase on acetaldehyde derived from pyruvate. Blood levels of endogenous alcohol in the human are very low, ranging only up to about 7.5 mg in total.

Studies on alcohol and exercise are notoriously difficult to control, as most subjects will recognize the taste of the experimental treatment. Most experimenters use vodka in orange juice as the alcohol beverage: the placebo can include enough vodka to taste but not enough to produce a measurable blood alcohol concentration. Another strategy is to put a noseclip on the subject, who is then given anaesthetic throat lozenges. Subjects vary in their responses to alcohol, as does the same subject from day to day, making inferences from laboratory studies difficult. As the effects of alcohol differ with body size, dosage is usually administered according to body weight. Effects also vary with the level of blood alcohol induced, but there is not general international agreement on acceptable maximum levels for day-to-day activities such as driving. Alcohol doses that render subjects intoxicated or drunk have little practical relevance in exercise studies and so experimental levels are usually low to moderate. Additionally, experiments that entail alcohol ingestion should be approved by the local human ethics committee, and high alcohol dosages are unlikely to gain acceptance in experimental protocols.

6.3.2 ACTION OF ALCOHOL ON THE NERVOUS SYSTEM

The effects of ethanol administration on central nervous tissue are due to direct action rather than to acetaldehyde, its first breakdown product. Following ethanol ingestion, very little acetaldehyde crosses the blood–brain barrier, despite elevated levels in the blood. Alcohol has a general effect on neural transmission by influencing axonal membranes and slowing nerve conductance. The permeability of the axonal membrane to potassium and sodium is altered by the lowering of central calcium levels that results from ingesting alcohol (Wesnes and Warburton, 1983). Alcohol has differential effects on the central neurotransmitters, acetylcholine, serotonin, noradrenaline and dopamine.

Alcohol blocks the release of acetylcholine and disrupts its synthesis. As a result, transmission in the central cholinergic pathways will be lowered. The ascending reticular cholinergic pathway determines the level of cortical arousal and the flow of sensory information to be evaluated by the cortex. The lowering of electro-cortical arousal reduces the awareness of stressful information and the ability of the individual to attend to specific stimuli. These de-arousing changes are reflected in alterations in the electroencephalogram with moderate to large doses of alcohol. The obvious results are impairments in concentration, attention, simple and complex reaction times, skilled performance and, eventually, short-term memory.

Alcohol decreases serotonin turnover in the central nervous system by inhibiting tryptophan hydroxylase, the enzyme essential for seritonin's biosynthesis. Activity in the neurones of serotonergic pathways is important for the experience of anxiety; output of corticosteroid hormones from the adrenal cortex increases the activity in these neurones. Alcohol has an opposing action and so may reduce the tension that is felt by the individual in a stressful situation.

An effect of alcohol is to increase activity in central noradrenergic pathways. This is transient and is followed, some hours later, by a decrease in activity. Catecholaminergic pathways are implicated in the control of mood states, activation of these pathways promoting happy and merry states. The fall in noradrenaline turnover as the blood alcohol concentration drops ties in with the reversal of mood that follows the initial drunken euphoric state. This is exacerbated by large doses of alcohol as these tend to give rise to depression.

Alcohol also has an effect on cerebral energy metabolism: the drug decreases glucose utilization in the brain. As glucose is the main substrate furnishing energy for nerve cells, the result is that the lowered glucose level may induce mental fatigue. This will be reflected in failing cognitive functions, and a decline in concentration and in information processing. It is unlikely that exercise, *per se*, will offset these effects.

The disruption of acetylcholine synthesis and release means that alcohol acts as a depressant, exerting its effect on the reticular activating system, whose activity represents the level of physiological arousal. It also has a depressant effect on the cortex: it first affects the frontal centres of the cortex before affecting the cerebellum. In large quantities it will affect speech and muscular coordination, eventually inducing sedation. In smaller doses it inhibits cerebral control mechanisms, freeing the brain from its normal inhibition. This release of inhibition has been blamed for aggressive and violent conduct of individuals behaving out of character when under the influence of alcohol. Undoubtedly, alcohol has been a factor in crowd violence and football hooliganism on the terraces. The belief led to the banning of alcohol at football grounds in Scotland, severe restriction of alcohol sales at English league grounds following the crowd control problems at the European Cup final in Brussels in 1985 and restriction of alcohol at cricket grounds in England after riots at an England–Pakistan match in 1987. These restrictions were extended to other sporting events in the years that followed.

Clearly, alcohol will have deleterious effects on performance in sports that require fast reactions, complex decision making and highly skilled actions. It will also have an impact on hand–eye coordination, on tracking tasks, such as driving, and on vigilance tasks such as long-distance sailing. An effect on tracking tasks is that control movements lose their normal smoothness and precision and become more abrupt or jerky. In vigilance tasks, some studies show a deterioration in performance with time on task (Tong, Henderson and Chipperfield, 1980). At high doses of alcohol, meaningful sport becomes impractical or downright dangerous. Progressive effects of alcohol at different blood alcohol concentrations are summarized in Table 6.1. An important effect of alcohol, not listed, is that it diminishes the ability to process appreciable amounts of information arriving simultaneously from two different sources.

The most frequently cited study that reported facilitatory effects of alcohol on human performance was the classical experiment of Ikai and Steinhaus (1961). They showed that in some cases moderate alcohol doses could improve isometric muscular strength. This result was similar to that obtained by cheering and loud vocal encouragement. They explained the effect on the basis of central inhibition of the impulse traffic in the nerve fibres of the skeletal muscles during maximal effort. This depression of the inhibitory effect of certain centres in the central nervous system may allow routine practices to proceed normally without any disturbing effects. It should be noted that this finding has not generally been replicated when other aspects of muscular performance are considered. These are reviewed in a later section.

Table 6.1 Demonstrable effects of alcohol at different blood alcohol concentrations

Concentration level (mg/100 ml blood)	Effects
30	Enhanced sense of well-being; retarded simple reaction time; impaired hand–eye coordination
60	Mild loss of social inhibition; impaired judgement
90	Marked loss of social inhibition; coordination reduced; noticeably 'under the influence'
120	Apparent clumsiness; loss of physical control; tendency towards extreme responses; definite drunkenness is noted
150	Erratic behaviour; slurred speech; staggering gait
180	Loss of control of voluntary activity; impaired vision

6.3.3 ALCOHOL AND HEALTH

The effects of alcohol on health are usually viewed in terms of chronic alcoholism. Persistent drinking leads to a dependence on alcohol so that it becomes addictive. Most physicians emphasize that alcoholism is a disease rather than a vice and devise therapy accordingly. The result of excessive drinking is ultimately manifested in liver disease: cirrhosis, a serious hardening and degeneration of liver tissue, is fatal for many heavy drinkers. Cancer is also more likely to develop in a cirrhotic liver. There is evidence of increased susceptibility to breast cancer in women who drink alcohol regularly (Willett et al., 1987). Cardiomyopathy or damage to the heart muscle can result from years of heavy drinking. Other pathological conditions associated with alcohol abuse include generalized skeletal myopathy, pancreatitis and cancers of the pharynx and larynx. Impairment of brain function also occurs, alcoholic psychoses being a common cause of hospitalization in psychiatric wards.

Alcohol was formerly used as an anaesthetic until it was realized that it was too dangerous to supply in large quantities for that purpose. The result of applying alcohol to living cells is that the protoplasm of the cells precipitates as a consequence of dehydration. Long-term damage to tissue in the central nervous system may be an unwanted outcome of habitual heavy drinking.

Heavy drinking is not compatible with serious athletics. For the athlete, drinking is usually done only in moderation, an infrequent respite for the ascetic regimens of physical training, though the odd end of season binge is customary. Nevertheless, drinking is a social convention in many sports, such as rugby, squash and water-polo, where there may be peer-group pressure to take alcohol following training or competition or at club functions. The sensible athlete drinks moderately and occasionally, avoiding alcohol for at least 24 hours before competing. Hangovers may persist for a day and disturb concentration in sports involving complex skills. The attitude of the retired athlete may be very different. If his active career is terminated abruptly and the free time that retirement releases is taken up by social drinking, the result may well be a gradual deterioration in physical condition, with body weight increasing and fitness declining. In this context, the effect of alcohol on the ex-athlete will be quite harmful. The case of the great Kenyan distance runner, Henry Rono, is a salutary example. Six years after setting world records at 3000 m, 3000 m steeplechase, 5000 m and 10000 m, he was referred for treatment to a rehabilitation clinic for chronic alcoholics.

Various institutions within sports medicine have addressed the problems of alcohol and exercise. In 1982 the American College of Sports Medicine set out a position statement on alcohol which was unequivocally against any indulgence. It underlined the adverse effects of alcohol on health and condemned the resort to alcohol by athletes. Its estimate was that there were 10 million adult problem drinkers in the United States and an additional 3.3 million in its 14–17 years age range. Any evidence of the beneficial aspects of alcohol was not mentioned.

There is a belief that moderate drinking has some positive benefits for health. Small amounts increase the flow of gastric juices and thereby stimulate digestion: in large doses, alcohol irritates the stomach lining, causing gastritis and even vomiting of blood. A national survey of lifestyles in England and Wales provided support for the view that healthy people tended to drink a little. Amongst men under 60, the likelihood of high blood pressure was found to increase with the amount of alcohol consumed. For older men and for women, light drinking was associated with lower blood pressure, even when effects due to body weight were taken into account (Stepney, 1987).

It is thought also that moderate drinking provides a degree of protection against coronary heart disease. This may have been nurtured in the vineyards of France where a habitually modest consumption of wine is associated with a low incidence of heart disease. One report claimed that myocardial infarction rates were lower in moderate drinkers than in non-drinkers (Willett *et al.*, 1980). A possible mechanism is the reduction in hypertension and the relaxation from business cares that drinking can bring. A link has been shown by an increase in high-density lipoprotein cholesterol levels with moderate levels of drinking alcohol. High-density lipoprotein particles remove cholesterol from the tissues and transfer it into other particles in the blood; low-density lipoprotein, on the other hand, obtains its cholesterol from these other particles and transfers it to the tissues. A high ratio of high-density to low-density lipoprotein fractions is generally found in well-trained endurance athletes, a low ratio being indicative of poor cardiovascular health. The effect is apparent in autopsies of alcoholics whose blood vessels are in good condition despite pathological changes in other tissues. The mechanism by which alcohol would raise the high-density lipoprotein cholesterol has not been fully explained.

It seems that for a healthy athlete in a good state of training, occasional drinking of alcohol in moderation will have little adverse effect. It is important to emphasize that any such occasional bouts of drinking should be restrained and should follow rather than precede training sessions, whose training stimulus is likely to be lowered by the soporific influence of drinking alcohol before strenuous exercise.

6.3.4 ALCOHOL AND PHYSIOLOGICAL RESPONSES TO EXERCISE

Alcohol ingestion has been shown to lower muscle glycogen at rest compared with control conditions. As pre-start glycogen levels are important for sustained exercise at an intensity of about 70–80% VO_2max., such as marathon running, taking alcohol in the 24 hours before such endurance activities is ill-advised. Effects of alcohol on the metabolic responses to submaximal exercise seem to be small. Juhlin-Dannfelt and co-workers (1977) reported that alcohol does not impair lipolysis or free fatty acid utilization during exercise. It may decrease splanchnic glucose output, decrease the potential contribution of energy from liver gluconeogenesis, cause a more pronounced decline in blood glucose levels and decrease the leg muscle uptake of glucose towards the end of a prolonged (up to 3-hour) run. The impairment in glucose production by the liver would lead to an increased likelihood of hypoglycaemia developing during prolonged exercise.

Some studies have shown an increase in oxygen uptake (VO_2) at a fixed sub-maximal exercise intensity after alcohol ingestion. This may be due to a poorer coordination of the active muscles as the decrease in mechanical efficiency, implied by the elevation in VO_2, is not a consistent finding. Related to this is an increase in blood lactate levels with alcohol; metabolism of alcohol shunts lactate away from the gluconeogenic pathway and leads to an increase in the ratio of lactate to pyruvate. It is possible that elevated blood lactate concentrations during exercise, after taking alcohol, may reflect impairment in clearance of lactate rather than an increase in production by the exercising muscles. A failure to clear lactate would militate against performance of strenuous exercise.

Alcohol does not seem to have adverse effects on maximum oxygen consumption (VO_2max.) or on metabolic responses to high intensity exercises approaching VO_2max. levels. At high doses (up to 200mg%, i.e 0.20% blood alcohol level) it is understandable that athletes may feel disinclined towards maximal efforts that elicit VO_2max. values and a reduction in peak VE is usually observed (Blomqvist, Saltin and Mitchell, 1970). Similarly, they may be poorly motivated to sustain high intensity exercise for as long as they would normally do. In middle-distance running events with an appreciable aerobic component, performance was found to be detrimentally affected in a dose-related manner, with increasing blood alcohol concentration (BAC) levels from 0.01 to 0.10% (McNaughton and Preece, 1986).

Although it has not been shown conclusively that alcohol alters VE, stroke volume or muscle blood flow at sub-maximal exercise levels, it does decrease peripheral vascular resistance. This is because of the vasodilatory effect of alcohol on the peripheral blood vessels, which would increase heat loss from the surface of the skin and cause a drop in body temperature. This would be dangerous if alcohol is taken in conjunction with exercise in cold conditions. Sampling from a hip-flask of whisky on the ski slopes may bring an immediate inner glow and feeling of warmth but its disturbance of normal thermoregulation may put the recreational skier at risk of hypothermia. Frost-bitten mountaineers especially should avoid drinking alcohol as the peripheral vasodilation it induces would cause the body temperature to fall further. In hot conditions, alcohol is also inadvisable as it acts as a diuretic and would exacerbate problems of dehydration.

Studies of maximum muscular strength, in the main, show no influence of moderate to medium doses of alcohol on maximum isometric tension. Similar results apply to dynamic functions, such as peak torque measured on isokinetic dynamometers. Muscular endurance is generally assessed by requiring the subject to hold a fixed percentage of maximum for as long as possible. Here, too, the influences of moderate alcohol doses are generally found to be non-significant. This may be because the tests represent gross aspects of muscular function and, as such, are insensitive to the effects of the drug.

6.3.5 ALCOHOL IN AIMING SPORTS

In aiming sports, a steady limb is needed to provide a firm platform for launching the missile at its target or to keep the weapon still. Examples of such sports are archery, billiards, darts, pistol shooting and snooker. Two pistol shooters were disqualified during the 1980 Olympics due to taking alcohol in an attempt to improve their performance. There are also aiming components in sports such as fencing and modern pentathlon, especially in the rifle-shooting discipline of the latter. In some of these sports alcohol levels are now officially monitored, whilst in others, notably darts, drinking is a conventional complement of the sport itself.

The Grand National Archery Society in the UK has not yet banned the use of alcohol in its competitions, and so alcohol is taken in small doses in the belief that it relaxes the archer, thereby steadying the hands as well as the nerves. In order to avoid fluctuating blood alcohol concentrations, the archer, like the dart thrower, tries to keep topping up the levels to prevent them from falling down the descending limb of the curve.

To understand how alcohol might affect the archer, it is useful to look at the task *in toto*. The competitive player has to shoot three dozen arrows at each of four targets – 90, 70, 60 and 50 m away – to complete a FITA (the world governing body) round. The highest possible score is 1440, 10 points being the maximum for each perfect shot. A world record score of 1342 was achieved by 1984 Olympic Games champion, Darrel Pace, back in 1979: this record has since been improved and the system of scoring has been modified for different competitive levels. Technological improvements in bow design have helped to produce such outstanding scores, leaving the gap to perfection due to human factors. The modern bow has two slot-in limbs which insert into a magnesium handle section and stabilizers which help to minimize vibration and turning of the bow. Muscle strength is needed to draw the bow, whilst muscle endurance is called for to hold it steady, usually for about 8 seconds for each shot, whilst the sight is aligned with the target. Deflection of the arrow tip by 0.02 mm at 90 m causes the arrow to miss the target, which gives some idea of the hand steadiness required. The archer, before release or loose, pulls the arrow towards and through the clicker (a blade on the side of the bow which aids in measuring draw length). The archer reacts to the sound of the clicker hitting the side of the bow handle by releasing the string which, in effect, shoots the arrow. Archers are coached to react to the clicker by allowing the muscles to relax; a slow reaction to the clicker is generally recognized as hesitation. This affects the smoothness of the loose and is reflected in muscle tremor causing a 'snatched loose'. For these reasons, the effects of alcohol on reaction time, arm steadiness, muscle strength and endurance, and the electromyogram of one of the arm muscles were selected as appropriate parameters to isolate and study under experimental conditions (Reilly and Halliday, 1985).

In the experiment, nine subjects underwent a battery of tests under four conditions: sober, placebo, 0.02% blood alcohol level and 0.05% blood alcohol level. The alcohol doses were administered in three equal volumes to total 500 ml over 15 minutes, 45 minutes being allowed for peak blood alcohol levels to be attained. The doses to elicit the desirable blood alcohol levels were calculated according to the formula of Hicks (1976) which was shown to be effective:

$$A = \frac{(454)(W)(R)(BAC + 0.0002)}{(0.8)(0.95)}$$

where

A	=	ml 95% ethanol
W	=	body weight (lb)
R	=	distribution coefficient of 0.765
BAC	=	desired blood alcohol concentration (0.05% = 0.0005)

A summary of the results for the performance measurement appears in Table 6.2. There was no effect of alcohol on the muscular strength and muscular endurance measures; the holding time in the endurance test was about the same time as the archer normally holds the bow drawn before shooting, so that this test turned out to be reasonably realistic.

Table 6.2 Effects of the alcohol treatments on four experimental tests (mean ± s.d.) (from Reilly and Halliday, 1985)

Variables	Sober	Placebo	0.02% BAC	0.05% BAC
Arm steadiness:				
Time-off-target(s)	2.64 ± 0.89	3.05 ± 0.74	3.24 ± 1.01	8.17 ± 1.49
Isometric strength (N)	546 ± 48	560 ± 37	541 ± 56	523 ± 78
Muscular endurance (s)	11.4 ± 2.1	12.0 ± 2.5	12.0 ± 2.0	10.8 ± 2.0
Reaction time (ms)	211 ± 6.5	209 ± 8.5	223 ± 9.6	226 ± 11.2

Reaction time was significantly slowed by the lower alcohol dose, a further small delay occurring at the higher blood alcohol dose. The more sensitive response of auditory reaction time to alcohol would mean, in practice, a slower reaction to the clicker and a faulty loose. Another adverse effect noted was the impairment in steadiness of the extended arm. Performance was degraded, especially at the 0.05% blood alcohol level, and the variability in arm steadiness also increased with alcohol. This effect contradicts the conventional wisdom in archery and may have been due to the high load on the arm muscles when holding the bow drawn. It is possible that alcohol only operates to advantage in steadying the limb in contexts more competitive than laboratory experiments.

Some benefits were noted in the electromyographic profile (Figure 6.3). A clearer loose was observed at the low alcohol levels which would be valuable in promoting a smoother release. This was supplemented by a tendency towards a reduced tremor in the muscle with both alcohol treatments. Together, these effects would indicate a greater muscle relaxation, the tremor being normally associated with a snatched loose. These factors were partly offset by the longer holding time prior to loose induced by the alcohol treatments. The overall conclusion was that alcohol has differential effects on tasks related to archery, depending on the concentrations, the components of the performance analysed and individual reactivity to the drug.

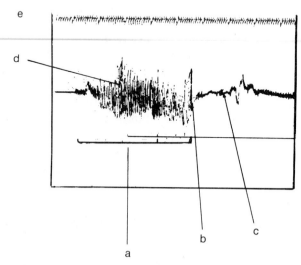

Figure 6.3 The electromyographic profile of an arm muscle whilst holding the bow down: (a) holding time; (b) the point of loose; (c) post-loose muscular activity; (d) tremor; (e) the time-scale of events marked in 100 ms.

The deleterious effects of alcohol on some aspects of archery would not apply to other aiming sports, such as darts and pistol shooting. In these the loading on the arm muscles is light, so a greater arm steadiness is likely to be induced by the drug. Another consideration is that the timing of the release is at the discretion of the subject and also is unaffected by a retarded reaction time. Reactions will have importance where the target is moving: it is noteworthy that the discipline of clay-pigeon shooting, for example, is not steeped in a history of alcohol use.

The bar-room sports, such as snooker, billiards and darts, have the alcohol industry as an adjunct to their matches. At the highest level of competition these sports are popular television spectacles. Although it is widely thought that the top performers swig large quantities of alcohol, this is not the case. Imbibition is regular but in small doses so that a moderate blood alcohol level is continually maintained (needless to say, at high blood alcohol levels, 0.15% or more, whole-body stability and mental concentration would be degraded and any possible erogenic effect would be swamped). Alcohol is not prohibited in these sports though other drugs are.

A study of the effects of elevating blood alcohol levels on tasks related to dart throwing (Reilly and Scott, 1993) confirmed the finding in archery. Whilst there were negative effects from the light alcohol dose (BAC 0.02%) on hand–eye coordination, effects were positive for balance and dart throwing. A higher level of 0.05% led to a fall-off in performance on all tasks. Results indicated some improvement with a light dose of alcohol for dart throwers, but performance deteriorated when BAC levels reached 0.05%.

In those sports that discourage alcohol for competition there is a disharmony in standards for what constitutes legality. (Alcohol is banned in several sports, for example modern pentathlon, fencing and shooting.) It is worthy of note that the legal limit for driving differs between countries: in Norway and Greece the limit is 50 mg/100 ml, in Ireland it is twice that level, whilst in the UK, France and Germany the safety limit is intermediate at 80 mg/100 ml. In Sweden the legal limit is 20 mg/100 ml, whilst in Turkey any measurable alcohol level is illegal. These values refer to alcohol in blood: the corresponding (to 80 mg/100 ml) levels for breath and for urine are 35µg/100 ml and 107 mg/100 ml respectively. The Amateur Fencing Association in Britain has adopted the Norwegian value as its limit for competition and has incorporated dope testing at its contests since 1984. At the request of the international governing body for fencing, alcohol tests are now carried out at the Olympic Games, although it is generally accepted that alcohol abuse is not a major problem in this sport.

Beckett and Cowan (1979) described drug testing for alcohol as a two-stage process. A breath sample is analysed immediately after competition using a standard breathalyser. If the result indicates a level greater than 50 mg/100 ml a blood sample is obtained. This is analysed by gas chromatography which is more sensitive than the breath test. It is possible to obtain accurate and reliable results with a spectrophotometer.

Testing for alcohol is also performed on competitors in the shooting event of the modern pentathlon. Here, participants are disadvantaged by losing time in settling down to prepare for taking their shots. Recovering from their prior activity is important if the shots are to be on target. Although alcohol might help competitors to relax whilst taking aim, it has little ergogenic benefit in the other disciplines of the pentathlon. For various reasons, tranquillizers and beta-blocking agents have been preferred. These are considered in the sections that follow.

6.4 BENZODIAZEPINES

Benzodiazepines, derivatives of benzodiazepine, are widely employed as tranquillizers in the population at large and have been used for calming or sedative purposes in sports. They are included in the list of drugs that may be taken by sports competitors. There are now over two dozen benzodiazepine drugs and these form over 90% of the tranquillizer market. More than 20 doses of these drugs per head of the USA population are prescribed annually, giving an idea of the vast scale of consumption.

The first benzodiazepine drug was synthesized in the mid-1950s, the best known of those that followed being Librium (chlordiazepoxide hydrochloride), introduced in the USA in 1960, and Valium (diazepam), introduced in 1963. The benzodiazepines have systematically replaced the barbiturates and the propranediol derivatives as drugs of clinical choice in treating stress and anxiety. There is little evidence that the barbiturates had a major use amongst active athletes as an ergogenic aid in the years when they were being widely prescribed, although they may have been used in more recent years.

Benzodiazepines decrease stress response indices, such as skin conductance and plasma corticosterone levels. They have been found to reduce anxiety in psychiatric and non-psychiatric patients and have demonstrated a superiority over barbiturates in clinical conditions. The drugs affect various neurotransmitters, the cholinergic and serotonergic effects having importance in reducing the stress response.

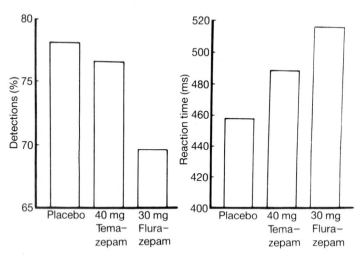

Figure 6.4   The effects of temazepam (40 mg) and flurazepam (30 mg) on the percentage of correct detections and the reaction time in a rapid information-processing task. The tasks were performed the morning after nightly administration of drugs. (From Wesnes and Warburton, 1983: reprinted with permission of John Wiley and Son Ltd.)

The benzodiazepines decrease the turnover in hemispheric cholinergic neurones by blocking the release of acetylcholine. By thus lowering the activity in cholinergic pathways, the drugs should have an adverse effect on human performance. Deterioration in the detection of sensory signals and in reaction time in a rapid information-processing task with nightly doses of flurazepam and temazepam have been found the morning after taking the drugs (Figure 6.4). The carry-over effects are due to the long half-lives of these particular drugs. Other types of performance which are affected include the rate of tapping, motor manipulation and complex coordination tasks, as well as real and simulated driving.

The function of one particular cholinergic pathway is to trigger the release of corticotrophic releasing factor from the hypothalamus into the pituitary blood vessels and produce a spurt of adrenocorticotrophic hormone (ACTH) from the anterior pituitary. The benzodiazepines would lower the emission of corticosteroid hormones from the adrenal cortex by affecting the ACTH release as a result of blocking cholinergic activity.

The benzodiazepines have been found to decelerate the turnover of noradrenaline. This effect is more apparent in conditions where the noradrenaline levels have been increased by stress. This change is not the basis of the drugs' anti-anxiety action, as repeated dosing with oxazepam results in a rapid tolerance to the decrease in noradrenaline turnover, whilst the drug maintains its anti-anxiety properties (Wesnes and Warburton, 1983). Similarly, dopamine turnover is retarded by benzodiazepines, but this effect is unrelated to the drugs' anti-anxiety properties.

The main anti-anxiety action of benzodiazepines seems to stem from the reduction in serotonergic activity which the drugs produce. Serotonergic neurones are important in the experience of anxiety so that this feeling is attenuated by the drugs. The effects of the benzodiazepines on serotonergic neurones may be mediated by a primary action of the drugs on gamma-aminobutyric acid (GABA). (It is thought that administration of GABA has been tried by some sports competitors.) The GABA-releasing neurones are primarily inhibitory and it is possible that when these are stimulated by the benzodiazepines the release of serotonin is inhibited. The GABA system is recognized as playing a crucial role in anxiety: some anxiety-related states may be due to diminished transmission at the level of GABA receptors which are functionally linked to benzodiazepine recognition sites (Corda, Concas and Biggio, 1986).

The effects of benzodiazepines on components of human performance will depend on the dosage and on the particular drug. Oxazepam, diazepam, nitrazepam, flurazepam and chlordiazepoxide are all 1,4 derivatives. Clobazam, a 1,5 benzodiazepine derivative, does not seem to impair psychomotor performance but does retain its anti-anxiety properties

(Wesnes and Warburton, 1983) and so may have more applications than the others in sport and exercise contexts.

Following the bans on alcohol overuse in the modern pentathlon, athletes at the 1972 Olympic Games in Munich were found to have used benzodiazepines and other tranquillizers, such as meprobamate, as anti-anxiety agents. They were thought preferable to alcohol as they might reduce anxiety without the potential adverse effects on judgement and coordination associated with alcohol. Meprobamate acts as a mild tran-quillizer without producing drowsiness. It is highly addictive and reduces tolerance to alcohol. The benzodiazepines are relatively safe in that they have low toxicity and few side-effects. They can induce a depen-dence in chronic users and severe withdrawal symptoms are experienced when patients are taken off them abruptly. They are highly dangerous when used in overdoses combined with other central nervous system depressants, such as alcohol. Benzodiazepines are banned in the sport of modern pentathlon, though not on the list banned by the International Olympic Committee (IOC).

One of the primary effects of the GABA-mediated reaction to benzo-diazepines is that the drugs act as muscle relaxants. For this reason, they can be beneficial in aiding recovery from spastic-type muscle injuries. The effect is associated with a feeling of freedom from 'nerves' and tension. There are repercussions for muscle function in both sub-maximal and extreme efforts. Spontaneous activity of animals is reduced under the influence of these drugs. A study of alprazolam by Cabri et al. (1990) demonstrated that the effects were dependent on the dose. Maximal torque on an isokinetic dynamometer was unaffected by a low dose (0.5 mg). Moderate doses of the drug (1.5 and 3.0 mg) caused a reduction in muscle performance during brief bouts of maximal effort, both 90 and 360 minutes after ingestion. The metabolic effects were reflected in a decrease in amplitude and integrated electromyogram, but these effects were reduced after 360 minutes. It was thought that GABA-ergic activity induced alterations both in central nervous system and in peripheral (neuromuscular) receptor sites for benzodiazepines. Different benzo-diazepine drugs vary in their pharmacokinetic profiles and so their influence on muscle performance may also be variable. For this reason, Zinzen et al. (1994) compared the effects of therapeutic doses of flunitrazepam (plasma half-life of 31 hours) and triazolam (half-life of 8 hours) on performance, utilizing an isokinetic dynamometer. (Triazolam is banned from prescription in the UK and in other European countries due to its potential for dependence.) No hangover effects were noted after an 8-hour sleep with triazolam; in contrast, flunitrazepam was shown to impair muscle force production after the night's sleep and sub-jects were reported as having a 'sleepy impression' throughout the following day.

Various stimulants, including caffeine, have been used to offset the depressant effects of benzodiazepines on psychomotor skills. Caffeine interacts with the GABA–benzodiazepine system and so may reverse some adverse effects of these tranquillizers. Collomp *et al.* (1993) showed that moderate benzodiazepine intake (1 mg lorazepam) significantly impaired performance on an all-out 30 second exercise test. Moderate caffeine intake (250 mg caffeine in combination with 1 mg lorazepam) antagonized the metabolic but not the performance effects of the tranquillizer.

Diazepam is frequently prescribed in the treatment of muscle spasm. As doses used for relaxation of skeletal muscle, the drug could cause drowsiness and impair intellectual as well as motor function. Diazepam would generally be used on a short-term basis for treating muscle spasm due to injury. Consequently it does not entail withdrawal symptoms when treatment is complete.

The effects of benzodiazepines on sustained exercise performance are poorly documented. In the resting normal human, coronary blood flow is increased by 22.5% by diazepam but more so (73%) in persons with coronary artery disease. Whether the drugs are of benefit in the treatment of angina associated with effort is unknown (Powles, 1981).

Barbiturates and sedatives have long been used in sleeping pills. Such a use, to facilitate the sleep of athletes the night before competition, is likely to be counterproductive because of a residual de-arousing effect the following day. The 'hangover' effect of benzodiazepines was found to be greater for flurazepam (30 mg) than for temazepam (40 mg). Although the former produced better sleep, it resulted in lowered clearheadedness on waking and impaired performance on a rapid visual information-processing task (Wesnes and Warburton, 1984).

The 'hangover' effect of sleeping tablets, including benzodiazepines, is likely to disturb complex skills more than simple motor tasks performed early the following day, and, depending on the sport, an increase in errors may promote a higher risk of injury. Similarly, the prescription of sleeping pills to assist adaptation to time-zone changes is likely to have limited success in combating jet-lag symptoms. Use of behavioural methods of adaptation is more productive, whilst orally ingested melatonin may be a practical method of countering jet-lag in the future. Low doses of benzodiazepines may benefit shift workers who have difficulty in sleeping during the day after a nocturnal shift. In a study of simulated shift work, Wesnes and Warburton (1986) found that 10–20 mg doses of temazepam helped daytime sleep without detrimental residual effects on subsequent information processing.

The circadian or 24-hour rhythm in arousal may have implications for the pharmacological effects of anti-anxiety drugs. The optimum dosage of drugs affecting the nervous system differs with the time of day at which they are administered. The barbiturate dose that is safe in the evening may have exaggerated effects in early morning (Luce, 1973). The same is true for alcohol and this is reflected in social drinking habits: usually only alcoholics drink before breakfast and in the late morning. Alcohol taken at lunch time has a much more detrimental effect on psychomotor performance than if taken in the evening (Horne and Gibbons, 1991). The diurnal variation in responses to benzodiazepines and the implications this has for the dosage at different times of day for effective pre-contest tranquillization does not seem to have been the subject of any serious research attention.

6.5 MARIJUANA

Marijuana is obtained from the hemp plant *Cannabis sativa*. It contains the compound tetrahydrocannabinol which accounts for its psychological effects. These include a sedating and euphoric feeling of well-being and relaxation, with a sensation of sleepiness. Balance may be disturbed; aggression and motivation to perform may be blunted. Maximum muscular strength is reduced, probably because of the reduced drive towards all-out effort.

Largely because of its promotion of happy and euphoric mood states, marijuana has been prominent amongst the drugs of abuse, notably by youngsters and college students in the USA and Europe. It was the main recreational drug used by later adolescents and young adults in the 1970s. A report of the US Department of Health and Human Services, *Student Drug Use in America 1975 to 1980*, claimed that nearly one-third of students had tried marijuana before entering high school. This background of experience with the drug might explain its popularity amongst young athletes as a mode of release from tension during the competitive season.

Persistent marijuana smoking is incompatible with serious athletic training. The single-mindedness of the athlete will be disturbed by the demotivating influence of the drug. A few cigarettes of marijuana may cause minor changes in personality, while high doses can induce hallucinations, delusions and psychotic-like symptoms. The major abuse of marijuana has been by collegiate games teams, playing basketball and football, in the USA. The practice of smoking marijuana is generally condemned by athletic trainers and coaches in that country.

The active ingredient in marijuana is 1-5-9-tetrahydrocannabinol (THC). About 60 to 65% of the THC in a marijuana cigarette is absorbed through the lungs when it is smoked. Effects of drug action are noted within 15 minutes of smoking and last for 3 hours or so. The primary effects are produced by changes in central nervous system function. Motivation for physical effort is decreased and motor coordination, short-term memory and perception are impaired. Chronic marijuana abuse has been found to decrease circulating testosterone levels amongst its toxic effects (Nuzzo and Waller, 1988).

In addition to the psychological effects, marijuana induces tachycardia, bronchodilation and an increase in blood flow to the limbs. The bronchodilation effect does not lead to substantial alteration of the respiratory pattern during exercise. A pre-exercise increase of heart rate by 25 beats/minute is sustained during exercise up to about 80% of maximal effort. This means that maximal heart rate is attained at a lower intensity during a graded exercise test and the maximal work capacity is decreased after marijuana smoking (Renaud and Cormier, 1986).

6.6 NICOTINE

The tobacco leaf, *Nicotiana tabacum*, is the source of the cigarettes on which the massive tobacco industry is based. As the tobacco burns it generates about 4000 different compounds, including carbon monoxide (CO), ammonia, hydrogen cyanide, many carcinogens, DDT and tar. CO reduces the oxygen transport capacity of the blood by combining with haemoglobin (Hb) and so takes the place of oxygen in the bloodstream, adversely affecting aerobic exercise performance. The affinity of CO for Hb is 230 times that of oxygen. Tobacco smoke contains about 4% CO; smoking 10–12 cigarettes a day results in a blood COHb level of 4.9%, 15–25 a day raises the value to 6.3%, whilst 30–40 each day takes the level to 9.3%. Adverse effects are noticeable only during physical exertion, and after smoking it may take 24 hours or more for blood CO levels to return to normal. The smoke also paralyses the cilia in the respiratory passages so that their filtering becomes ineffective and the individual is more susceptible to respiratory tract infections.

The anti-smoking argument is centred around the links between smoking and cancer. Another strong link has been shown between smoking and hardening of the peripheral arteries and deterioration of the circulation to the limbs. Other long-term health hazards associated with heavy smoking are acceleration of coronary atherosclerosis, pulmonary emphysema and cerebral vascular disease.

About 30% of the adult population throughout the world smoke cigarettes and it is likely that double this number have sampled cigarettes at some time or another. As passive inhalation of smoke by non-users of tobacco – especially in crowded public places – has similar effects to those in smokers, smoking in public facilities is now restricted in many countries. About 20% of the smoke exhaled can be recirculated in passive inhalation.

The psychological and addictive effects of smoking are attributable to nicotine. Smokers report that cigarettes help them to relax, and the intensity of smoking increases at times of stress. They also report that smoking has a tranquillizing effect when they are angry. These influences on subjective states do not tally with the neurochemical and physiological responses to nicotine.

Nicotine is a cholinergic agonist and so by acting as a brain stimulant is likely to enhance arousal. In this respect it differs from alcohol and the benzodiazepines. There is a secondary rise in plasma corticosteroids, and an increase in central release of noradrenaline and in urinary cate-cholamine output. These changes are normally associated with the stress response, so that the relaxing characteristics of nicotine present a paradox. A few theories attempting to resolve this conflict have been reviewed by Wesnes and Warburton (1983), though none fits all the experimental evidence satisfactorily. They argued that it is the action of nicotine on cholinergic pathways controlling attention that reduces stress by enabling individuals to concentrate more efficiently. Neurotic individuals, who comprise the majority of smokers, are helped by the drug to filter out distracting thoughts; this enables them to perform more effectively, increasing their self-confidence in the process.

Smokers tend to experience stress when trying to give up cigarettes. For this reason, games players and other athletes who smoke pre-competition need astute counselling in attempting to overcome the habit. This would be best done during non-critical periods of the week and the pre-match smoking could be replaced unobtrusively by behavioural techniques of relaxation. However, resort to smoking may be easily replaced by an increase in snacks between meals, leading to unwanted weight gain. This occurs because the appetite centre in the brain is released from the depressant effect that smoking has on it. This problem will be greatest in the casual recreationist whose energy expenditure during physical activity will generally be low.

Quite apart from the effects on health and on human performance, smoking may also have repercussions for sports injury, particularly under conditions of cold. An acute effect of smoking is peripheral vaso-constriction which decreases blood flow to the limbs. For this reason, the frost-bitten climber should avoid any temptation to smoke until after recovery through hospitalization where alternatives therapies are ensured.

Clearly cigarette smoking has few advocates in sport and the sports sciences. Advertising of cigarettes is prohibited in some Scandinavian countries and top athletes are frequently prominent in anti-smoking campaigns. Smoking is rare amongst élite athletes, so that there are few models for youngsters taking up smoking to cite as examples. Those sports stars that do smoke might ultimately benefit from adopting alternative strategies to ease their troubled minds at times of emotional stress.

6.7 BETA BLOCKERS

Sympathetic adrenergic nerve fibres are classified according to their alpha and beta receptors. Effects of these receptors are sometimes contradictory.

In the blood vessels of muscle and skin, alpha adrenergic receptors cause vasoconstriction, whereas beta receptors induce vasodilation. The beta receptors are further divided into $beta_1$ and $beta_2$ categories according to the responses to sympathomimetic drugs. Functions of $beta_1$ receptors include cardiac acceleration and increased myocardial contractility; $beta_2$ receptors cause bronchodilation and glycogenesis. The action of these receptors is blocked by the activities of inhibitory drugs, the so-called beta blockers. These include, for example, atenolol, a cardioselective beta blocker with selectivity for $beta_1$ adrenoceptors; propranolol, which blocks both types of beta receptors, and labetalol which is a combined alpha and beta blocker. A more detailed description of sympathomimetic amines and their antagonists is given in Chapter 3.

Besides decreasing heart rate and myocardial contractility, the beta-blocking agents also reduce cardiac output, stroke volume and mean systemic arterial blood pressure. These effects explain the use of beta blockade in hypertension and in individuals with poor coronary health. Because of the effects on the circulation, beta blockade in clinical doses reduces maximal oxygen uptake and endurance time in normal individuals, but increases maximal work capacity in patients with angina pectoris. At sub-maximal exercise levels a decrease in heart rate and contractility is balanced by a decrease in coronary blood flow and an increased duration of myocardial contraction. The fall in exercise heart rate is not matched by a corresponding drop in perceived exertion rating, so that the usual close correlation between these variables is dissociated by beta blockade.

The effects of beta blockers on metabolism have implications for the performance of sub-maximal exercise. By inhibiting the enzyme phosphorylase, beta blockade may decrease the rate of glycogenolysis in skeletal muscle. Breakdown of liver glycogen is also likely to be inhibited, so that in sustained exercise blood glucose levels may decline. This fall is noted with propranolol but is not so evident with atenolol or metoprolol, two cardioselective beta blockers. Kaiser (1982) showed that jogging was markedly influenced only by propranolol at the low dose of 40 mg: at doses of 80 mg and above, atenolol had a similar adverse effect. Selective beta blockade inhibits lipolysis which may reduce the availability of free fatty acids as a substrate for prolonged exercise and cause an earlier onset of fatigue.

The effect of beta blockade on short-term high intensity performance was examined by Rusko *et al.* (1980). The subjects performed a range of anaerobic tasks after taking the beta blocker oxprenolol, and results were compared with performances after being given an inert placebo. The drug had no effect on isometric strength of leg extension, vertical jumping and stair running. Power output over 60 seconds on a cycle ergometer was reduced under the influence of the drug, whilst peak lactates and heart rates were also decreased. It seems that the beta blocker caused a reduction in anaerobic capacity as well as in heart rate.

Use of beta blockers has implications for thermoregulation if exercise is conducted in the heat. Gordon *et al.* (1987) showed that a non-selective beta blocker (propranolol) produced greater sweating than did a beta$_1$-selective blocker (atenolol). In this study, both drugs produced equivalent reductions in exercise tachycardia, a similar decrease in skin blood flow and a similar rise in rectal temperature. The authors suggested that beta$_1$-selective adrenoceptor blockers should be the preferred therapy during prolonged physical activity when adequate fluid replacement cannot be guaranteed. The findings indicated an increased need for persons treated with propranolol to stick to a strict fluid replacement regimen during sustained exercise.

Another consideration is whether the physiological adaptations to a fitness training programme are altered by the use of beta blockers. Propranolol, even in low doses of 80 mg daily, does blunt the effects of exercise training in normal individuals. At higher doses of 160–320 mg/day this impairment is more pronounced. The apparent mechanism is a prevention of the normal peripheral circulatory and metabolic responses to exercise (Opie, 1986). Although beta blockade permits patients with angina to exercise more easily, the chronic effects of physical training in patients with ischaemic heart disease may still be attenuated. Indeed, Powles (1981) considered that the many physiological effects of beta blockade meant that for each patient there may be an optimal dosage. This optimal point is that at which adverse effects on the functioning of the left ventricle, the myocardial perfusion and metabolism did not outweigh the benefits associated with decreased heart rate.

Beta blockers cross the blood–brain barrier to varying extents, depending on their lipid solubility (Table 3.5); for example propranolol does so to a greater degree than atenolol. Their anti-anxiety effect may not necessarily be centrally mediated. The suppression of cardiac activity which would result in a reduction in the afferent information from the heart may be the cause. Inhibition of the beta receptors, through which glycogenolysis is stimulated by adrenaline and lactic acid production is increased, is an alternative mechanism. Low levels of lactic acid tend to be associated with a state of relaxation, free from anxiety. On balance, however, the evidence favours the interpretation that the anti-anxiety effects of these drugs are due to direct action within the central nervous system.

As beta-blocking agents are not addictive they tend to be preferred over the benzodiazepines and alcohol in combating anxiety. They attenuate emotional tachycardia, limb tremor and unpleasant manifestations of anxiety, such as palmar sweating, pre-competition. High-risk sports, such as ski-jumping, motor-racing and bobsleighing, provide especially suitable contexts for their use. Undesirable effects might be produced by beta blockers in athletes suffering from asthma and in individuals with reduced cardiac function.

The beta blockers have been banned by the International Shooting Union as they are believed to be of potential use to marksmen in reducing anxiety before competitions and enhancing performance. Nevertheless, they were repeatedly used by many competitors in shooting events at the 1984 Olympic Games (and to a lesser extent at the subsequent Games), being prescribed by team physicians for health reasons. Similar practices by top professional snooker players were disclosed at the 1987 World Championship. They are unlikely to be used in endurance events where the aerobic system is maximally or near-maximally taxed. They would have an ergogenic effect in the shooting discipline of the modern pentathlon, an event in which they have been allegedly used for a steadying influence before shooting.

The use of beta blockers in selected sports was reflected in the IOC Medical Commission's decision to test for beta blockers only in the biathlon, bob sled, figure-skating, luge and ski-jump competitions at the 1988 Winter Olympic Games in Calgary. In the 1988 Summer Olympic Games in Seoul, and the 1992 Summer Games in Barcelona, the IOC Medical Commission tested for beta blockers in the archery, diving, equestrian, fencing, gymnastics, modern pentathlon, sailing, shooting and synchronized swimming events only.

In the March 1993 revision of the IOC list of doping classes and methods, beta blockers were transferred from Section I, Doping Classes to Section III, Classes of Drugs Subject to Certain Restrictions, indicating that they should be tested for only in those sports where they are likely to enhance performance, as listed in the previous paragraph. Tests for beta blockers are performed at the request of an international federation and at the discretion of the IOC Medical Commission.

Studies of the effects of beta blockers on pistol shooters suggest that they are mainly of benefit to the less competent and less experienced shooters, as well as those most anxious prior to competition (Siitonen, Solnck and Janne, 1977). A study of the British national pistol squad found that significant improvement in shooting scores was restricted to slow-fire events, the ergogenic effect being slightly greater for an 80 mg dose than for 40 mg of oxprenolol (Antal and Good, 1980). The effect of a 40 mg dose of oxprenolol was matched by an effect of alcohol equivalent to a half pint (284 ml) of beer (S'Jongers et al., 1978). There appeared to be a substantial placebo effect which applied equally to alcohol and beta blockers.

6.8 OVERVIEW

Stress and anxiety are inescapable corollaries of contemporary professional activities and participation in top-level sport. Indeed, a high degree of competitiveness seems to be a prerequisite for success in both spheres, and those without the essential coping mechanism fail to climb to the top of the ladder. The relationship between sport and anxiety is paradoxical in that sport, as a recreational activity, offers release from occupational cares, whilst at a highly competitive level it becomes a strong stressor. Indeed, exercise is effective therapy for highly anxious individuals, though this function was not central to the present topic. Neither has the role of behaviour modification strategies been considered here, either as a replacement for or complement to anti-anxiety drugs, although behavioural techniques have promise for the future in treating anxiety.

In the recent decade or so, sports officials and governing bodies in sport have assumed increasing responsibility for attempts to eliminate the use of drugs for ergogenic purposes. It is likely that the process of adding new pharmacological products to the list of banned substances will continue in spite of a running contest with those practitioners prepared to grasp at any means of improving their performances. The risks and benefits of anti-anxiety drugs, as described, demonstrate that regulations for their use in sport must be set down with care and circumspection. Legislation must ensure that, for the sport in question, participants especially prone to anxiety are not endangered by being deprived of their genuine prescriptions, whilst at the same time allowing fair competition to all entries.

6.9 REFERENCES

Antal, L.C. and Good, C.S. (1980) Effects of oxprenolol on pistol shooting under stress. *The Practitioner*, **224**, 755–60.

Beckett, A.H. and Cowen, D.A. (1979) Misuse of drugs in sports. *Br. J. Sports Med.*, **12**, 185–94.

Blomqvist, G., Saltin, B. and Mitchell, J. (1970) Acute effects of ethanol ingestion on the response to submaximal and maximal exercise in man. *Circulation*, **62**, 463–70.

Cabri, J., Clarys, J.P., Vanderstappen, D.V. and Reilly, T. (1990) Les influences de différentes doses d'alprazolam sur l'activité musculaire dans des conditions de mouvements isocinétiques. *Archives Internationales de Physiologie et de Biochemie*, **98**(4), c 48.

Collomp, K.R., Ahmaidi, S.B., Caillaud, C.F. *et al.* (1993) Effects of benzodiazepine during a Wingate test: interaction with caffeine. *Med. Sci. Sports Exerc.*, **25**, 1375–80.

Corda, M.G., Concas, A. and Biggio, G. (1986) Stress and GABA receptors, in *Biochemical Aspects of Physical Exercise*, (eds G. Benzie, L. Packer and N. Siliprandi), Elsevier, Amsterdam, pp. 399–409.

Gordon, N.F., van Rensburg, T.P., Russell, H.M.S. *et al.* (1987) Effect of beta-adrenoceptor blockade and calcium antagonism, alone and in combination, on thermoregulation during prolonged exercise. *Int. J. Sports Med.*, **8**, 1–5.

Hicks, J.A. (1976) An evaluation of the effect of sign brightness and the sign reading behaviour of alcohol impaired drivers. *Human Factors*, **18**, 45–52.

Chintu sat in silence.

'All right, now tell me first. Did you truly see a gun beside Dawkins memsahib when you heard the sound of that shot and went running to look inside bungalow?'

'Yes. Yes, I did. I did.'

And at the moment into Ghote's head came the sight of Primrose Cottage as he had seen it earlier walking up the path beside the cannas bed. The house had looked as if it was fast asleep in the noonday heat, the *chiks* at every window, all rolled right down.

'You are lying,' he told Chintu.

'No. No, Inspector sahib, why would I lie? I saw her body. I saw that gun.'

'You saw it through the *chiks* rolled down at that time of day? You are very-very clever if you were able to do that.'

But, even before he had fully brought out the jibe, he saw it had in no way thrown the boy.

'Inspector, I am not so clever. It is just that on that day it was not hot. *Khansamah* had not told the servants to roll down the *chiks*. *Mali* had not told me to water them.'

Ghote heard this denial with mixed feelings. Had his ruse been successful, it would have made the differing descriptions he had heard of Iris memsahib's body, Chintu's and Bullybhoy's, less of a complication. He could have passed over Chintu's account as nothing more than an invention produced to make himself look important. On the other hand he felt — he scarcely knew why — distinctly pleased that Chintu was turning out to be honest. Amid the daily turmoil back in Dadar he had encountered few people, old or young, who could be relied on invariably to give an honest answer to a police question. So it was a source of warm pleasure to find a wretched, shirtless boy like Chintu saying, at this moment, something with plainly the ring of truth about it.

But he put him to the test once more.

'Very well. But tell me again now: on which side of Memsahib's body did the gun lie?'

'Inspector, on her left.'

'But if *Khansamah* was telling Inspector Barrani it was on the right . . . ?'

'Inspector, on the left.'

Ghote thought for a moment.

All right, Chintu could genuinely have remembered wrongly. He might not even know his right from —

'Raise your right hand.'

Up came the boy's right hand. Unhesitatingly.

'But something more I must ask.'

The anabolic steroids and peptide hormones   7

Alan George

7.1 SUMMARY

The conclusions reached in surveying anabolic steroid use in male and female athletes are that anabolic steroids probably do increase muscle bulk and body weight in all anabolic steroid takers, but that increases in strength are certain to occur only in those undertaking regular training exercise. The long-term side-effects of anabolic steroids are severe and will depend on dosage and duration. In particular, early death from cardiovascular disease, sterility in men and, in women, masculinization and possible foetal effects constitute the most serious hazards. More recently, studies have suggested that psychological and behavioural changes and addiction may result from chronic anabolic steroid abuse. There is evidence of increased abuse of steroids for cosmetic reasons.

7.2 INTRODUCTION

For centuries, it was popularly believed that symptoms of ageing in men were caused by testicular failure. This stimulated a search for an active principle of the testicles which, when isolated, would restore sexual and mental vigour to ageing men. The testicular principle, we now know, is the male sex hormone testosterone, which was first synthesized in 1935.

Experimental studies in both animals and humans soon showed that testosterone possessed both **anabolic** and **androgenic** actions. The androgenic actions of testosterone are those actions involving the development and maintenance of primary and secondary sexual characteristics, whilst the anabolic actions consist of the positive effects of testosterone in inhibiting urinary nitrogen loss and stimulating protein synthesis, particularly in skeletal muscle.

Drugs in Sport, 2nd edn. Edited by David R. Mottram. Published in 1996 by E & FN Spon, London. ISBN 0 419 18890 8

7.3 THE TESTOSTERONE FAMILY

Testosterone is a so-called C-19 steroid hormone. The steroid hormones are derived in the body from the substance cholesterol. The structure of testosterone is closely related to the steroid substance androstane, and the structure of androstane is used as a reference when naming most of the compounds related to or derived from testosterone (Figure 7.1).

7.3.1 BIOCHEMISTRY AND PHYSIOLOGY OF TESTOSTERONE

Testosterone, the most important naturally occurring compound with androgen and anabolic activity, is formed in the Leydig cells of the testis but also in the adrenal cortex. Adrenocortical and ovarian testosterone is important in women as it is responsible for some secondary sexual characteristics, such as pubic and axillary hair growth, and in some cases for its influence on sexuality. Mean testosterone production in men is approximately 8 mg per day, of which 90–95% is produced by the testis and the remainder by the adrenal cortex. When testosterone is synthesized in the body, for every 30 molecules of testosterone formed, one molecule of its isomer, epitestosterone, is formed. Epitestosterone has exactly the same number of atoms as testosterone but the –H and –OH groups at C^{19} are oriented differently (Figure 7.1). However, approximately 1% of this testosterone is excreted in the urine unchanged compared to 30% of epitestosterone. As a result, the ratio of testosterone to epitestosterone in the urine is approximately 1:1.

The testis also produces 5α-dihydrotestosterone (DHT), which is approximately equal in androgenic and anabolic activity to testosterone, and also two compounds with much weaker biological activity, androstenedione and dehydroepiandrosterone. After puberty, plasma testosterone levels are approximately 0.6 µg/dl in males and 0.03 µg/dl in women. Of testosterone in the blood, 95% is bound to protein, mainly sex hormone-binding globulin; 2–3% of testosterone remains free, i.e. unbound, whilst the remainder is bound to serum albumin.

Mode of action

Like most other steroid hormones, testosterone produces its principal effect on tissues by altering cellular biochemistry in an interaction with the cell nucleus. Testosterone diffuses into the cell as it is lipid soluble and thus readily crosses cell membranes. It combines with a testosterone binding protein which transports it to the cell nucleus. Here, the testosterone interacts on a particular chromosome with one or more specific binding sites, called hormone receptor elements, and activates the synthesis of one or more proteins which may be either enzymes or structural proteins. In

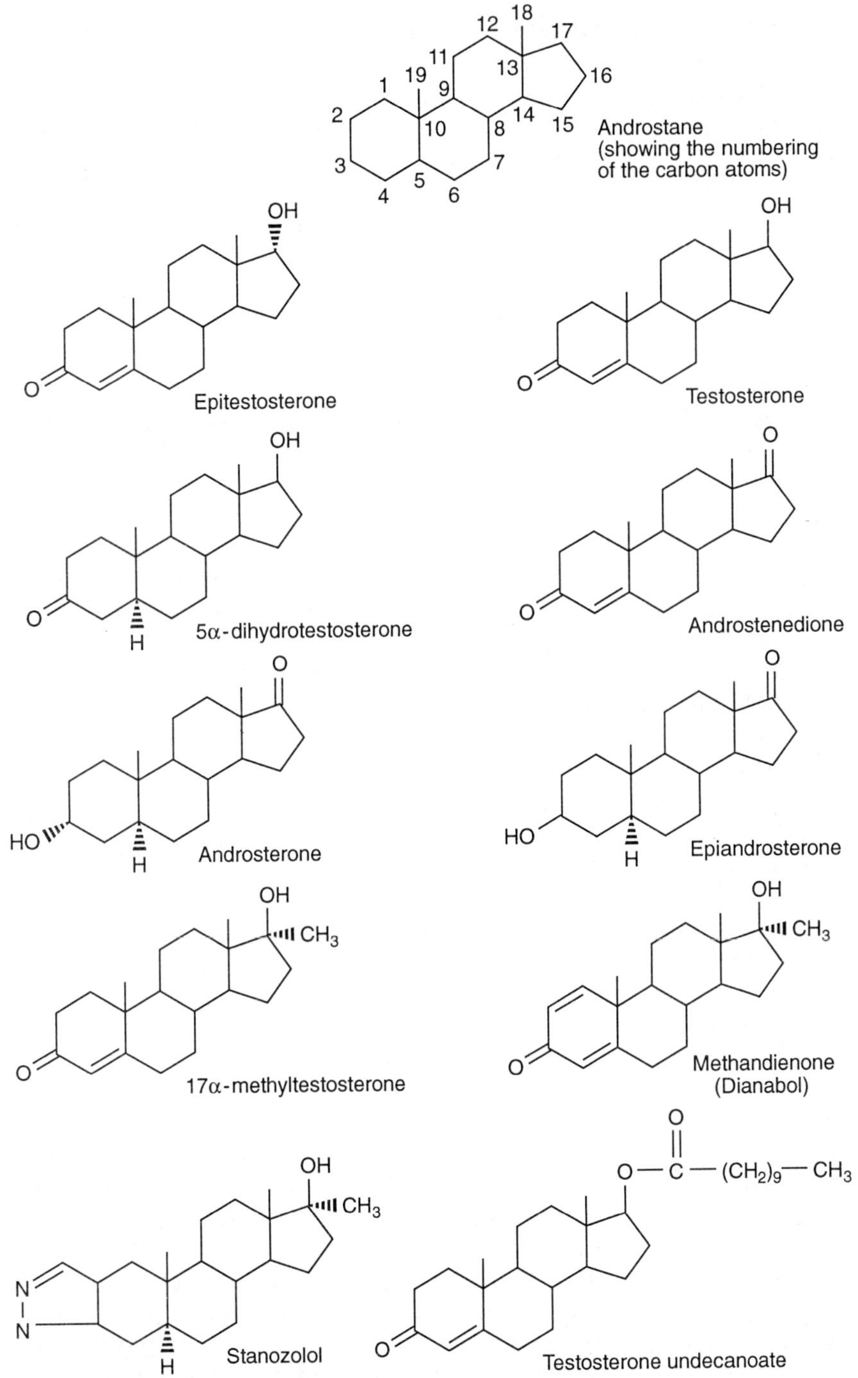

Figure 7.1 The structure of testosterone, its derivatives and some anabolic steroids.

some tissues testosterone is first converted to DHT, also called androstanolone, by the enzyme 5-α-reductase. The DHT is then transported to the nucleus and produces similar biochemical changes to those of testosterone. In many testosterone-sensitive tissues, it is now thought that the anabolic effects of testosterone are mainly produced by the action of DHT. DHT can be formed from testosterone in the testes, liver, brain, prostate gland and external genitalia, but there is little 5-α-reductase activity and therefore little **direct** formation of DHT in human skeletal muscle. Generally, in the liver and locally in brain areas, such as the hypothalamus, testosterone can be converted to oestradiol by the aromatase enzyme system. DHT is primarily androgenic; oestradiol antagonizes some androgenic actions whilst enhancing others. The full details of testosterone synthesis and metabolism have been expertly reviewed by Wilson (1988) and Lukas (1993).

Metabolism

Apart from conversion to DHT in various tissues, testosterone is metabolized in the liver mainly to DHT and androstenedione and then to either androsterone or one of its two isomers, epiandrosterone or etiocholanolone. All five metabolites are present in plasma and urine. Androsterone and epiandrosterone have weak androgen activity, whilst etiocholanolone has none. Some testosterone is converted in the testis to oestradiol. Significant amounts of oestradiol are also thought to be formed from testosterone in the brain.

7.3.2 THE PHYSIOLOGICAL ROLE OF TESTOSTERONE

Testosterone and its structurally related analogues possess androgenic and anabolic activity.

Androgenic effects

Testosterone is responsible for the development of primary sexual characteristics in males. Normally, in a genetically male foetus, i.e. one with the XY sex chromosome configuration, the embryonic testis begins to differentiate under the influence of H-Y antigen, the production of which is directed by the Y chromosome. As the male gonad differentiates, Leydig cells are formed which begin to secrete testosterone. Testosterone and a polypeptide factor, MRF (Mullerian regression factor) together stimulate the formation of the male genitalia. The external genitalia develop solely under the influence of testosterone. From birth until puberty the Leydig cells which secrete testosterone produce small amounts of testosterone. From the age of approximately 10 years, increased testosterone secretion occurs principally from the testicular Leydig cells. The pubertal changes induced by this increase in testosterone are the secondary sexual characteristics, which include changes in hair distribution, musculoskeletal configuration, genital size, psychic changes and induction of sperm production. The chronology of male puberty and adolescence has been described in detail by Tanner (1962), and the Tanner index provides a useful guide for the assessment of the progress of puberty and the attainment of maturity.

Anabolic effects

The anabolic effects of testosterone and anabolic steroids are usually considered to be those promoting protein synthesis and muscle growth, but they also include effects such as stimulation and inhibition of skeletal growth in the young. Attempts to produce purely anabolic, synthetic testosterone derivatives have been unsuccessful. It should be remembered that, though the anabolic action of anabolic steroids may be much greater than testosterone, all anabolic steroids also possess androgenic activity.

7.3.3 STRUCTURAL ANALOGUES OF TESTOSTERONE:
THE ANABOLIC STEROIDS

To the dismay of clinical scientists, it was soon discovered that when the newly isolated testosterone was given orally or injected into patients it was ineffective. When taken by mouth, testosterone is absorbed from the

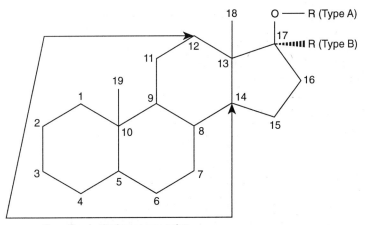

Figure 7.2 The three major types of testosterone modification. (After Wilson, 1988.)

small intestines and passes via the portal vein to the liver where it is rapidly metabolized, mostly to inactive compounds. Injected testosterone also passes rapidly into the blood and then to the liver where it is inactivated. In the late 1940s, medicinal chemists began to develop analogues of testosterone which might be degraded less easily by the body. Forty years of intensive research have yielded three major types of testosterone modification, each of which gives rise to a class of anabolic steroids (Figure 7.2). Addition of an alkyl group at position 17α renders the structure orally active (B). A type (A) modification makes the compound suitable for 'depot' injection, whilst type (C) modifications allow oral dosing and sometimes increased potency. A more detailed account of the medicinal chemistry of the currently available anabolic steroids is provided by Wilson (1988), whilst a description of their development is described by George (1994).

7.3.4 CLINICAL USES OF ANDROGENS/ANABOLIC STEROIDS

Replacement therapy in men

Anabolic steroids may be given to stimulate sexual development in cases of delayed puberty. The therapy is then withdrawn gradually once full sexual maturity is reached. They may also be given in cases where the testicles have been surgically removed, either because of physical injury or because of a testicular tumour. In this case the replacement therapy must be continuous for life.

Replacement therapy in women

Testosterone production is necessary in women as well as men. In the rare condition known as sexual infantilism, a young female fails to secrete oestradiol, progesterone and testosterone. As a consequence she suffers from amenorrhoea and a lack of libido and pubic and axillary hair. Only when she is treated with testosterone does libido appear. Some post-menopausal women suffer from loss of libido. In both these cases administration of testosterone restores sex drive and sexual characteristics (Greenblatt *et al.*, 1985).

Gynaecological disorders

Anabolic steroids are occasionally used to treat gynaecological conditions in women, though long-term usage produces severe side-effects, such as erratic menstruation and the appearance of male secondary characteristics. In the USA, they have sometimes been used to repress lactation after childbirth. They are also sometimes used to combat breast tumours in pre-menopausal women.

Protein anabolism

The initial use of anabolic steroids in the early 1940s was to inhibit the loss of protein and aid muscle regeneration after major surgery, and to stimulate muscle regeneration in debilitating disorders, such as muscular dystrophy and diabetes. Many concentration camp survivors owe their early recovery from debilitation to the skilled use of dietary measures coupled with anabolic steroids.

Anaemia

Anabolic steroids are sometimes used in large doses to treat anaemias which have proved resistant to other therapies: this therapy is not recommended in women because of masculinizing side-effects.

Osteoporosis

There is some evidence that combined oestrogen/androgen therapy is able to inhibit bone degeneration in this disorder.

Growth stimulation

Anabolic steroids may be used to increase growth in prepubertal boys who have failed to reach their expected height for their age. The treatment must be carried out under carefully controlled conditions so that early fusion of the epiphyses does not occur.

7.3.5 SIDE-EFFECTS OF ANDROGENS

Principally in women

These include acne, growth of facial hair and hoarsening or deepening of the voice. If the dose given is sufficient to suppress gonadotrophin secretion, then menstrual irregularities will occur. Chronic, i.e. long-term, treatment with androgens, as for example in mammary carcinoma, may produce the following side-effects: male pattern baldness, prominent musculature and veins and clitoral hypertrophy.

In children

Administration of androgens can cause stunting of growth, a side-effect directly related to disturbance of normal bone growth and development. The enhancement of epiphyseal closure is a particularly persistent side-effect which can be present up to three months after androgen withdrawal.

In males

Spermatogenesis is reduced by testosterone treatment with as little as 25 mg testosterone per day over a 6-week period. Anabolic steroids will produce the same effect, since they will suppress natural testosterone secretion. The inhibition of spermatogenesis may persist for many months after anabolic steroid withdrawal.

General side-effects

Oedema

Oedema, or water retention, related to the increased retention of sodium and chloride ions, is a frequent side-effect of short-term androgen administration. This may be the major contribution to the initial weight gain seen in athletes taking these drugs (see p. 194). Water and electrolyte gain is an unwanted side-effect in all normal individuals, but is particularly unhealthy in people with circulatory disorders or in those with a family background of such disorders.

Blood volume

Significant increases in steroid-induced water retention are likely to produce an increase in the blood volume. It should be noted that any expansion of the blood volume is likely to be a result of the simultaneous increase in water retention plus the increased erythropoiesis caused by anabolic steroid administration (Rockhold, 1993).

Jaundice

Jaundice is a frequent side-effect of anabolic steroid therapy and is caused mainly by reduced flow and retention of bile in the biliary capillaries of the hepatic lobules. Hepatic cell damage is not usually present. Those anabolic steroids with a 17α methyl group are most likely to cause jaundice.

Hepatic carcinoma

Patients who have received androgens and/or anabolic steroids for prolonged periods may develop hepatic carcinoma. This is also particularly prevalent in people who have taken 17α methyl testosterone derivatives.

7.4 ANABOLIC STEROIDS AND SPORT

The desire to increase sporting performance and athletic prowess by means other than physical training has been experienced for at least 2000 years. Ryan (1981) quotes the observation of the Greeks that a high protein diet was essential for body-building and athletic achievement. The Greeks, of course, knew nothing of protein structure or biosynthesis but they felt that by eating the flesh of a strong animal, such as the ox, the athlete would gain strength himself. We have seen previously that one of the first therapeutic uses of anabolic steroids was in treating the protein loss and muscle wasting suffered by concentration camp victims. Following the publication of the results of these treatments it was natural that anabolic steroids should be used in an attempt to increase muscle strength in athletes. Many early studies on the effect of anabolic steroids often involved self-administration and were necessarily anecdotal with no attempt at scientific or controlled investigation of the effect of the steroid drugs. Several studies relied on subjective feelings and lacked any objective measure of increased strength or stamina. Also, side-effects were never admitted to or were simply omitted from the results.

Subsequent studies, many of which were carried out in the late 1960s and early 1970s, were more scientifically based but often entirely contradictory in their results. In this chapter we will discuss what any physician, student or lay person would wish to know about the use of an anabolic steroid: where is it obtained; how is it used; does it work; does it confer any advantage over normal training practices; what are the side-effects; what are the long- and short-term consequences? In addition the athlete needs to know whether the practice is ethical and the sports administrator how to discover whether anabolic steroids are being taken. Finally we will consider future trends.

7.4.1 SOURCES, SUPPLY AND CONTROL

The increased usage of anabolic steroids by athletes and the spread of usage from sport to the general population has prompted governmental intervention in several countries and stimulated investigation into the illicit supply of anabolic steroids and the control of their abuse.

In Great Britain anabolic steroids are licensed by the Department of Health's Medicine Control Agency as prescription only medicines within the meaning of the Medicines Act (1968). This means that it is illegal for a doctor or pharmacist to **supply** them other than by a doctor's prescription and there are recorded cases of individual prosecution for illegal supply (Report, 1989). However, **possession** of anabolic steroid drugs is not yet illegal. The UK government has been under pressure recently to legislate to classify anabolic steroids as controlled drugs under the Misuse of Drugs Act (1971). In November 1994 they finally decided to reclassify anabolic steroids as controlled drugs, with effect from late 1995. This made both supply without prescription **and** possession illegal, but this view has been contested by many experts on addiction and those closely associated with counselling and treating anabolic problems in gyms and sports clubs. Denmark has recently raised anabolic steroids to 'controlled' status and has made possession a criminal offence punishable by two years in jail.

In the USA, anabolic steroids were recently added to Schedule III of the Controlled Substances Act, making supply and possession of the drugs a federal offence. However, the American Medical Association opposed this legislation because it contends that most of the anabolic steroids are illegally smuggled in or manufactured and such legislation, when enacted for cocaine, led to an **increase** in its illegal supply (Daigle, 1990).

There are numerous sources of anabolic steroids, which vary between nations. In the USA, the major external sources appear to be Panama and Mexico, whilst illegal synthesis by 'street traders' is another major source. Both these internal and external sources provide drugs which are untested, unstandardized, contain potentially toxic impurities and have not been produced in the stringently hygienic conditions of the modern pharmaceutical industry. Surveys show that the majority of steroid abusers in the USA are supplied by the black market (Lamb, 1991), with the remainder coming from physicians, pharmacists and illicit postal supplies (Catlin *et al.*, 1993). Counterfeit supplies of stanozolol were recently discovered in the UK (*Pharmaceutical Journal*, 1994).

7.4.2 PATTERNS OF ADMINISTRATION AND USE

No two groups of athletes who abuse anabolic steroids seem to use the same pattern of drug administration. It is this observation that above all so confounds attempts to make scientific comparisons between various studies of anabolic steroid efficacy (7.4.5). There are a number of administration regimes in use (Wilson, 1988; Rogol and Yesalis, 1992), though each has its variations and often combinations of regimes may be used concurrently:

Cycling

A period of administration is followed by a similar period of abstinence before the administration is recommenced. Typical cycling patterns are short – 6–8 weeks on drug, 6–8 weeks' abstinence – or long – 6–8 weeks on drug with up to 12 months' abstinence. The rationale here is that the periods of abstinence may reduce the incidence of side-effects. This regime is preferred by body-builders.

Pyramiding

This is a variation of cycling in which the dose is gradually built up in the cycle to a peak and then gradually reduced again towards the end of the cycle. This regime is said to cause fewer behavioural side-effects, such as lowered mood, caused by the withdrawal of the drug.

Stacking

Stacking involves the use of more than one anabolic steroid at a time. In its simplest form, this regime involves the simultaneous use of both an orally administered steroid and an injectable one. More 'sophisticated' patterns involve intricate schedules of administration using many different steroids, each with supposedly different pharmacological profiles. The aim of this technique is to avoid **plateauing**, the development of tolerance to a particular drug. According to the amateur pharmacologists of locker rooms and gymnasia, these 'super stacking' programmes allow more receptor sites to be stimulated. This is very dubious pharmacology since the number of intracellular testosterone/DHT steroid receptors is stable and all are probably saturated under normal physiological conditions. Exact doses tried by abusers are almost impossible to establish. What is certain is that doses used by weightlifters and body-builders are at least 100 times those indicated for therapeutic use (Rogol and Yesalis, 1992) and also those used in most scientific studies (Elashoff *et al.*, 1991). The dose–response studies of Forbes (1985) also indicate that the doses used in 'ethical/clinical' studies of anabolic steroid effects on athletic performance are only sufficient to cause modest improvements in lean body mass. It is claimed that endurance and sprint athletes who abuse steroids may use doses closer to clinical recommendations (Rogol and Yesalis, 1992).

7.4.3 EXTENT OF USAGE

It is difficult to calculate which anabolic steroid is most often abused world-wide. Some anabolic steroids are not available in every country, some are stolen veterinary preparations and some have been illicitly manufactured. Many athletes will also be 'stacking' several preparations at once. The most popular of abused drugs in the US college survey of Pope, Katz and Champoux (1988) is shown in Table 7.1 whilst in a survey of US power-lifters the most popular drugs were methandrostenolone (93%) and testosterone esters (80%). The first British survey of anabolic steroid usage (Table 7.2) showed also that Dianabol (methandrostenolone) at 69% was the most frequently administered anabolic steroid (Perry, Wright and Littlepage, 1992). In their study, published in 1994, Pope and Katz found that the majority of abusers reported taking testosterone, whilst 54% admitted taking nandrolone. When the urine of the same athletes was tested, only 41% were found to be abusing testosterone and 57% nandrolone. This study illustrates the possible confusion of different drugs by abusers or the possibility of deception by drug suppliers. The study showed the tendency towards testosterone abuse. The supply, administration and abuse of the veterinary steroid Equipoise (Table 7.2), has been identified by Perry, Wright and Littlepage (1992). In 1994, Chinese athletes were alleged to be abusing dihydrotestosterone.

Table 7.1 The most popular anabolic steroids abused by a sample of 17 US college men (Pope *et al.*, 1988)

Drug	No. using drug*
Methandrostenolone	8
Testosterone esters	6
Nandrolone	5
Oxandrolone	4
Stanozolol	1
Methenolone	1

*More than one drug abused by some subjects.

Table 7.2 The most frequently abused anabolic steroids amongst 62 male gymnasia attenders in West Glamorgan, UK (Perry *et al.*, 1992)

Drug	No. abusing drug*
Dianabol	43
Deca Durabolin	37
Testosterone esters	32
Stanozolol	19
Equipoise	10

*More than one drug abused by some subjects.

7.4.4 THE EPIDEMIOLOGY OF ANABOLIC STEROID ABUSE

In response to the widespread view that anabolic steroid abuse was rife in the sporting population, several American investigators began surveys of athletes in order to establish the distribution and prevalence of anabolic steroid abuse. In a summary of these (1976–1984) findings, Pope, Katz and Champoux (1988) reported that as many as 20% of intercollegiate athletes and fewer than 1% of non-athlete students reported using anabolic steroids. This prevalence was much higher than the 2.5% usage rate reported in a 1971 study. The review by Pope, Katz and Champoux (1988) also records a survey of students at a Florida high school where 18% of male students but no females reported using anabolic steroids. This high prevalence of usage was suggested to be peculiar to Florida and could be related to so-called cosmetic factors discussed below.

From their own survey of 1010 college males, Pope, Katz and Champoux (1988) found that 2% reported taking anabolic steroids, with university-standard athletes more likely to be taking steroids than non-athletes. Of this 2%, 42% reported that body-building and appearance were their main reasons for anabolic steroid abuse and 58% reported various reasons connected with sport for their abuse. High degrees of prevalence of abuse (6.6%) were found by Buckley *et al.* (1988) in 1700 US high school students, whilst Windsor and Dumitru (1988) found a 3% abuse level in 800 US college students. In this survey, 5% of males and 1.4% of females admitted abusing steroids. Williamson (1993) has carried out the major British study of anabolic steroid abuse (4.4% in males, 1% in females) at a college of technology in Scotland.

When surveys of non-college athletes are conducted the percentage of abusers is much higher. Yesalis *et al.* (1988) found a current prevalence of 33% amongst US power-lifters which rose to 55% when previous usage amongst non-users was included. In the UK, Perry, Wright and Littlepage (1992) reported a 38.8% prevalence amongst weight-trainers in private gymnasia in their West Glamorgan survey area. The figures for young abusers in the UK and the USA (3–6%) may vary in different locations. In Britain, there is anecdotal evidence to suggest that anabolic steroid abuse is higher in areas with a macho culture, ample male leisure time (i.e. unemployment), low self-esteem and proximity to sandy beaches. Thus, abuse may be said to be led by cultural pressure, feelings of social inadequacy and a suitable location to parade the results of your body-building. The higher prevalence of steroid abuse in Florida (18% according to Pope, Katz and Champoux, 1988) may well reflect this latter theory!

The prevalence of anabolic steroid abuse in international competition is difficult to judge. At the 1972 (pre-testing) Munich Olympics, 68% of interviewed athletes in middle- or short-distance running or in field events admitted taking steroids. At the Mexico Olympics, all the US weightlifters admitted taking steroids (Wilson, 1988). Perhaps the introduction of mandatory testing for the 1976 Olympics in Montreal has led to a decline in steroid abuse rather than a switching to less detectable doping agents, such as human growth hormone (hGH). The official International Olympic Committee (IOC) figures in 1992 show that, though anabolic steroid abuse at IOC accredited events as a percentage of total positive results was 48.6% compared to 65.3% in 1986, the actual numbers of positive anabolic steroid tests was up from 439 in 1986 to 611 in 1989. In the UK, the number of positive steroid tests fell from 14 in 1990 to seven in 1991, but rose again to 22 in 1992 and 20 in 1993 (Sports Council Doping Control Report, 1993). Perhaps in the UK we are just witnessing the full impact of stringent regular testing. We may also have to regard the current generation of athletes as a lost cause and, instead, concentrate education and deterrent resources on the young. Recent progress in the USA (education programmes, legislation) has encouraged some experts to suggest that the availability and usage of steroids in the US is decreasing (Catlin *et al.*, 1993). However, the suspension of three members of the University of Maine football team after positive steroid tests in early 1993 is not encouraging (Leach, 1993).

7.4.5 EFFICACY OF ANABOLIC STEROIDS

Whether anabolic steroid treatment 'works' is perhaps the most difficult question of all to answer satisfactorily since the known investigations which have been carried out are, in the main, poorly designed scientifically, clinically and statistically (see Ryan, 1981). Increases in muscle strength are proportional to increases in the cross-sectional diameter of the muscles being trained, but there is no way of showing conclusively, *in vivo*, that any increase in muscle diameter consists of increased muscle protein rather than increased content of water or fat. It is also apparent that different groups of athletes may wish to increase their muscle bulk for different purposes. For example the American footballer or the wrestler may wish simply to increase bulk and weight, whereas a weightlifter may want increased dynamic strength and the long-distance runner may wish to accelerate muscle repair after an arduous and taxing run.

Studies into the efficacy of anabolic steroids

The first serious investigator of the question as to whether anabolic steroids work seems to be Ryan (1981) who reviewed a total of 37 studies from 1968 to 1977. He was confounded by the many different measurements being taken as indices of anabolic steroid activity. Some studies attempted to measure gains in strength of experimental subjects over controls, other studies measured the change in circumference of a limb. One study attempted to measure change in lean body mass. In 12 studies which claimed that athletes taking anabolic steroids gained in strength, the gains reported in these studies were often quite small. The majority of these 12 studies were not 'blind': that is either the investigator or the subject (or perhaps both!) knew when an active principle was being taken. In only five of the studies were protein supplements given, and in none of the studies examined was there any dietary control or at least a listing of total protein and caloric intake for each subject. Other features of these studies were their poor design in matching control and experimental subjects, and there were also errors in calculating the results.

Ryan then examined 13 other studies in which valid matching of controls and experiments **had** occurred. Ten of these 13 studies were double-blind (neither experimenter nor subject knew when an active substance was being administered), the control and experimental groups contained at least six subjects in each and the average period of experimentation was some 50% longer than in the early studies in which improvements were claimed. Also, in this second group of experiments, five different steroid groups were investigated compared to only two in the earlier group. Ryan's conclusion from examining these two groups of studies was that there was no substantial evidence for an increase in lean muscle bulk or muscle strength in healthy young adult males receiving anabolic steroids.

Comparison of these studies is difficult because the various parameters used to assess improvement in strength were not the same. Though the majority of studies assessed by Ryan measured changes in gross body weight and 'improvement' in standard strength tests, the other tests employed included VO_2 max., limb circumference, lean body mass and 'changes in blood chemistry'. One reason for the variety of measurements used and a possible explanation for the lack of agreement in assessing anabolic steroid efficacy is that different athletic groups each sought different parameters for improvement. As I have mentioned before, the American footballer or wrestler may be seeking increased bulk, and the weightlifter or thrower an increase in strength or perhaps both.

Experiments with anabolic steroids since 1975 have tended to be more carefully carried out, controlled and more sophisticated than those reviewed by Ryan. An example of a well-conducted trial is the frequently quoted study by Freed et al. (1975). In this study, six standard strength exercises were used as a measure of increased strength. The study was carried out over a 6-week period in weightlifters who were given either 10 mg or 25 mg per day of methandienone. Drug treatment increased strength by 0.3–13% during the 6-week study, whilst those taking placebo showed strength gains of 0.3–2.3%. Body weight increased only in the drug-treated athletes and those on the 25 mg dose showed no greater strength increase than those on 10 mg. A significant finding was that withdrawal of the anabolic steroid caused a loss of weight but no loss in strength gained. This suggested that anabolic steroid taking amongst athletes might be harder to detect since the drug could be withdrawn from an athlete well in advance of a meeting without significant loss of performance, thus allowing the athlete to evade detection in any post-competition doping test but not in out-of-competition testing. Further analysis of Freed's study shows that the doses of methandienone are some 75% lower than those claimed to be used by some athletes. It might have been more useful to tailor the dose of the drug to the athlete's initial body weight, i.e. calculate the dose in terms of mg/kg body weight and also to measure the actual free and bound plasma concentration of the drug. It is reasonable to conclude from Freed's work that only a proportion of people show a significant improvement in strength as a result of steroid treatment.

Further studies should determine the types of athlete or individual which 'benefit' from anabolic steroids. Another factor absent from the analyses of this and previous experiments is consideration of the subject's body build. The bodily changes induced by testosterone at puberty and, indeed, those that are produced *in utero* occur as a result of an interaction-between testosterone and the individual genetic 'constitution' or genotype. The individual emerging from puberty with a lean, well-muscled body (the classical mesomorph somatotype) does so because of the expression of the genes controlling muscularity rather than because of having higher testosterone levels than the more lightly muscled ectomorph. Thus, only certain somatotypes may benefit from anabolic steroid treatment.

The importance of athletic experience and pre-training on the response of athletes to anabolic steroid treatment has been researched by Wright (1980). He noted that inexperienced weightlifters showed no increase in strength or lean muscle mass whilst simultaneously taking anabolic steroids and protein supplements and undergoing short-term training. In contrast, weightlifters who trained regularly, i.e. to nearly their maximum capacity, did show increased strength compared to their pre-treatment level. Though his results did not show consistent increases in strength amongst the steroid-treated trained athletes, Wright claimed to show that the trained athletes responded better to anabolic steroid treatment, a finding he could not explain adequately. However, the presence of a greater initial muscle mass in the trained athletes before anabolic steroid treatment might have been a factor. Another possibility is that trained muscles **are** different, i.e. they may produce some endogenous factor which enhances anabolic steroid action. It is already known that the muscles of trained athletes can increase their uptake of glucose by the production of an endogenous factor and that regular exercise regimes increase the responsiveness of skeletal muscle to insulin.

Training and anabolic steroids

If the results of these studies produce such inconsistent results, why do athletes continue to take anabolic steroids? One possible explanation is that the steroid trials published so far are based on dose levels which, whilst medically and ethically acceptable, are considerably less than those commonly taken by athletes. This factor, coupled with the necessity of pre-drug intensive training and a high protein diet, might explain the failure of anabolic steroids to produce a consistent increase in strength and performance.

The importance of training during and before a period of steroid treatment is apparently emphasized in a sophisticated series of experiments carried out by Hervey and colleagues between 1976 and 1981, and reviewed by Hervey (1982). The experimental design involved the administration of the anabolic steroid Dianabol, 100 mg per day during one 6-week period and a placebo during the other 6 weeks. The two treatment periods (drug and placebo) were separated by a 6-week treatment-free period. The experiments were carried out double-blind. All volunteers were athletes, one group being professional weightlifters. In each group, body weight, body fat, body density and the fat and lean tissue proportion were measured.

The non-weightlifting group of athletes showed the same improvement in weightlifting performance and leg muscle strength during both placebo and drug administration periods. In the group containing experienced weightlifters there was a significant improvement during drug administration when compared to the placebo period. Both weightlifters and other athletes exhibited weight gain and increases in limb circumference. Though the weightlifters were heavier than their non-weightlifting counterparts, the proportion of lean body mass was the same in both groups.

Hervey *et al.* (1981) concluded from these experiments that, in athletes engaged in continuous hard-training regimes, anabolic steroids in the doses athletes claim to use cause an increase in muscle strength and athletic performance. The experimental design could be criticized in that it is possible that those subjects taking the drug in the first 6-week period were not completely drug-free at the start of the placebo period 6 weeks later. Thus, the residual effect of the steroid could have affected measurements during the placebo period of evaluation and could have masked any apparent difference between the placebo and treatment periods.

These are two examples of well-conducted trials carried out in the early 1980s. Summarizing the evidence gained from these and earlier trials, Haupt and Rovere (1984) concluded that abuse of anabolic steroids will consistently result in a significant increase in strength if all of the following criteria are satisfied:

- they are given to athletes who have been intensively trained in weightlifting immediately before the start of the steroid regimen and who continue this intensive weightlifting training during the steroid regimen;

- the athletes maintain a high protein diet;

- the changes in the athletes' strength are measured by the single repetition–maximal weight technique for those exercises with which the athlete trains.

Studies demonstrating significant increases in body size and body weight during the anabolic steroid regimen were consistently those studies that demonstrated significant increases in strength. These consistencies were statistically significant.

Studies that did not demonstrate significant increases in body size and body weight during the anabolic steroid regimen were consistently those studies that did not demonstrate significant increases in strength. These consistencies were statistically significant.

Janet Elashoff and her colleagues at Cedars Sinai Medical Centre, Los Angeles, have provided an even more sophisticated analysis of 30 studies in which athletes received two or more doses of anabolic steroid and in which changes in muscular strength were measured. They made use of the statistical technique known as meta-analysis and also analysed for the statistical power of the study. In addition to the study defects described previously, Elashoff *et al.* (1991) found marked evidence of poor statistical design and computation in many of the 30 studies examined. They queried whether any of the studies were truly blind and whether checks for compliance were carried out properly. Their conclusions were that it must be obvious to both experimenter and athlete who is on an active preparation, since it should be possible to see who develops greater acne, beard growth and weight gain, and the athletes will almost certainly experience the psychopharmacological effects of 'being on steroids'. As in previous reviews, the authors question whether further analysis of these studies is worthwhile since the amounts administered are obviously below those normally abused. Referring to the studies of Forbes (1985) quoted previously, it is obvious that the maximum dose of 7245 mg used in the experiments reviewed by Elashoff is at the start of the dose/lean body mass curve and thus only just at the threshold of producing an observable improvement in lean body mass.

This latest review, then, questions whether further analysis of studies carried out using these low doses is worthwhile, and whether more consideration should be given in studies to those anabolic steroid effects which are not directly concerned with increases in muscle strength, that is lean body mass, psychological changes and even physical appearance. Again it must be emphasized that increases in lean body mass in runners and increased aggressiveness in American footballers and ice-hockey players may be far more important to them than improved muscle strength.

Because anabolic steroids increase haemoglobin concentration, it has been suggested that they may be able to enhance aerobic performance by improving the capacity of the blood to deliver oxygen to the exercising muscle. However, only two out of 10 recent studies support this hypothesis, and one actually suggests that steroids may reduce aerobic power.

If anabolic steroid administration does produce these increases in muscle strength, should this not be reflected in the progression of athletic records? Howard Payne (1975) analysed UK and world sporting records from 1950 to 1975. The trend in all the events analysed, namely the 10 000 metres, pole vault, discus and shot, shows a steady improvement year by year without a sudden upsurge in any event. Thus, anabolic steroids cannot be shown to have significantly improved performances in field events nor in the 10 000 metres where competitors are erroneously assumed not to be steroid takers.

If even in the most careful experiments the positive effects of anabolic steroids are seen only in maximally exercising individuals, why is it that so many claims are made for them? One possible reason is that steroids make athletes 'feel better'. Some athletes claim they feel more competitive and aggressive, others may feel they **should** run faster as they are on anabolic steroids. The increase in body weight and in circumference of leg and arm muscles may improve the athlete's self-image. Whether anabolic steroids enhance aggression or competitiveness is hard to assess. It is difficult to demonstrate conclusively that steroids, or indeed testosterone, are responsible for aggressiveness since many behaviours are probably learnt. It is quite likely that behaviour, if it is hormonally influenced, is imprinted soon after birth. However, both male and female sexual behaviour is strongly influenced by androgens (7.3.2).

If it is agreed that anabolic steroids do increase athletic performance, albeit in strictly defined circumstances, what advantages do they confer on the taker? Obvious advantages are that the steroid taker may have stronger muscles with greater endurance, and a greater body mass with which to endure impact in sports like rugby, ice hockey or wrestling.

A further advantage conferred on the anabolic steroid taker is that muscles and associated tissues **may** have greater reparative powers and so the athlete may be able to undertake more events in a short time. This observation has led to the increased use of steroids by both middle- and long-distance runners and marathon runners.

How does the anabolic steroid produce these effects?

The original idea that anabolic steroids simply stimulate muscle growth needs to be revised following the results of the studies carried out in exercising individuals. From the results quoted previously it is possible to deduce that anabolic steroids may simply allow more intense exercise to take place, thus stimulating muscle growth. Again, it could be that muscle produces an endogenous factor which stimulates further muscle growth, or that exercise induces increased production of hormones such as insulin, growth hormone and somatomedins, each of which is able to increase protein synthesis, particularly in muscle. It is interesting that most major studies involving anabolic steroids, with the exception of that by Hervey *et al.* (1981), have failed to measure other hormones simultaneously.

The study by Hervey *et al.* measured testosterone and cortisol during the treatment of athletes with methandienone. They showed that as testosterone was suppressed by methandienone treatment by the end of the experiment, so plasma cortisol concentration rose. It is not clear whether this is the free or total cortisol in the plasma, but the deduction made was that anabolic steroid effects are possibly mediated via a rise in cortisol concentration. The authors claimed that the puffy facial and thoracic features produced by anabolic steroids are similar to those occurring in Cushing's Disease (CD), in which plasma cortisol is abnormally high as the result of either a pituitary or adrenocortical tumour producing adrenocortical overproduction of cortisol. There are many objections to this ingenious theory. The symptoms of CD and anabolic steroid administration are far from similar: CD patients have a characteristic moon face, abnormal fat distribution and distended abdomen. The limb muscles are thin and wasted, producing the characteristic 'lemon on sticks' appearance of CD. More importantly, the plasma cortisol levels in CD are much greater than those quoted by the authors at the end of the study.

Following Hervey's original hypothesis, other theories have suggested that the anabolic steroids may block the action of cortisol and corticosterone on muscle by competing with them for their intracellular receptors. Cortisol and corticosterone inhibit muscle protein synthesis and enhance muscle protein catabolism. If this action were inhibited then muscle protein anabolism would be enhanced. Evidence for anabolic steroid binding to glucocorticoid (GC) receptors has been summarized by Rockhold (1993). Such theories of anabolic effects produced by antagonism of GC receptors may account for the observation that androgen and GC receptor numbers increase during training regimes that increase muscle mass but not during those that increase endurance.

7.4.6 THE STRANGE CASE OF CLENBUTEROL

Just before the start of the Barcelona Olympics in 1992, two British weightlifters, Andrew Saxton and Andrew Davis, tested positive for the drug clenbuterol. During the Games the IOC acted swiftly to confirm that it was a banned substance.

Clenbuterol is classed as a beta$_2$ agonist; it is structurally related to salbutamol (Chapter 3) and in some EU countries (but not the UK) is similarly licensed for the treatment of asthma. However, the reason for banning the drug was associated with claims that it increases muscle mass whilst simultaneously reducing body fat.

Beta$_2$ agonists can promote normal skeletal muscle growth and experiments with clenbuterol show that it can increase muscle weight in rats by 10–12% after 2 weeks of treatment (Yang and McElliott, 1989) and can reduce amino acid loss from incubated muscle. It has been shown that clenbuterol can reverse experimentally induced muscle fibre atrophy by increasing muscle protein synthesis, as well as inhibiting amino acid loss. In contrast, salbutamol has no significant effect on muscle protein, though this difference may be related to the short half-life of salbutamol since continuous infusion of salbutamol causes similar anabolic effects to clenbuterol.

Clenbuterol does not produce its anabolic effects by interacting with testosterone, growth hormone or insulin (Choo *et al.*, 1992) but via beta$_2$ receptor stimulation. Similarly, the fat mobilizing action of clenbuterol is also mediated via beta$_2$ receptors. However, the dose of clenbuterol required in animal studies to bring about an 'anabolic' effect is approximately 100 times the maximum dose that humans can tolerate.

Therapeutic use

Clenbuterol is not licensed in the UK, but in some EU countries it is licensed for the treatment of asthma. The fact that it increases lean body mass, decreases fat and may increase muscle protein synthesis suggests that the drug may be useful in weaning anabolic steroid abusers off their drugs.

Should clenbuterol be banned?

Most recent evidence suggests that clenbuterol does reduce body fat and increase muscle mass, though whether this leads to increased strength does not seem to have yet been tested. The important point to be considered here is whether clenbuterol confers any athletic advantage. It is assumed that reductions in body fat and increases in lean body mass will confer advantages to most athletes. The positive 'anabolic' effects, while not yet associated with increases in strength, may be advantageous in **maintaining** the anabolic effects of anabolic steroids when these are withdrawn before an athletic event to avoid detection by doping tests. The association between clenbuterol, other beta$_2$ agonists and gains in muscle strength in athletes warrants further investigation.

7.5 ANABOLIC STEROID SIDE-EFFECTS WITH PARTICULAR REFERENCE TO ATHLETES

In the introductory section, the general side-effects of anabolic steroids were discussed. Of these side-effects some are of particular significance to athletes taking steroids, namely cardiovascular side-effects since exercise imposes a particular stress on the cardiovascular systems, and hepatic side-effects because anabolic steroids, particularly those with C^{17} alkyl substituents, are suspected hepatic carcinogens in the doses in which they are taken by athletes.

7.5.1 CARDIOVASCULAR AND HEPATIC SIDE-EFFECTS

Blood volume

Rockhold (1993) has examined nine studies on the effect of anabolic steroids on blood volume. Eight of these studies were carried out on non-athletes and produced variable results. Some studies showed increases in blood volume whilst others demonstrated no change. In the single study carried out in athletes, a 15% increase in total blood volume in athletes taking methandienone was recorded. This study did not measure haematocrit and so any effect of the steroid on erythropoiesis could not be determined.

Salt and water retention

In the previous section, the effect of anabolic steroids on salt and water retention was discussed in relation to steroid-induced gains in body weight and muscle circumference. The increase in salt and water retention responsible for these changes has a deleterious effect on the cardiovascular systems. Thus, the increased blood sodium concentration causes a rise in blood osmotic pressure. Since sodium ions cannot diffuse into cells, they remain in the extracellular fluid and blood unless excreted by the kidney, thus raising osmotic pressure and withdrawing water from the tissues. An expansion of the blood volume then occurs which imposes an increased workload on the heart. The heart increases its output and the blood pressure rises. The increased sodium concentration may also directly stimulate vasoconstriction, thus enhancing the hypertensive effect of the increased blood volume.

Hypertension

An increased incidence of potentially fatal hypertension in athletes on anabolic steroids is frequently mentioned in early reviews of anabolic steroid abuse in sport (Goldman, 1984; Wright, 1980). According to Rockhold (1993), the evidence for this is equivocal. He mentions three studies, two in athletes and one in healthy men, in which administration of either testosterone or oxandrolone for 3 months failed to cause an increase in blood pressure. An earlier study by Holma (1979) found a 15% increase in blood volume in men taking methandienone but no increase in blood pressure. However Kuipers et al. (1991) found mean increases in blood pressure of 12 mmHg in athletes self-administering various anabolic steroids. In a second double-blind study, using only nandrolone decanoate, no increase in blood pressure could be detected. The association between blood pressure and anabolic steroid abuse warrants further careful investigation, particularly in relation to the suggestion by

Rockhold (1993) that an increased hypertensive effect might be associated with specific types of anabolic steroid molecule.

Ventricular function

Studies in animals of the effect of anabolic steroids on ventricular function and morphology have indicated an association between steroids and ventricular pathology which may have significance for humans (Lombardo, Hickson and Lamb, 1991), particularly as the autopsy of an American footballer who was abusing anabolic steroids revealed significant cardiomyopathy. The technique of echocardiography has revolutionized non-invasive investigation of cardiac function and allows clinicians to measure accurately the dimensions of the ventricles during exercise and at rest at each stage of the cardiac cycle. A survey of six studies of ventricular function in athletes from different disciplines abusing anabolic steroids has been conducted by Rockhold (1993). The overall conclusion was that in intensely training athletes steroid administration induced left ventricular thickening and increases in end diastolic volume and relaxation index. Deligiannis and Mandroukas (1992) have shown that such changes occur in relation to increases in skeletal muscle mass. It should be noted that all the above studies were carried out in weightlifters and so may not be relevant to all athletes. The fact that, so far, only isolated cases of cardiomyopathy have occurred in athletes abusing steroids should serve as a warning rather than a comfort.

Effects on blood lipids and lipoproteins

Anabolic steroids have important effects on the plasma levels of triglycerides, cholesterol and lipoproteins.

Lipoproteins are large molecular conglomerates of lipids and specialized proteins called apolipoproteins. Their presence in the blood is to carry water-insoluble lipids from their site of production to tissues where they are utilized or stored. Anabolic steroids have been shown to increase blood triglyceride and cholesterol levels. They decrease the blood levels of high-density lipoprotein (HDL), especially the HDL_2 and HDL_3 fractions, whilst increasing the level of low-density lipoprotein (LDL). In addition, there is a significant rise in the ratio of free cholesterol to HDL-bound cholesterol following anabolic steroid administration, though the effect is less pronounced with testosterone (Alén and Rahkila, 1988). These changes appear to be induced by an action of anabolic steroids on key liver enzymes, such as lipoprotein lipase and hepatic lipase, associated with lipoprotein metabolism. Several studies, especially the widely quoted Framingham study in the USA, have shown that a reduction of just 10% in the blood concentration of HDL could increase the chances of coronary disease by 25%

(Kannel, Castelli and Gordon, 1979). A more recent study by Costill, Pearson and Fink (1984), has shown that in athletes taking anabolic steroids, HDL fell by 20% after only 102 days of treatment, whilst cholesterol concentration was unchanged. Rockhold (1993) reports even greater percentage reductions, i.e. HDL down 52%, HDLb down 78%. In normal males 22% of cholesterol is in the form of HDL, whilst in steroid takers only 7.8% of cholesterol is found combined in this way.

There is wide agreement that anabolic steroids cause a reduction in the serum HDL cholesterol (Alén and Rahkila, 1988), and that this phenomenon is particularly associated with the abuse of orally administered steroids (Lombardo, Hickson and Lamb, 1991). At least two recent reviews of the literature concluded that this effect of HDL is reversible, i.e. HDL levels return to normal within 3–5 weeks of cessation of steroid administration (Lukas, 1993; Rockhold, 1993).

These reductions in HDL levels have been associated with increased incidence of cardiovascular disease (Alén and Rahkila, 1988; Wagner, 1991) in the general population. Low serum HDL is recognized as a risk factor for cardiac and cerebrovascular disease (Wagner, 1991). There are several well-documented cases of coronary heart disease in apparently fit, healthy athletes aged under 40 who have been taking anabolic steroids (Goldman, 1984). However, according to Lukas (1993), so far only one case has been reported of an athlete dying of coronary heart disease whilst abusing anabolic steroids. It could be interpreted that low serum HDL is not a significant risk factor for steroid abusers, but it is also possible that such individuals may be fitter than the rest of the population so that any pathological changes are delayed. The statistics are also complicated by the different drug administration regimes used by abusers. This subject requires intensive long-term study.

Blood clotting

The increased risk of coronary and cerebrovascular disease in anabolic steroid abusers has prompted some physicians to consider whether there is increased risk of platelet aggregation leading to increased blood clot formation. Animal studies suggest that there is such a relationship, but so far there is only one report of an athlete taking steroids dying of a stroke (Lombardo, Hickson and Lamb, 1991). However, there is an association between increased platelet aggregation and age in weightlifters taking steroids (Lukas, 1993).

Carcinomas

The association between anabolic steroid administration and tumour formation, particularly of the liver and kidney, is now firmly established.

Significant changes in liver biochemistry have been found in 80% of otherwise healthy athletes taking anabolic steroids but without any signs of liver disease. In 1965, a detailed case study was published linking the death of an anabolic steroid-taking athlete with hepatocellular cancer (HC). Since then, 13 other athletes taking anabolic steroids have been demonstrated to have HC and all were taking 17-alkylated androgens. A second more insidious liver pathology, petiocis hepatis, was associated with anabolic steroids in 1977 (Goldman, 1984). In this disorder hepatic tissue degenerates and is replaced by blood-filled spaces. Anabolic steroids have also been suspected of causing death from Wilm's tumour of the kidney in two adult athletes. The tumour is very rare in post-adolescent individuals.

7.5.2 SEX-RELATED SIDE-EFFECTS

Fertility

Earlier it was noted that spermatogenesis in human males is under the control of gonadotrophins and testosterone. Administration of anabolic steroids caused inhibition of gonadotrophin secretion followed by inhibition of testosterone. Holma (1979) administered 15 mg methandienone to 15 well-trained athletes for 2 months. During the administration period, sperm counts fell by 73% and in three individuals azoospermia (complete absence of sperm) was present. Even in those individuals with sperm present there was a 10% increase in the number of immotile sperm and a 30% decrease in the number of motile sperm. Thus, fertility was severely reduced in males in this study, which provides confirmation of many clinical reports of the same phenomena. Though it is obviously unethical to test this, many clinical data suggest that long-term anabolic steroid-induced infertility might be permanent.

Effects on libido

The suppression of testosterone secretion in both males and females may well have effects on libido. As previously discussed, libido in males and females is thought to be influenced, at least in part, by testosterone. Thus, high levels of anabolic steroids in the blood suppress testosterone secretion and reduce libido.

Gynaecomastia

This is a paradoxical condition occurring in athletes attempting to increase their muscle mass, as it involves the development of mammary tissue. The most common cause of this condition in anabolic steroid abusers is that the agent they are administering is converted by liver aromatase enzymes to oestradiol which then induces development of mammary tissue. Thus, athletes who abuse anabolic steroids, testosterone or human chorionic gonadotrophin (hCG) (which releases testosterone) are all at risk from developing gynaecomastia (Friedl and Yesalis, 1989). It is widely assumed by steroid abusers that use of an anabolic steroid which cannot be aromatized will reduce the incidence of gynaecomastia, but there is no evidence for this. Concurrent administration of the anti-oestrogen, tamoxifen, is thought by many abusers in both the US and Britain to be an effective antidote to gynaecomastia induced by steroids (Perry, Wright and Littlepage, 1992). Though it is sometimes effective in reducing the pain associated with this condition, tamoxifen has little effect on the size of breast tissue in steroid abusers (Friedl and Yesalis, 1989).

Specific actions in female athletes

Considering the side-effects mentioned in the introduction, people often wonder why female athletes should take anabolic steroids. The simple answer is that women's athletics is now as competitive as men's and, according to some reports, the effects of anabolic steroids on muscle strength and bulk in a female athlete are considerably greater than in men. This has been explained by the lower normal circulating level of testosterone in females as compared to men. Thus, some female athletes take anabolic steroids in the knowledge that they may produce greater muscle strength and bulk at the expense of irreversible change, such as deepening of the voice and clitoral enlargement.

7.5.3 TENDON DAMAGE

Several researchers have noted the increased incidence of tendon damage in athletes taking anabolic steroids. A summary of the various tendon pathologies associated with anabolic steroid abuse has been provided by Laseter and Russell (1991). These include the quadriceps and rectus femoris tendons and the triceps. The four cases cited by Laseter and Russell all involved powerlifters. This phenomenon has been explained in at least three different ways. Firstly, that the increase in muscle strength acquired by a course of steroids, plus training, produces a greater increase in muscle power than in tendon strength, since tendons respond slowly to strength regimes and anabolic steroids have little or no effect on tendon strength. Secondly, it is thought that anabolic steroids have, in common with corticosteroids (such as cortisol), the ability to inhibit the formation of collagen, an important constituent of tendons and ligaments. Thirdly, anabolic steroids appear to induce changes in the arrangement and contractility of collagen fibrils in tendons, leading to critical alterations in physical properties known as the 'crimp angle'. The overall effect is to reduce the plasticity of the tendons. It should be pointed out that tendon ruptures also occur in athletes not abusing steroids. Weightlifters taking anabolic steroids appear to be particularly prone to muscle and tendon injuries. This has been explained by apologists for anabolic steroid abusers as evidence of greater weights being lifted. Sports doctors say it is the bio-chemical effects of anabolic steroids previously discussed, whilst others say that the increased aggressiveness and competitiveness induced by anabolic steroid administration causes athletes to attempt more and greater lifts with an increasingly reckless attitude to the actual mechanics of the lifting.

7.5.4 GLUCOSE REGULATION

Anabolic steroid abuse has been shown to reduce glucose tolerance and increase insulin resistance. This can lead to the induction of diabetes (Cohen and Hickman, 1987).

7.5.5 IMMUNOLOGICAL EFFECTS

Transient decreases in immunoglobulin IgA and IgG have been reported during steroid use.

7.5.6 BEHAVIOURAL EFFECTS AND ADDICTION

Since the late 1940s it has been known that anabolic steroids have impor-tant influences on behaviour, but these have usually been acknowledged to be the stimulatory effects which anabolic steroids have on libido in both males and females (Greenblatt et al., 1985). More recent studies, in the 1980s, have suggested that anabolic steroids have reduced the depres-sion symptoms in a number of groups of depressed patients (Williamson and Young, 1992). Research by Alder et al. (1986) has shown that some women suffering from postnatal depression have abnormally low testos-terone levels.

Given the frequency of anecdotal reports from athletes using steroids that they experienced euphoria, general feelings of well-being, and increased confidence, self-esteem, libido and energy, it is surprising that until the late 1980s little systematic research into the behavioural effects of anabolic steroids had been carried out. A review by Kashkin and Kleber (1989) cites many documented cases of increased aggression and violent behaviour, many of them reported by the abusers themselves. The same authors also report detailed cases of mild to severe psychiatric distur-bances occurring in those abusing anabolic steroids, ranging from impaired judgement, insomnia and agitation to panic attacks, grandiose ideas and paranoid delusions. Pope and Katz (1988) interviewed 41 body-builders and football players who had used anabolic steroids. Nine of these fulfilled the DSMIIIR criteria for mood disorder and five displayed psychotic symptoms associated with steroid use. In a larger study comparing 88 anabolic steroid abusers with 68 non-abusers, Pope and Katz (1994) found that 23% of abusers and 6% of non-abusers had some form of mood disorder. Clinical depression which persisted after abuse, suffered by 13% of abusers, had stopped in 55 of the subjects. Manic episodes were significantly reduced in individuals who withdrew from steroid abuse. Pope and Katz also identified a condition they named as 'reverse anorexia nervosa', defined as individuals who considered their body build to be too small. This 'condition' was present in 7% of abusers but rose to 11% in those who withdrew from steroid abuse. Williamson and Young (1992) describe several cases of manic episodes in athletes taking anabolic steroids. In a number of instances depressed steroid abusers, attempting to withdraw from steroid administration, became manic when treated with antidepressant drugs.

Since the mid-1980s, there have been increasing reports of abusers maintaining steroid administration despite repeated attempts to stop them. There are similar reports in the literature of patients on high glucocorticoid doses being unable to stop their medication or suffering depressive symptoms upon withdrawal of the drugs. Kashkin and Kleber (1989) also produce evidence of withdrawal symptoms in some individuals who stop taking steroids and cite several studies where steroid withdrawal had resulted in clinical depression. Of a sample of men who stopped taking steroids, 12.2% were diagnosed as depressed within 3 months of abstinence. In Britain, the suicide of a Royal Marine guardsman whose anabolic steroids were withdrawn was reported (*Guardian*, 1994).

There are a number of reports of steroid cravings associated with increased sympathetic nervous system activity in some abusers who attempt to refrain from anabolic steroids. There is also widespread fear, real and imaginary, of what I call 'muscle melt down', in those considering or attempting to withdraw from steroid abuse. This appears from the literature to involve feelings of loss of esteem, both social and sexual, if the well-developed torso is seen to 'melt away' after steroid withdrawal. Kashkin and Kleber (1989) consider that all the clinical evidence so far suggests the existence of a 'sex steroid hormone dependence disorder' which obeys the following established criteria for addiction:

- the hormones are used over longer periods than desired;

- attempts are made to stop without success;

- substantial time is spent obtaining, using or recovering from the hormones;

- use continues despite acknowledgement of the significant psychological and toxicological problems caused by the hormones;

- characteristic withdrawal symptoms occur;

- hormones (or their supplements) are taken to relieve the withdrawal symptoms.

The evidence assembled by Kashkin and Kleber (1989) and Williamson and Young (1992) is substantial and convincing, but, as Lukas (1993) has emphasized, the majority of athletes and body-builders do not report major psychiatric symptoms, or perhaps refrain from doing so.

One of the major reasons proposed by steroid abusers for the use of these drugs in their sport is that it increases their aggression. A number of studies have failed to find any relationship between endogenous testosterone levels and aggression (Archer, 1991), and a review of aggression and hostility in anabolic steroid v. placebo studies in several groups of athletes revealed both positive and equivocal results (Williamson and Young, 1992).

Perhaps the most disturbing reports of all are those linking anabolic steroids with serious crime, including murder. Lubell (1989) has documented three cases of murder where anabolic steroids were cited by the defence as the cause of their clients' behaviour, and one case in Florida where the defence (unsuccessfully) entered a plea of 'not guilty by reason of insanity' for a client who committed murder whilst abusing anabolic steroids. The effects of anabolic steroids on behaviour and their association with psychiatric illness and criminality appears strong, but most studies reviewed here have not demonstrated clear or quantitative relationships and none has been prospective. It is therefore impossible to know the personality or even the psychiatric profile of the person **before** they began abusing steroids. It is possible that body-builders and even some athletes may have psychological problems and/or abnormal personalities before they begin steroid abuse. Thus body-builders may suffer from body dysmorphic syndromes (feelings that their body size/shape is inadequate). Athletes may form obsessional/perfectionist desires to be the best at all costs.

We also know very little about the cultural, social and psychological influences which affect both the developing and the adult athlete and which of these influences may lead to psychiatric disturbance and/or drug abuse. In 1992, David Begel reviewed the most recent research in sport psychiatry and concluded that the close relationship between mental and physical phenomena in sport may account for the psychiatric problems associated with poor performance. Amongst American athletes a decrease in athletic performance is termed a 'slump'. It would be interesting to know what the relationship was between 'slump' and anabolic steroid taking and whether abuse of the drugs was associated with attempts to pre-empt it.

The association between anabolic steroid abuse and all aspects of behaviour, personality and psychiatric disorder in sport should be the subject of further careful study.

7.6 INDIRECT CONSEQUENCES OF ANABOLIC STEROID ABUSE

Many of the surveys quoted (Perry, Wright and Littlepage, 1992; Lamb, 1991; Pope, Katz and Champoux, 1988) suggest that abuse of orally active steroids is declining in favour of the injectable varieties, particularly testosterone. This may be due to better awareness of the toxicity of the oral compounds or to the supposedly lower risk of detection with injectable compounds once treatment is stopped. It is surely no coincidence that this switch appears to be associated with the appearance of HIV amongst steroid abusers, the first case of which was reported in the USA 10 years ago (Sklarek et al., 1984). There have been several further cases reported subsequently in body-builders in the USA (Yesalis et al., 1988). The potential for the spread of HIV by this route in Great Britain has been highlighted by Perry, Wright and Littlepage (1992), who reported high-risk behaviour in their sample of body-builders in Swansea, i.e. needle sharing and drug sample sharing with all the attendant risks of cross-contamination of drug supplies and abusers' blood.

Another unforeseen consequence of anabolic steroid abuse by injection is tissue and organ damage caused by inexperienced and untrained injectors. Several anecdotal cases have been reported to me by a local GP of 'steroid limp'. This condition is characterized by the patient who can only raise the affected leg to walk by using the abdominal adductor muscles. It is caused by damage to the sciatic nerve by injection of anabolic steroids in the buttocks either into or close to the nerve, resulting usually in permanent neuromuscular impairment. Other complications involving adulterated or inappropriate drugs have been reported to me. These included the supply of stolen veterinary stilboestrol, an oestrogen used in Europe to stimulate flesh growth in poultry. The abusers concerned suffered significant mammary development!

7.7 EDUCATIONAL AND SOCIAL ASPECTS OF ANABOLIC STEROID ABUSE

Though the number of positive steroid tests at Olympic events appears to be falling (7.4.4), the high level of anabolic steroid usage by body-builders and weightlifters and the disturbing level of abuse by the young in the USA and Britain shows that much remains to be done to counteract the anabolic steroid problem. The imposition of mandatory testing, whilst possibly contributing to the decline in anabolic steroid usage in top class athletes, will have little influence on the school or college abuser. In the USA mandatory testing measures have been introduced at school and college level, resulting in a number of positive tests (Leach, 1993). How can the abuse be combated and how should the abuser be treated? It seems that we must first understand who is abusing and why. Though it cannot be condoned, it is easy to understand why athletes are tempted to cheat in order to run faster or throw further, particularly with the substantial financial rewards that go with winning. It is less easy to understand why athletes will risk disqualification and gamble on their own health to achieve this. In contrast, European soccer, at least in the UK, appears to be steroid-free. Here, individual financial rewards can make successful players millionaires. Perhaps it is the potential loss of all this, consequent on being tested positive, which is a disincentive. The abuse of anabolic steroids by body-builders and others for cosmetic reasons is also difficult to understand, especially when they are well acquainted with the long- and short-term side-effects and have even expressed concern about them recently (Yesalis *et al.*, 1988).

In the USA, the problem has been tackled by utilizing educational programmes in colleges, schools and gymnasia and encouraging medical practitioners to adopt a sympathetic attitude towards steroid abusers, particularly by advising on and treating side-effects of anabolic steroids (Frankle and Leffers, 1992). Central to this has been a planned intervention for abusers proposed by Frankle and Leffers (1992), including psychiatric intervention, group education at gyms, schools and colleges, drug testing for competitive athletes at all levels and a problem-related counselling approach emphasizing the relationship between steroid use and side-effects. They concluded that legal restraints on anabolic steroid supply are necessary but that more stringent legislation should be kept in the background. A similar approach has been adopted in the UK. Perry, Wright and Littlepage (1992) have described a local project in West Glamorgan in which powerlifters in private gymnasia have been counselled in order to prevent the spread of HIV by the sharing of contaminated drug samples and infected needles. They also advocate a sympathetic approach by GPs, involving counselling, advice and support, the option of routine health checks and the admission of steroid abusers to needle-exchange schemes.

In November 1994, the UK government decided to reclassify anabolic steroids as controlled drugs, probably as Class C, the category including the least dangerous drugs of abuse. This may not be the answer to the UK problem. A sensible compromise might be the compulsory licensing of all local authority leisure centres and private gymnasia. The worrying trend of increasing anabolic steroid abuse in schools and colleges in the USA has been noted (Buckley *et al.*, 1988; Pope, Katz and Champoux, 1988), but until recently has been unrecognized in Great Britain. The recent survey in Scotland by Williamson (1993) emphasizes that such complacency is misplaced as 56% of those admitting to steroid abuse began doing so when 17 or younger. It is also important that this survey identified a significant number (50%) who were regular rugby union players, athletes who are not usually recognized as steroid abusers. However, in November 1994, Jamie Bloem became the first rugby league player in the UK to test positive for steroids. In Great Britain, at least, soccer appears to be 'steroid-free' – the latest statistics from the Football Association show no positive tests for steroids since testing began (Hodson, 1994).

More studies in Great Britain need to be carried out and an immediate education programme centred on schools and colleges should be instigated.

7.8 HUMAN GROWTH HORMONE

This was described in the previous edition of this book as the 'next potential drug of abuse' in sport (George, 1988). Its illicit use and potential was then being recognized in the USA (Taylor, 1988).

hGH is one of the major hormones influencing growth and development in humans. Such is the complexity of human growth, a period extending from birth to the age of 20 years, that a very large number of hormones influence it, producing many complex interactions. Besides hGH, the hormones testosterone, oestradiol, cortisol, thyroxine and insulin have important roles at different stages of growth and development. The exact role of hGH is difficult to evaluate because of the many different developmental and metabolic processes which hGH can influence.

Secretion of hGH is episodic, the highest levels (0.5–3.0 /mg) occurring 60–90 minutes after the onset of sleep. hGH is metabolized in the liver; the plasma half-life is 12–45 minutes. The physiological regulation of hGH release is complex: systemic factors stimulating secretion include hypoglycaemia, a rise in blood amino acid concentration, stress and exercise, whilst, conversely, hGH secretion is inhibited by hyperglycaemia.

Release of hGH from the somatotroph cells of the anterior pituitary is under the control of the hypothalamic hormones, somatostatin which inhibits secretion and somatocrinin which stimulates its secretion. Oestradiol also stimulates hGH secretion, whilst testosterone has very little effect. Various brain neurotransmitter systems also influence hGH secretion. This is thought to occur via a controlling influence on the hypothalamic production of somatostatin and somatocrinin, but direct effects on the somatotroph cells cannot be ruled out. Drugs such as clonidine, which stimulate $alpha_2$ adrenergic receptors, cause increases in hGH secretion, while drugs which stimulate beta$_2$ receptors, such as salbutamol, decrease hGH secretion. The factors influencing hGH secretion have been reviewed in detail by Macintyre (1987).

7.8.1 ACTION AND EFFECTS OF hGH

The most obvious action of hGH is that it stimulates somatic growth in pre-adolescents, but it also has metabolic effects. The importance of these metabolic actions in homeostatic regulation of fuel usage and storage is unclear, as is the overall role of hGH in the adult, discussed in detail by Macintyre (1987). Discussion of the actions of hGH is further complicated by the involvement of the plasma growth factors, or somatomedins, in the action of hGH. The release from liver and kidney of two polypeptides, somatomedin C (or insulin-like growth factor I(IGF-I)) and somatomedin A (insulin-like growth factor II(IGF-II)) is stimulated by hGH, and a full account of this is provided by Macintyre (1987) and Kicman and Cowan (1992).

Effects on muscle

Although hGH seems to have some effects on muscle growth, the effect of somatomedin C is greater. This action is similar to that of insulin in that it promotes amino acid uptake and stimulates protein synthesis resulting, in children, in an increase in the length and diameter of muscle fibres, whilst only the latter growth occurs in adults. This stimulation of muscle protein synthesis and growth is qualitatively different to that induced by work, since insulin is required for hGH-stimulated muscle growth but not for that induced by work (Macintyre, 1987).

Effects on bone

The elongation of bone in pre-adolescents is stimulated directly and via the somatomedins by hGH. This is achieved by a stimulation of cartilage proliferation in the epiphyseal plates situated at each end of each long bone. Cartilage cells possess receptors for hGH and somatomedins.

Effects on metabolism

The actions of hGH on metabolism are complex at both the cellular and organ level and appear to be biphasic. In the first or acute phase, which seems to involve the action of hGH alone, amino acid uptake into muscle and liver is stimulated, and there is increased glucose uptake into muscle and adipose tissue together with reduced fat metabolism (Smith and Perry, 1992). During the second, chronic phase, mediated by the somatomedins, there is increased lipolysis (triglyceride breakdown) in adipose tissue resulting in a rise in the plasma concentration of fatty acids and increased fatty acid utilization, thus sparing glucose.

Overall effects

Treatment with hGH causes a rise in blood free fatty acid levels and a rise in the blood glucose level and a reduction in the triglyceride content of adipose tissue which contributes to a decrease in adipose tissue mass and an increase in fat-free weight (Kicman and Cowan, 1992).

It is worth considering the hGH response to exercise in more detail. Within 20 minutes of beginning exercise to 75–90% VO_2max., hGH levels rise. The intensity of the response depends on age, level of fitness and body composition. The type of exercise undertaken also produces varying hGH responses. Intense exercise produces earlier hGH secretion, endurance exercise produces hGH peaks in mid-term, whilst intermittent intense exercise is claimed to result in the highest hGH levels (Macintyre, 1987).

According to Macintyre (1987) a number of artificial stimuli have been used to increase hGH secretion. The ones used most frequently in clinical situations are clonidine, arginine and insulin-induced hypoglycaemia.

7.8.2 ADMINISTRATION AND SUPPLY OF hGH

Since hGH is a peptide and must be injected, the same problems of possible contamination of samples and infection of needles apply as with injection of anabolic steroids. It is now produced synthetically, as hGH from human sources has been withdrawn because of possible contamination with the agent which spreads the degenerative brain disorder, Creutzfeldt Jakob disease. Initially, synthetic hGH when injected was associated with the stimulation in the recipient of hGH antibodies. This problem has been solved by increased purification procedures. Therapeutically, hGH administration is usually recommended as either three single intramuscular or subcutaneous injections or daily subcutaneous injections in the evening.

The supply of hGH is controlled by law in the UK under the Medicines Act 1968. In the USA, hGH is regulated by the Food, Drug and Cosmetic Act, but Congressional hearings have taken place with a view to making it a Schedule II controlled substance (Smith and Perry, 1992). One of the major limitations on hGH supply is its price. It is claimed that abusers in the US have had to spend $30 000 per year (£20 000) to obtain worthwhile effects (Smith and Perry, 1992). There is also some evidence that much of the hGH reaching the abuser is either counterfeit, adulterated, of animal origin or some other product (Smith and Perry, 1992; Cowart, 1988). Thus, abusers are being sold bovine growth hormone stolen from farms (useless in humans), other peptide hormones, such as hCG which actually stimulates testosterone production, or even anabolic steroids themselves (Taylor, 1988; Cowart, 1988; Smith and Perry, 1992).

Attempts to counteract the embargo on hGH have included administering drugs which stimulate hGH release, such as clonidine, propranolol and bromocriptine (Smith and Perry, 1992). More legitimate means include the ingestion of the amino acid, arginine. Arginine is the most potent of a number of amino acids which stimulate hGH secretion. As it is a normal constituent of protein and of a balanced diet, its 'abuse' would be difficult if not impossible to detect. Some dietary products for athletes claim to be rich in arginine so as to promote hGH secretion. The long-term effectiveness of arginine in promoting or maintaining increase in hGH levels remains to be investigated.

7.8.3 GROWTH HORMONE DISORDERS

Inadequate secretion of hGH gives rise to the condition known as dwarfism. This disorder is usually recognized in childhood when the rate of growth is below the 90% percentile for the child's age, race and sex. Further tests involve 'challenges' to the pituitary in the form of arginine, clonidine or insulin. If these fail to evoke adequate hGH secretion, then a diagnosis of dwarfism due to inadequate hGH can be made. The treatment is regular administration of synthetic hGH until the end of puberty. Treatment after adolescence is ineffective in stimulating growth in stature because by this time the epiphyseal plates in the long bones have fused, terminating any further bone growth. Overproduction of hGH as a result of a tumour may occur in puberty and adolescence when it gives rise to gigantism; the individual is well above average adult height for their age and sex, and the limbs and internal organs are also enlarged.

In late adulthood, a tumour of the anterior pituitary, causing increased hGH secretion, causes the condition known as acromegaly. The affected individual does not grow any taller because the epiphyses have fused, but their internal organs enlarge (especially the heart), the fingers grow and the skin thickens. Metabolic disorders occur which often precipitate diabetes.

7.8.4 THERAPEUTIC USE OF hGH

hGH is used to treat pituitary dwarfism, when it must be administered to the affected individual before the end of puberty. The administration must be carefully monitored to prevent diabetes and/or hyperplasia (overgrowth) of the skin. Synthetic growth hormone is now used instead of hGH obtained from human autopsies (7.8.2).

It has also been suggested by a number of geriatricians that hGH might be used to reverse some of the bodily changes occurring in old age. Normal ageing is associated with a reduction in lean body mass, an increase in fat mass and a reduction in skin thickness. Trials of hGH treatment in the elderly have shown that the hormone is able to reverse these changes (Jorgensen and Christiansen, 1993). Reviewing the recent trials of hGH in middle-aged and elderly men, Neely and Rosenfield (1994) reported a 7% rise in lean body mass, a 14% drop in fat mass and a 7% increase in the fasting blood glucose level. However, they also reported that at least one study indicated severe disturbances of carbohydrate metabolism and glucose homeostasis during a trial in which adults were treated with hGH 0.12 mg/day. The elevation of fasting glucose (+24%) and serum insulin (+25%) in this study are strongly indicative of a 'pre-diabetic state'. A possible role for the hormone in patients with severe burns and even AIDS is also under investigation.

7.8.5 THE ABUSE OF hGH IN SPORT

There appear to be four major abuses of hGH in sport: (1) to increase muscle mass and strength, (2) to increase lean body mass, (3) to improve the 'appearance of musculature' and (4) to increase final adult height. Scientific evidence from controlled trials that hGH increases muscle strength is negligible, and so most reports on hGH efficacy are either anecdotal or based on animal experiments. Several 'underground' advocates have recently withdrawn their support for growth hormone, stating that hGH treatment has no value in increasing muscle strength in the athlete (Kicman and Cowan, 1992). Smith and Perry (1992) concluded that there are no records of experiments examining the efficacy of hGH on muscle strength in athletes. They describe controlled animal experiments in which hGH increased the strength of atrophied rat muscle but produced no increase in strength in normal muscle.

There is some evidence to support the claim that hGH administration may increase lean body mass. Lombardo, Hickson and Lamb (1991) describe experiments where hGH administration has caused significant reductions in 'fat weight' and increases in fat free weight compared to placebo. A similar effect has been observed during hGH administration to elderly men (Kicman and Cowan, 1992).

It is claimed that hGH administration, because of the above effects, improves the appearance of the body-builder, making muscles more salient or 'sculpted' and improving their photogenicity. There is no way this can be measured, but it appears to be a logical development associated with loss of fat tissue.

The desire to produce tall offspring either for cosmetic reasons, 'so that their athletic potential is increased' where height is an advantage, or so that they can qualify for a vocation where there is a minimum height limit has prompted hGH abuse amongst children in the USA. Despite the ethical problems that it presents in relation to sport, the child may later resent his/her tallness, particularly if later failing to qualify as a professional sportsperson for other reasons. Also, it is difficult to gauge exactly how much hGH should be given so as not to produce an overly tall individual. Other potential problems of child treatment relate to side-effects discussed in the next section.

7.8.6 SIDE-EFFECTS ASSOCIATED WITH GROWTH HORMONE ABUSE IN SPORT

The potential risks of hGH therapy in children have been mentioned, together with the close monitoring required in paediatric patients. In the UK, the recommended standard **replacement** dose of hGH is about 0.6 IU/kg body weight per week. It is widely assumed that athletes who abuse the drug are taking 10 times this dose (Smith and Perry, 1992). Major side-effects include skeletal changes, enlargement of the fingers and toes, growth of the orbit and lengthening of the jaw. The internal organs enlarge and the cardiomegaly which is produced is often one of the causes of death associated with hGH abuse. Although the skeletal muscles increase in size, there are often complaints of muscle weakness. Biochemical changes include impaired glucose regulation (usually hyperglycaemia) and hyperlipidaemia. These changes contribute to the prevalence of diabetes in hGH abusers. Arthritis and impotence often occur after chronic hGH abuse (Kicman and Cowan, 1992).

A weird consequence of the increased protein synthesis during hGH abuse is thickening and coarsening of the skin. The so-called 'elephant epidermis' produced has been known to make the skin almost impenetrable by standard gauge syringe needles (Taylor, 1988). This combination of side-effects, particularly the cardiomegaly, hyperlipidaemia and hyperglycaemia, almost certainly contributes to the shortened lifespan seen in those suffering from overproduction of hGH (Smith and Perry, 1992).

7.8.7 WHO ABUSES GROWTH HORMONE AND WHY?

There are few scientific studies available on the prevalence of hGH abuse. Macintyre (1987) has identified American football players and bodybuilders as the most likely abusers, based on lab reports from accredited testing agencies. Significantly, the UK investigation into drug abuse by athletes in South Wales by Perry, Wright and Littlepage (1992) revealed no hGH abuse.

The reasons for hGH abuse appear to be based on false premises that it is as effective as anabolic steroids, with fewer side-effects, is less easily detected and may protect the athlete who has abused anabolic steroids and wishes to stop 'muscle meltdown'.

If abuse is difficult to identify in adults, this is not the case in adolescents. In a recent survey (Ricker *et al.*, 1992), 5% of adolescents admitted using hGH and 24.5% claimed to know of someone who was abusing it. Of the abusers, 50% could not name one side-effect of hGH. Those who abused hGH were most likely to be involved in wrestling or American football and to have obtained their information about hGH from another person, such as a coach. There was also some evidence of co-abuse of anabolic steroids and hGH in the same adolescent sample.

7.8.8 DETECTION OF hGH

It is beyond the scope of this chapter to discuss detection of hGH abuse in detail but some consideration of it is important because of the widespread belief that it is undetectable. This is based on the observations that administered hGH is indistinguishable from endogenous hGH, that the plasma half-life of hGH is only 15–28 minutes and less than 0.01% of hGH is excreted in urine (Kicman and Cowan, 1992). Despite this, there is a good correlation between plasma and urinary hGH concentrations, which might enable recent hGH abuse to be detected during random urine sampling.

The most promising means of detecting hGH abuse is by examining the ratio of urinary IGF-I to IGF-II. In normal adults the serum concentrations of IGF-I and II are much greater than the mean hGH concentration. The administration of hGH to normal adults causes a significant and chronic increase only in the serum concentration of IGF-I. Thus adults who abuse hGH would be expected to have an abnormal serum IGF-I/IGF-II ratio which recent research suggests would also be reflected in the urinary ratio. Further work is now being undertaken world-wide in IOC accredited laboratories to determine the accuracy and efficacy of this detection method, and also to investigate how age, gender, diet and exercise may influence IGF-I/II ratio.

7.8.9 SOCIAL FACTORS AND hGH ABUSE

The hGH 'problem' **appears** to be mainly confined to the US, but this may be because the US is the major source of information on hGH abuse in athletes. The prevalence of hGH abuse in the young (5% in the survey by Rickert *et al.*, 1992) suggests that hGH abuse is taking a hold in a small group of obsessed athletes. Educational programmes similar to those advocated for steroids (7.7) are obviously required. However, according to Cowart (1988) much pressure on physicians to prescribe hGH comes from parents, who will also need educating. In the USA, there have already been Congressional inquiries into the law relating to hGH, and a number of state legislatures, such as Texas, have enacted laws classifying hGH as a controlled drug (Taylor, 1988).

7.9 ADRENOCORTICOTROPHIC HORMONE (ACTH)

The use and abuse of corticosteroids in sport is discussed in Chapter 5. It is relevant here to discuss the abuse of the peptide hormone ACTH.

ACTH is produced and secreted by the corticotroph cells of the anterior pituitary. It is a polypeptide consisting of 39 amino acids, of which only the 24 N-terminal amino acids are necessary for its biological activity. ACTH stimulates the reticularis and fasciculata cells of the adrenal cortex to synthesize and secrete corticosteroids, such as cortisol and corticosterone.

7.9.1 ADMINISTRATION OF ACTH

ACTH is never used for treatment or abuse – instead a synthetic derivative, the peptide tetracosactrin consisting of the first 24 N-terminal amino acids, is administered by injection. Tetracosactrin administration stimulates a rise in blood cortisol and corticosterone concentration within 2 hours.

7.9.2 ABUSE OF ACTH

ACTH abuse is limited to short-term boosting of plasma cortisol and corticosterone in an attempt to reduce lethargy and produce 'positive' effects on mood during training and competition. It is for this reason that it is banned by the IOC along with corticosteroids. ACTH and corticosteroids are unsuitable for chronic use because they decrease muscle protein synthesis, leading to skeletal muscle wasting.

7.9.3 DETECTION OF ACTH

Tetracosactrin abuse and endogenous ACTH are difficult to detect in urine samples. In the blood a rise in ACTH levels, and therefore of corticosteroids, occurs naturally during exercise. However, IOC laboratories are currently refining a blood analysis for tetracosactrin which should enable abuse to be detected (Kicman and Cowan, 1992).

7.10 HUMAN CHORIONIC GONADOTROPHIN (hCG)

hCG is produced by placental trophoblast cells during pregnancy and also by a number of different types of tumour cell. Its major physiological role is stimulation of the corpus luteum, to maintain synthesis and secretion of the hormone progesterone during pregnancy. However, when injected into males, hCG also stimulates the Leydig cells of the testis to produce testosterone and epitestosterone, and so it can mimic the natural stimulation of testicular hormone production produced by luteinizing hormone (LH).

The Leydig cells of the testis possess receptors which when stimulated by LH or hCG bring about activation of testosterone synthesis. This increase in synthesis is rapid, a 50% increase in plasma testosterone concentration has been measured 2 hours after intramuscular injection of 6000 IU of hCG (Kicman, Brooks and Cowan, 1991).

7.10.1 THERAPEUTIC USE OF hCG

To stimulate ovulation, hCG is used in conjunction with FSH (follicle stimulating hormone) in infertile women. Occasionally, hCG is used to stimulate testicular hormone production when puberty is delayed.

7.10.2 ABUSE OF hCG IN SPORT

The increasingly successful identification of anabolic steroid abusers by various IOC approved tests has led abusers to switch to testosterone abuse, which itself may be detected by measurement of the testosterone:epitestosterone ratio (7.3.1). Abuse of hCG has become popular because it stimulates the secretion from the testes of both testosterone and epitestosterone, resulting in a urinary excretion ratio of less than 6:1, below the limit set by the IOC. This led to the banning of hCG by the IOC in 1987.

A standard doping regime for hCG has been described (Brooks *et al.*, 1989) in which the abuser firstly injects testosterone. Apart from any gains in strength or competitiveness, the testosterone causes inhibition of LH secretion from the pituitary. When testosterone is withdrawn before competition (to avoid detection) the athlete would be at a disadvantage with lower than normal plasma testosterone levels. However, administration of hCG stimulates testicular testosterone secretion and also that of epitestosterone, so that apparent compliance with IOC regulations occurs. In a small, elegant experiment, Kicman, Brooks and Cowan (1991) have reproduced this situation in three normal men and shown that hCG can stimulate the testosterone substitution claimed by abusers and retain the testosterone/epitestosterone ratio within the IOC limits. In all three cases, the hCG could be detected in the urine by radioimmunoassay as long as plasma testosterone levels were raised. Despite the availability of a highly specific radioimmunosassay for hCG, it does not yet reproduce the discriminating power of gas chromatography and mass spectrometry and so it is as yet unaccepted by the IOC.

7.10.3 SIDE-EFFECTS OF hCG IN SPORT

The side-effects of hCG will be similar to those described for anabolic steroids (7.5). However, the incidence of gynaecomastia may be greater as hCG also stimulates oestradiol production by the Leydig cells.

7.11 LUTEOTROPHIC HORMONE

LH is produced by the gonadotroph cells of the anterior pituitary in both males and females. In males, LH stimulates testicular sperm production and the synthesis and secretion of testosterone, whilst in females it stimulates ovulation and the production of progesterone. There are structural similarities between LH and hCG and a detailed comparison is made by Kicman and Cowan (1992). LH secretion is subject to negative feedback control by testosterone, i.e. as plasma testosterone levels rise, so LH secretion is reduced.

LH is a **potential** drug of abuse because its stimulation of testosterone production by the testis also produces epitestosterone, such that the normal testosterone to epitestosterone ratio is maintained in plasma and urine. Its abuse is limited by its scarcity and its high cost and because its plasma half-life is 50% less than hCG (Kicman and Cowan, 1992). 'Designer' synthesis of LH, a dual-chain peptide, is probably impossible owing to the complexity of its structure.

The detection of LH is probably more important than its potential abuse. When testosterone is abused LH secretion falls and the ratio of testosterone to LH rises. Computation of the testosterone:LH ratio in normal male athletes and its comparison to that in males abusing testosterone is a potentially important test in addition to the testosterone:epitestosterone ratio. This is because a very small number of males are low epitestosterone secretors.

There is also some evidence that epitestosterone may soon be synthesized by 'underground' laboratories, enabling testosterone and epitestosterone to be administered together and so negating detection of abuse by measurement of testosterone:epitestosterone ratios. It has already been mentioned that administration of hCG provides a potential means of obscuring the testosterone:epitestosterone ratio test. However, simultaneous measurement of testosterone:LH ratios would detect abuse because the testosterone:LH ratio is increased by administration of testosterone or testosterone plus epitestosterone.

Measurement of testosterone:LH ratios are precluded for female athletes because the oestrogen and progesterone ingredients of oral contraceptives suppress LH secretion, leading to erroneous testosterone:LH ratios (Kicman and Cowan, 1992).

7.12 THE FUTURE

Unfortunately, all the predictions made in the first edition of this book have come true (George, 1988). Future trends for abuse would seem to be the obvious ones of LH and epitestosterone administration in order to escape detection by measurement of testosterone:LH and testosterone:epitestosterone ratios. The scope for this will depend on the ability of 'underground' laboratories to supply the drugs, though it is conceivable that LH may eventually be produced commercially. A possible development in the confirmation of manipulation of testosterone levels is the use of the drug ketoconazole (Kicman *et al.*, 1993).

This compound is an antifungal agent which inhibits testosterone secretion by the testis. When 400 mg ketoconazole is administered to a normal male, the plasma testosterone level declines by approximately 50% within 8 hours causing a fall in the testosterone/epitestosterone ratio. However, when administered to someone who has self-injected with testosterone, the plasma levels of the hormone remain unchanged or may rise, thus increasing the ratio of testosterone to epitestosterone. The ketoconazole test was proposed in 1994 for the defence of the UK 800 m champion, Diane Modahl, who was alleged to have an abnormally high testosterone level and testosterone:epitestosterone ratio. In this controversial case, bacterial decomposition of the test sample had been proposed as a cause of the abnormal findings. My colleague, Rod Bilton (1995), has recently suggested that the conversion of urinary steroids to testosterone by urinary bacteria is possible, and has emphasized that **all** urine samples collected on behalf of the IOC and affiliated organizations should be frozen immediately to prevent bacterial degradation.

A possible future countermeasure is the collection and registration of 'hormone profiles' from all competitive athletes by the IOC. Some progress on the utility of hormone profiles in weightlifters has recently been outlined by Donike, Greyer and Routh (1993). It is quite likely that abusers may change their tactics and switch to hGH. Despite the equivocal or even negative effects that chronic administration of hGH may have on muscle physiology, its short-term effects on lean body mass make it a popular choice for abusers. Juvenile abuse of hGH may also increase so that its positive effects on growth, which will only occur before the end of puberty, will be undetectable during an adult athletic career. This will encourage those who would like to introduce the universal testing of juvenile athletes, as is mandatory in some American colleges (Taylor, 1988). The best hope for combating hGH abuse is probably the development and accreditation of the urinary IGF-I/II test. However, the recent development of orally active hGH-releasing peptides with similar actions to somatocrinin have been described (Jorgensen and Christiansen, 1993). If these compounds are developed successfully, they will further complicate the picture. Future alternatives to hGH are the somatomedins. These are not available commercially, but, being much smaller and simpler molecules than hGH or LH, their synthesis by 'designer' chemists is more feasible. They could be used to circumvent hGH:somatomedin ratio tests or by themselves.

A final possibility is negative doping or 'spiking', as happens in horseracing. This would involve either administering a negative ergogenic aid to an athlete without their knowledge so as to reduce their performance or secretly to administer a banned substance so that the person is disqualified. An alleged case of 'spiking' was reported recently involving the Australian weightlifter, Ron Laycock.

Keep on testing!

7.13 REFERENCES

Alder, E.M., Cook, A., Davidson, D. *et al.* (1986) Hormones, mood and sexuality in lactating women. *Br. J. Psychiat.* **148**, 74–9.

Alén, M. and Rahkila, P. (1988) Anabolic–androgenic steroid effects on endocrinology and lipid metabolism in athletes. *Sports Med.*, **6**, 327–32.

Archer, J. (1991) The influence of testosterone on human aggression. *Br. J. Psychol.*, **82**, 1–28.

Begel, D. (1992) An overview of sport psychiatry. *Am. J. Psychiat.*, **149**, 606–14.

Bilton, R.F. (1995) Microbial production of testosterone. *Lancet*, **345**, 1187.

Brooks, R.V., Collyer, S.P., Kicman, A.T. *et al.* (1989) HCG doping in sport and methods for its detection, in *Official Proceedings of Second IAF World Symposium on Doping in Sport*, (eds P. Bellot, G. Benzi and A. Ljungavist), London, pp. 37–45.

Buckley, W.E., Yesalis, C.E., Friedl, K.E. *et al.* (1988) Estimated prevalence of anabolic steroid use among male high school seniors. *J. Am. Med. Assoc.*, **260**, 3441–5.

Catlin, D., Wright, J., Pope, H. and Kiggett, M. (1993) Assessing the threat of anabolic steroids. *Physician and Sports Medicine*, **21**, 37–44.

Choo, J.-J., Horon, M.A., Little, R.A. and Rothwell, N.J. (1992) Clenbuterol and skeletal muscle are mediated by β_2 adrenoceptor activation. *Am. J. Physiol.*, **263**, 50–56.

Cohen, J.C. and Hickman, R. (1987) Insulin resistance and diminished glucose tolerance in powerlifters ingesting anabolic steroids. *J. Clin. Endocr. Metab.*, **64**, 960–63.

Costill, D.L., Pearson, D.R. and Fink, W.J. (1984) Anabolic steroid use among athletes. Changes in HDC-C levels. *Physician and Sports Medicine*, **12**, 113–17.

'Counterfeit steroid found'. News item. *Pharmaceutical Journal*, **252**, 26 March, p. 431.

Cowart, V. (1988) Human growth hormone: the latest ergogenic aid? *Physician and Sports Medicine*, **16**, 175–85.

Daigle, R.D. (1990) Anabolic steroids. *J. Psychoact. Drugs*, **22**, 77–80.

Deligiannis, A.P. and Mandroukas, K. (1992) Noninvasive cardiac evaluation of weight-lifters using anabolic steroids. *Scand. J. Med. Sci. Sports*, **3**, 37–40.

Donike, M., Greyer, H. and Routh, S. (1993) Development of steroid profiles and performance in weightlifting after introduction of strict dope controls. *Sportmedz.*, **44**, 329–30.

Elashoff, J.D., Jacknow, A.D., Shain, S.G. and Braunstein, G.D. (1991) Effects of anabolic–androgenic steroids on muscular strength. *Annals Int. Med.*, **115**, 387–93.

Forbes, G.B. (1985) The effect of anabolic steroids on lean body mass. The dose response curve. *Metabolism*, **34**, 571–3.

Frankle, M. and Leffers, D. (1992) Athletes on anabolic androgenic steroids. *Physician and Sports Medicine*, **20**, 75–87.

Freed, D.L.J., Banks, A.J., Longson, D. and Burley, D.M. (1975) Anabolic steroids in athletes: cross-over double-blind trial in weightlifters. *Br. Med. J.*, **2**, 471–3.

Friedl, K.E. and Yesalis, C.E. (1989) Self-treatment of gynaecomastia in body-builders who use anabolic steroids. *Physician and Sports Medicine*, **17**, 67–79.

George, A.J. (1988) Anabolic steroids, in *Drugs in Sport*, (ed. D.R. Mottram), E. & F.N. Spon, London, p. 75.

George, A.J. (1994) Drugs in sport – chemists v. cheats, score draw! *Chem. Review*, **4**, 10–14.

Goldman, B. (1984) *Death in the Locker Room: Steroids and Sports*, Century Publishing, London.

Greenblatt, R.B., Chaddha, J.S., Teran, A.Z. and Nezhat, C.H. (1985) Aphrodisiacs, in *Psychopharmacology: Recent Advances and Future Prospects*, (ed. S.D. Iverson), British Association for Psychopharmacology Monograph No. 6, Oxford University Press, Oxford, pp. 290–302.

Haupt, H.A. and Rovere, G.D. (1984) Anabolic steroids: a review of the literature. *Am. J. Sports Med.*, **12**, 469–84.

Hervey, G.R. (1982) What are the effects of anabolic steroids?, in *Science and Sporting Performance: Management or Manipulation?*, (eds B. Davies and G. Thomas), Oxford University Press, Oxford, pp. 121–36.

Hervey, G.R., Knibbs, A.V., Burkinshaw, L. *et al.* (1981) Effects of methandienone on the performance and body composition of men undergoing athletic training. *Clin. Sci.*, **60**, 457–61.

Hodson, A. (1994) Football Association. Personal communication.

Holma, P.K. (1979) Effects of an anabolic steroid (methandienone) on spermatogenesis. *Contraception*, **15**, 151–62.

Jorgensen, J.O.L. and Christiansen, J.S. (1993) Brave new senescence. hGH in adults. *Lancet*, **341**, 1247–8.

Kannel, W.B., Castelli, W.P. and Gordon, T. (1979) Cholesterol in the prediction of atherosclerotic disease, new perspectives based on the Framingham Study. *Annals of Internal Medicine*, **90,** 85–91.

Kashkin, K.B. and Kleber, H.D. (1989) Hooked on hormones? An anabolic steroid addiction hypothesis. *J. Amer. Med. Assoc.*, **262,** 3166–70.

Kicman, A.T., Brooks, R.V. and Cowan, D.A. (1991) Human chorionic gonadotrophin and sport. *Br. J. Sport Med.*, **25**, 73–80.

Kicman, A.T. and Cowan, D.A. (1992) Peptide hormones and sport: misuse and detection. *Br. Med. Bul.*, **48**, 496–517.

Kicman, A.T., Oflebro, H., Walker, C. *et al.* (1993) Potential use of ketoconazole in a dynamic endocrine test to differentiate between biological outliers and testosterone use by athletes. *Clin. Chem.*, **39**, 1798–1803.

Kuipers, H., Wijnen, J.A.G., Hartgens, F. and Willems, S.M.M. (1991) Influence of anabolic steroids on body composition, blood pressure, lipid profile and liver functions in body-builders. *Int. J. Sports Med.*, **12**, 413–18.

Lamb, D.R. (1991) Anabolic steroids and athletic performance, in *Hormones and Sport*, (eds Z. Laron and A.D. Rogol), Raven Press, New York, pp. 259–73.

Laseter, J.T. and Russell, J.A. (1991) Anabolic steroid-induced tendon pathology: a review of the literature. *Med. Sci. Sports Exc.*, **23**, 1–3.

Leach, R.E. (1993) Anabolic steroids – round 4. *Am. J. Sports Med.*, **21**, 337.

Lombardo, J.A., Hickson, P.C. and Lamb, D.R. (1991) Anabolic/androgenic steroids and growth hormone, in *Perspectives in Exercise Science and Sports Medicine, Vol. 4: Ergogenics – Enhancement of Performance in Exercise and Sport*, (eds D.R. Lamb and M.H. Williams), Brown and Benchmark, New York, pp. 249–78.

Lubell, A. (1989) Does steroid abuse cause – or excuse – violence? *Phys. Sport Med.*, **17**, 176–85.

Lukas, S.E. (1993) Current perspectives on anabolic–androgenic steroid abuse. *Trends in Pharmacological Sciences*, **14**, 61–8.

Macintyre, J.G. (1987) Growth hormone and athletes. *Sports Med.*, **4**, 129–42.

Neely, E.K. and Rosenfield, R.G. (1994) Use and abuse of human growth hormone. *Ann. Rev. Med.*, **45**, 407–20.Payne, A.H. (1975) Anabolic steroids in athletics. *Br. J. Sports Med.*, **9**, 83–8.

Payne, A.H. (1975) Anabolic steroids in athletics. *Br. J. Sports Med.*, **9**, 83–8.

Perry, H.M., Wright, D. and Littlepage, B.N.C. (1992) Dying to be big: a review of anabolic steroid use. *Br. J. Sports Med.*, **26**, 259–61.

Pope, H.G. and Katz, D.L. (1988) Affective and psychotic symptoms associated with anabolic steroid use. *Am. J. Psychiat.*, **145**, 487–90.

Pope, H.G. and Katz, D.L. (1994) Psychiatric and medical effects of anabolic–androgenic steroid use. *Arch. Gen. Psychiat.*, **51**, 375–82.

Pope, H.G., Katz, D.L. and Champoux, R. (1988) Anabolic–androgenic steroid use among 1010 college men. *Physic. Sports Med.*, **16**, 75–81.

Report of the Statutory Committee of the Pharmaceutical Society of Great Britain (1989) *Pharmaceutical Journal*, 4 February, p. 144.

Rickert, V.I., Pawlak-Morello, C., Sheppard, V. and Jay, M.S. (1992) Human growth hormone: a new substance of abuse among adolescents? *Clin. Paediat.*, **31**, 723–6.

Rockhold, R.W. (1993) Cardiovascular toxicity of anabolic steroids. *Ann. Rev. Pharmac. Tox.*, **33**, 497–520.

Rogol, A.D. and Yesalis, C.E. (1992) Anabolic–androgenic steroids and athletes: what are the issues? *J. Endocr. Metab.*, **74**, 465–9.

Ryan, A.J. (1981) Anabolic steroids are fool's gold. *Fedn. Proc.*, **40**, 2682–8.

Sklarek, H.M., Mantovani, R.P., Erens, E. *et al.* (1984) AIDS in a body-builder using anabolic steroids. *N. Engl. J. Med.*, **311**, 861–2.

Smith, D.A. and Perry, P.J. (1992) The efficacy of ergogenic agents in athletic competitors. Part II: Other performance-enhancing agents. *Annals Pharmacother.*, **26**, 653–9.

Sports Council (1993) *Doping Control in Sport*, Sports Council, London.

Tanner, J. (1962) *Growth at Adolescence*, Blackwell, Oxford.

Taylor, W.N. (1988) Synthetic human growth hormone. A call for federal control. *Physic. Sports Med.*, **16**, 189–92.

Wagner, J.C. (1991) Enhancement of athletic performance with drugs. *Sports Med.*, **12**, 250–65.

Williamson, D.J. (1993) Anabolic steroid use among students at a British college of technology. *Br. J. Sports Med.*, **27**, 200–201.

Williamson, P.J. and Young, A.H. (1992) Psychiatric effects of androgenic and ana-bolic–androgenic steroid abuse in men: a brief review of the literature. *J. Psychopharmac.*, **6**, 20–26.

Wilson, J.D. (1988) Androgen abuse by athletes. *Endocr. Revs.*, **9**, 181–99.

Windsor, R.E. and Dumitru, D. (1988) Anabolic steroid use by athletes. *Postgrad. Med.*, **84**, 37–49.

Wright, J.E. (1980) Anabolic steroids and athletics. *Exercise and Sport Science Reviews*, **8**, 149–202.

Yang, Y.T. and McElliott, M.A. (1989) Multiple actions of β adrenergic agonists on skeletal muscle and adipose tissue. *Biochem. J.*, **261**, 1–10.

Yesalis, C.E., Herrick, R.T., Buckley, W.E. *et al.* (1988) Self-reported use of anabolic–androgenic steroids by elite powerlifters. *Physc. Sports Med.*, **16**, 91–100.

Blood boosting and sport

8

David J. Armstrong and Thomas Reilly

8.1 INTRODUCTION

In sports events or strenuous exercise lasting more than 1 minute, the predominant mode of energy production is aerobic. This means that performance is limited by the oxygen that is delivered and utilized by the active muscles. The level of performance is determined by the level of training which affects both central and peripheral factors. When the muscles are well trained, as in the case of élite endurance athletes, the limiting factors in determining the maximal oxygen uptake are the cardiac output and the oxygen-carrying capacity of the blood. The maximal cardiac output is also highly important when exercise is conducted in the heat since it then subserves two functions – the distribution of blood to the skin for thermoregulatory purposes and the supply of oxygen to the active muscles for energy metabolism.

The oxygen-carrying capacity of the blood is determined by the haemoglobin content which helps bind oxygen within the red blood cells. It is the total body haemoglobin rather than its relative concentrations which is correlated with the maximal oxygen uptake. When haemoglobin levels fall, exercise performance is impaired. Athletes and their mentors are cognizant of this and many performers regularly take iron supplements to prevent anaemia. It is also well recognized by sports practitioners that 'blood boosting' can enhance endurance performance. Consequently, various ways have been devised of augmenting the oxygen-carrying capacity of the blood of athletes. These methods include the so-called procedures of 'blood doping' as well as altitude training.

The mechanisms by which blood doping and altitude might work are analogous. They operate by elevating the number of red blood cells, either by infusion or increased production via the process of erythropoiesis. The

Drugs in Sport, 2nd edn. Edited by David R. Mottram. Published in 1996 by E & FN Spon, London. ISBN 0 419 18890 8

haematological background to erythropoiesis is first presented before the practice of blood boosting is described in an exercise context.

8.2 ERYTHROPOIESIS

Erythropoiesis, the production of the red blood cells takes place in haemopoietically active bone marrow. Nearly all bones contain haemopoietically active 'red' marrow for the first 2–3 years of life. In a normal adult the only sites of haemopoietically active marrow are to be found in the skull, bony thorax, vertebrae, iliac crests and the upper ends of the femur and humerus. The majority of bone marrow consists of fatty or yellow marrow which is haemopoietically inactive. It can become active once more in times of pathologically elevated demand for production of red blood cells.

Although erythropoiesis takes place within the bone marrow (i.e. medullary) it is extravascular, that is it occurs outside the blood vessels that supply and drain the bone marrow. The most primitive stem cells which are found in the endothelial lining of the medullary sinusoids are pluripotential haematopoietic stem cells (HSC) which can develop into any type of blood cell. The HSCs give rise to multipotent myeloid stem cells or colony-forming unit spleen (CFU-S) (Figure 8.1). These in turn are stimulated to mature into committed precursor cells, burst-forming units-erythroid (BFU-E) by interleukin-1 (IL-1), interleukin-6 (IL-6) and granulocyte colony-erythroid stimulating factor (G-CSF). Under the influence of interleukin-3 (IL-3), granulocyte-macrophage colony-stimulating factor (GM-CSF) and erythroid promoting factor (distinct from erythropoietin), which are produced in the bone marrow and act locally, BFU-E cells become committed to the formation of erythrocytes. They then give rise to discrete colony-forming unit-erythrocyte (CFU-E) cells which, in turn, generate discrete colonies of developing erythrocytes. The CFU-E is the first red cell precursor to possess receptors for erythropoietin.

The BFU-E compartment contains thousands of erythroblasts. The cells reach a maximum size by 14 days and produce 3–6 CFU-E. Each CFU-E forms clusters of erythrocytes (approximately 20–25) within 7 days. The BFU-E cells develop as islands of erythroblasts centred about a single histiocyte or macrophage. This cell, which has processes extending between the developing erythroblasts, is responsible for engulfing the extruded nuclei of the late normoblasts as they mature into reticulocytes (see below).

The first recognizable precursor of an erythrocyte is a pronormoblast (Figure 8.2). This cell is 15–20 µm in diameter, with a nucleus containing 1–2 nucleoli, mitochondria but no haemoglobin. It divides mitotically three times, giving three generations of normoblasts: early or basophilic, intermediate or neutrophilic, and late or eosinophilic. The terms baso-neutro- and eosinophilic refer to the affinity for histological stains. As the normoblasts develop they synthesize haemoglobin which stains with eosin and confers a pink tinge upon the cytoplasm. The development of normoblasts is also characterized by a decrease in cell diameter and condensation of nuclear material, such that the cytoplasm:nucleus ratio increases from early to intermediate to late normoblast. The late normoblast is approximately 10–12 μm in diameter, has a dense pyknotic nucleus and is almost fully haemoglobinized. It is incapable of mitotic division and further development occurs by maturation. Intramedullary development from pronormoblast to late normoblast takes approximately 3 days.

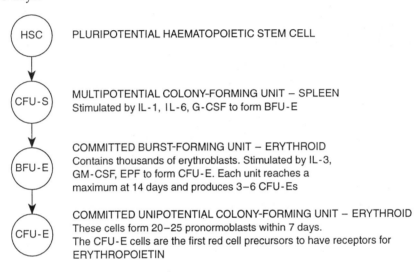

Figure 8.1 Early stages in the development of red cell precursors.

Development to this stage has been intramedullary but extravascular. The developing erythrocyte must now enter the circulation. The late normoblast loses its nucleus by extrusion. The residue of the cell passes between the junctions of the medullary capillaries by diapedesis (amoeboid-like movement) and enters the circulation as a reticulocyte. This cell is slightly smaller than a late normoblast (8–10 μm diameter) and lacks a nucleus. It contains residual ribosomal material and mitochondria which have an affinity for haematoxylin and which confer a blue reticular appearance upon the cytoplasm, hence the name of the cell. Final maturation to the mature erythrocyte involves completion of haemoglobinization and loss of reticular material. This occurs either during sequestration in the spleen or in the circulation and takes 24–48 hours.

The mature red blood cell is a biconcave disc, diameter 6.7–7.7 μm, volume 85 ± 8 fl containing an average of 29.5 ± 2.5 pg of haemoglobin. Mature

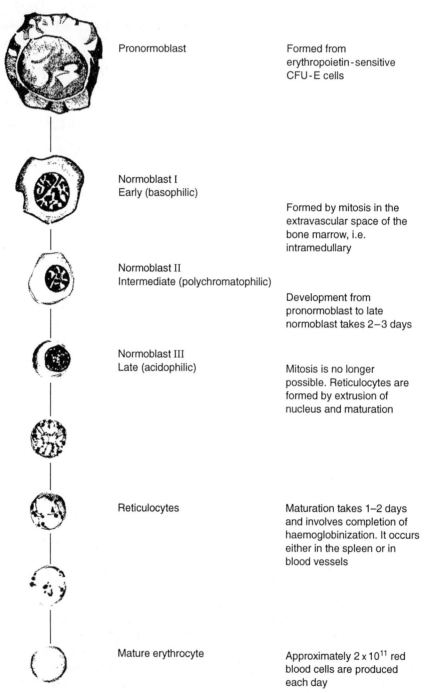

Pronormoblast — Formed from erythropoietin-sensitive CFU-E cells

Normoblast I
Early (basophilic)

Formed by mitosis in the extravascular space of the bone marrow, i.e. intramedullary

Normoblast II
Intermediate (polychromatophilic)

Development from pronormoblast to late normoblast takes 2–3 days

Normoblast III
Late (acidophilic)

Mitosis is no longer possible. Reticulocytes are formed by extrusion of nucleus and maturation

Reticulocytes

Maturation takes 1–2 days and involves completion of haemoglobinization. It occurs either in the spleen or in blood vessels

Mature erythrocyte

Approximately 2×10^{11} red blood cells are produced each day

Figure 8.2 Stages in development of committed red blood cells.

erythrocytes have neither a nucleus, RNA nor mitochondria. They have an inability to synthesize enzymes and to produce adenosine triphosphate (ATP) aerobically. They metabolize glucose by glycolysis, to produce ATP for maintenance of cationic pumps, and by the hexose monophosphate pathway for generation of reduced NAD^+P for maintenance of haemoglobin in the reduced state (Bick *et al.*, 1993). They have a finite lifespan of 120 days. After that time they are removed by the reticulo-endothelial system, principally the spleen. If anaemia is not to develop, the rate of production of new erythrocytes must equal the rate of destruction. Consequently, 0.83% of the circulating red cell mass must be replaced each day. Since the total red cell mass, the erythron, is approximately 3×10^{13} cells, that means that some 2.5×10^{11} erythrocytes must be produced and released each day, i.e. some 3×10^6 per second. The total body haemoglobin contained in 3×10^{13} cells is approximately 900 g.

The normal red cell indices by which anaemia is diagnosed and classified are shown in Table 8.1.

Table 8.1 Normal red cell indices

		Male	Female	Units
Red cell count	(RBC)	5.5 ± 1.0	4.8 ± 1.0	10^{12}/l
Haemoglobin concentration	(Hb%)	15.1 ± 2.5	14.0 ± 2.5	g/dl
Mean corpuscular volume	(MCV)	85 ± 8	85 ± 8	fl
Mean corpuscular haemoglobin	(MCH)	29.5 ± 2.5	29.5 ± 2.5	pg
Mean corpuscular haemoglobin conc.	(MCHC)	33 ± 2	33 ± 2	g/dl
Packed cell volume or haematocrit	(PCV or HCT)	0.47 ± 0.07	0.42 ± 0.05	l/l

8.2.1 REGULATION OF ERYTHROPOIESIS

Erythropoietin in health

The rate of production of red blood cells must be closely regulated because of the huge number of cells involved (3×10^6/s). Erythropoiesis is controlled by the circulating level of **erythropoietin**, a glycoprotein hormone which consists of 166 amino acids and has a molecular weight of 34 000. In adults, it is produced primarily in the kidney with a minor contribution from the liver. It has a half-life of 5 hours and is inactivated in the liver. Normal serum concentration is approximately 20 mU or 10 pM.

The stimulus for the production of erythropoietin is reduced oxygen delivery to the kidney. This may happen as a result of either altitude-induced hypoxia (including training-induced (8.3)) haemorrhage, cardiovascular disease, respiratory disease or anaemia. A reduction in tissue oxygen pressure can increase red cell production by as much as 6–9 times by stimulation of erythropoietin secretion. Secretion is facilitated by the action of catecholamines upon beta adrenergic receptors. Androgens increase erythropoiesis and have been used with some success to treat aplastic anaemia. Cobalt, thyroid hormone (by an indirect effect upon metabolic rate and oxygen requirement), adrenal corticosteroids (directly), growth hormone and stimulation of peripheral chemoreceptors all increase erythropoietin production (Hoffbrand and Lewis, 1989; Ganong, 1995).

The site of production of erythropoietin is the endothelial cells of the peritubular capillaries in the renal cortex. The hypoxaemia-sensitive receptor contains a haem moiety. The deoxy form of the haem moiety stimulates, and the oxy form inhibits, the transcription of the erythropoietin gene to form erythropoietin mRNA (Ganong, 1995). The system is extremely sensitive. A decrease in haematocrit below 20% results in a hundred-fold increase in erythropoietin.

Mode of action of erythropoietin

Erythropoietin stimulates proliferation of late BFU-E cells and controls the rate at which the erythropoietin-sensitive cells (CFU-E) give rise to pronormoblasts. The effect is receptor-mediated. Within minutes there is a burst of RNA synthesis. This is followed after several hours by an

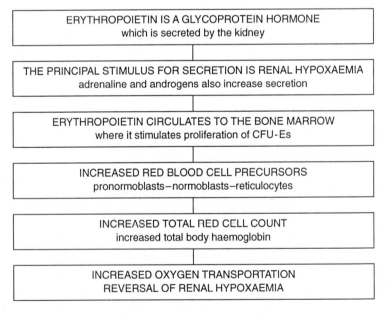

Figure 8.3 Regulation of erythropoiesis by erythropoietin.

increase in DNA synthesis. Stimulation of nucleic acid synthesis increases the number of committed stem cells, increases the rate of cell division, decreases the maturation time of more mature cells and increases haemoglobin synthesis. The net effect is an increase in the number of erythrocytes that are produced and the rate at which they are released into the circulation (Figure 8.3).

8.2.2 ERYTHROPOIETIN IN DISEASE

Increased secretion of erythropoietin causes an increase in the number of circulating erythrocytes, secondary polycythaemia, characterized by elevated haemoglobin and haematocrit. The increases can be of both renal and extra-renal origin. Renal causes include renal cell carcinoma, renal cysts, hydronephrosis and renal graft rejection. Extra-renal causes include hepatoma, phaeochromocytoma and cerebellar haemangioblastoma.

Secondary polycythaemia can also be caused by increased erythropoietin secondary to decreased tissue oxygenation, caused by low arterial oxygen saturation consequent upon chronic lung disease, right–left shunts and altitude exposure or, alternatively, normal oxygen saturation consequent upon sleep apnoea, high affinity haemoglobins and abnormal 2,3-bisphosphoglycerate (2,3-BPG) metabolism.

8.2.3 RECOMBINANT ERYTHROPOIETIN

The gene responsible for the synthesis of erythropoietin has been located and characterized on chromosome 7. Recombinant erythropoietin (rEPO) is licensed in the UK for the treatment of anaemia associated with chronic renal failure. Before erythropoietin is prescribed, other possible causes of anaemia or chronic renal failure should be excluded, e.g. iron and folate deficiency should be corrected. Erythropoietin can be administered either subcutaneously or intravenously. The dose is adjusted according to the patient's response. The aim is to increase haemoglobin concentration at a rate not exceeding 2 g/100 ml/month to a stable level of 10–12 g/100 ml (British National Formulary, 1995). A typical regimen for Epoetin Alfa (human rEPO) would be 50 units/kg three times weekly, increased according to response in steps of 25 units/kg at intervals of 4 weeks. The maximum dose is 600 units/kg weekly in three divided doses. The maintenance dose is usually 100–300 units/kg weekly in 2–3 divided doses.

Treatment requires careful supervision because of the risk of a dose-dependent increase in blood pressure. This may evoke an acute hypertensive crisis which necessitates urgent medical attention (British National Formulary, 1995).

8.3 EXERCISE AT ALTITUDE

As altitude increases, the barometric pressure falls. At sea level the normal pressure is 760 mmHg, at 1000 m it is 680 mmHg, at 3000 m it is about 540 mmHg and at the top of Mt. Everest (height 8848 m) it is 250 mmHg. So high-altitude conditions are referred to as low-pressure or hypobaric conditions.

The main problem associated with hypobaric environments is what we term hypoxia. Although the proportion of oxygen in the air at any altitude is constant at 20.93%, as ambient pressure decreases (with increase in altitude) the air is less dense. As a result there are fewer oxygen molecules in a given volume of air, and, if we were to inspire the same volume of air as at sea level, less oxygen would be inspired. Thus the uptake of oxygen into the body by the lungs is decreased and there is a decreased rate of oxygen delivery to the tissues where it is needed. However, the body is able to show some adaptive responses which compensate for the relative lack of oxygen in the air. Although these responses begin immediately on exposure to hypobaric conditions, for some people the full response is not manifested until weeks or months at altitude. It is to be noted, however, that even with complete acclimatization, the sea-level visitor to altitude is never as completely adapted as the individual born and bred at altitude. This becomes apparent with endurance sports events in particular.

The hypoxia of altitude is probably more widely recognized in mountaineering than in any other sporting activity. Mountaineers need to have very good aerobic fitness levels to climb the high peaks. The conventional practice has been to use oxygen to compensate for the reduced alveolar oxygen tension. In 1978, it was shown that Mt. Everest could be climbed without supplementary oxygen! This was possible with mountaineers who had a high VO_2max., were acclimatized and were favoured by the day-to-day variations in atmospheric pressure on the peak. At this level of altitude, prior acclimatization at medium altitude is essential. Nevertheless the ascents need to be planned so that the time above 6000 m is restricted to avoid inevitable high-altitude deterioration. Above an altitude of 5200 m (the highest permanent settlement in the Andes) acclimatization is replaced by a steady deterioration.

8.4 PHYSIOLOGICAL ADAPTATIONS TO ALTITUDE

An immediate physiological response to exercise in hypobaric conditions or lack of oxygen is respiratory compensation. This achieved by an increased tidal volume (depth of breathing) and/or an increased respiratory frequency. An increase in depth of respiration is the main response, especially relevant during sports such as swimming and running where the breathing rate is synchronized with stroke patterns.

The hyperventilation (increase in breathing) that occurs on exposure to altitude causes a problem in that more carbon dioxide is 'blown off' from blood passing through the lungs. Elimination of carbon dioxide, which is a weak acid in solution in the blood, leaves the blood more alkaline than normal because of an excess of bicarbonate ions. The kidneys compensate by excreting bicarbonate over several days, which helps return the acidity of the blood towards normal. The outcome is that the alkaline reserve is decreased, and so the blood has a poorer buffering capacity for tolerating entry of additional acids into it. Consequently lactic acid diffusing from muscle into blood during exercise at altitude will be more difficult to neutralize. High-intensity performance will decline earlier than at sea level because of this, and the intensity of aerobic exercise training will need to be reduced for training sessions to be sustained.

The low oxygen tension (partial pressure) does not significantly affect the uptake of oxygen by the red blood cells until the oxygen pressure declines to a certain point (Figure 8.4). However, with adaptation to altitude the critical oxygen pressure falls. This results from increased production of 2,3-BPG by the red blood cells, and is beneficial in that it aids the unloading of oxygen from the red cells at the tissues. The oxygen-carrying capacity of the blood is enhanced by an increase in the number of red blood cells. This process begins within a few days of altitude, and is stimulated by erythropoietin secreted by the kidneys which later causes increased red blood cell production by the bone marrow. As a result the bone marrow increases its iron uptake to form haemoglobin after about 48 hours at altitude. If the individual remains at high altitude, it takes 2–3 weeks to secure a true increase in total body haemoglobin and the red cell count continues to increase for a year or more but does not attain the values observed in high-altitude natives. The haemoglobin concentration also

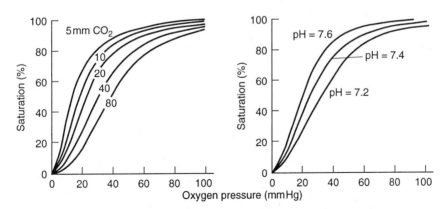

Figure 8.4   The oxygen–haemoglobin saturation curve: the influence of carbon dioxide is shown on the left and the effect of changes in pH on the right.

increases, and there is a rise in haematocrit, the percentage of blood volume occupied by red blood cells.

On first exposure to altitude there is an increase in heart rate. Later, successful adaptation to altitude results in a reduction in the heart rate to near normal level.

Within a few days of reaching an altitude location a rise in haemoglobin concentration is apparent, but this initial increase in haemoglobin is a result of haemoconcentration due to the drop in plasma volume. Nevertheless there is a gradual true increase in haemoglobin which is mediated by stimulation of the bone marrow to over-produce red blood cells in the course of erythropoiesis, as explained earlier. This requires that the body's iron stores are adequate and may, indeed, mean supplementation of iron intake prior to and during the stay at altitude.

Upon return to sea level it will take a few days for the acid–base status to be re-established. Hypoxia no longer stimulates erythropoiesis and the elevated red cell count will slowly come down. The decreased affinity of red blood cells for oxygen, which facilitated unloading to the active tissues by means of the activity of 2,3-BPG, is soon lost on return to sea level. Any exploitation of the haematological adaptation must be carefully timed to occur before the red blood cell count returns to normality: this may take up to 6 weeks. Otherwise, repeated sojourns to altitude are needed.

The use of altitude training camps for enhancement of sea-level performance has received renewed interest in the 1990s amongst British coaches. The outcome was a symposium convened by the British Olympic Association (1993). This was an attempt to coordinate the experiences of the various sports and provided an opportunity to consider the relevance of altitude training for games players.

Middle and distance runners used a range of altitude locations from Albuquerque (1500 m) to Mexico City (2300 m). The difference in these two exposures was reflected in a significant increase in haemoglobin concentration at Mexico and no change after Albuquerque. It does seem that an altitude in excess of 2000 m, when the reduction in ambient pressure takes the oxygen-saturation curve of haemoglobin into a steep decline, is needed to induce an appreciable effect.

The most comprehensive monitoring of athletes was of the rowers. Particular attention was given to reducing the training load on early exposure to avoid acute mountain sickness. Later, individuals were carefully programmed with increased training loads and metabolic responses were recorded (Grobler and Faulmann, 1993). The programme took into account the competitive schedule following return to sea level. There is not complete consensus on the timing of this return to sea level before participation in major competition.

A study of Swedish skiers was carried out for a similar 3-week period at 1.9 km with a subsequent long-term follow-up. Ingjer and Myhre (1992) reported that a strict liquid intake regimen was effective in reducing the fall in plasma volume associated with dehydration at altitude. The blood lactate response to a sub-maximal exercise test was lowered on immediate return to sea level. This decrease was correlated with the improvement in haemoglobin and haematocrit that occurred at altitude. It seems that those that benefit most from altitude training are those with the greatest room for elevating oxygen-carrying capacity.

The level of altitude seemingly influences the stimulatory effect of erythropoietin. At about 1900 m the rise in serum erythropoietin is about 30% higher than at sea level after 2–3 days, but at 4500 m this increase is about 300%. Serum erythropoietin concentrations decrease after approximately 1 week at altitude, and this may be associated with increased oxygenation of the tissues due to 2,3-BPG. The average true rise in haemoglobin approximates to 1% each week, at least at altitudes between 1.8 and 3 km (Berglund, 1992).

Best estimates are that optimal haematological adaptations to altitude take around 80 days. This may be accelerated by periodic visits to higher altitude (up to about 3 km) but not training there. The inability to tolerate high training loads at altitude may lead to a drop in aerobic fitness which offsets the positive effects of the altitude sojourn. The answer may be a combination of living at altitude for a sustained period but frequently returning to near-sea level (locally if possible) for strenuous exercise training.

8.5 BLOOD DOPING

Blood doping refers to artificial means of producing high concentrations of red blood cells. It is called 'blood boosting' also, and known physiologically as induced polycythaemia. It can be achieved in two ways: by transfusing matched blood from a donor, in much the same way as compatible blood for therapeutic transfusions is drawn from a blood bank; and by drawing an amount of blood from an athlete, storing the frozen red cells for 4 to 5 weeks or longer and later reinfusing them to augment the extra cells produced in the meantime to compensate for those withdrawn earlier.

Transfusional polycythaemia was used in the 1970s to correct for anaemia in a Finnish 3000 m steeplechaser who broke the world record soon after receiving a transfusion but otherwise made little impact on the track. Since that time a number of notable Finnish distance runners have admitted to using blood doping, whilst the ploy has also been linked with US cyclists at the 1984 Olympics and with Italian runners and cyclists. The improved performance capability is achieved virtually overnight. Once the excess fluid is excreted, the blood is left with a supranormally high red cell count. This elevates the oxygen-carrying capability of the blood which delivers more oxygen to the active muscles. The same end result is achieved from reinfusing one's own blood after a few weeks' storage, a ploy which avoids risks associated with any error in matching blood donations.

The early experiments on blood reinfusion did not all agree that this manoeuvre was effective as an ergogenic measure. The main reason for

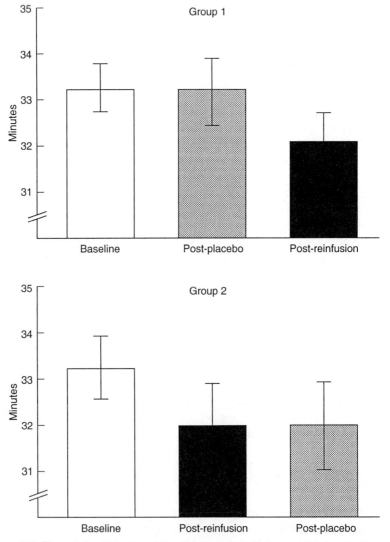

Figure 8.5 The relation between 10 km times and reinfusion or placebo. In Group 1, running time fell after infusion but not after placebo. In Group 2, time fell after reinfusion and the improvement was maintained 13 days afterwards at the time of a placebo infusion. (Brien and Simon, 1987.)

inconclusive findings was that the refrigerated blood cells aged in storage. Storage of packed cells from 900 to 1000 ml of blood with special freezing techniques can provoke a 10% increase in haemoglobin when the cells are reinfused. Some experimenters have reinfused up to 1.5 litres of freeze-preserved blood, but it is usual to infuse only the packed cells. Mostly, volumes of 800 to 900 ml have been withdrawn (usually two separate phlebotomies) but reinfused volumes of 400 to 500 ml have proved effective in enhancing performance; improvements have been shown in maximal oxygen uptake and in endurance performance of runners and skiers. Runners over 10 km have displayed improvements of over 1 minute in their times (Figure 8.5), whilst experiments have also indicated improvements in 1500 m running. The runners also showed a decrease in sub-maximal heart rate in response to a set treadmill run (Brien and Simon, 1987). The characteristic change in performance is that the runners do not slow down during the later parts of their races but can maintain a steady pace to the end without relenting. The improvement in performance was retained over at least a 2-week period.

8.6 THE USE OF ERYTHROPOIETIN IN BLOOD BOOSTING

The natural improvement in oxygen transport with acclimatization to altitude is due to increased synthesis of erythropoietin. The result on return to sea level is an increased oxygen-carrying capacity of the blood and an improved potential for endurance performance in trained individuals. It is possible to simulate the benefits of altitude training upon secretion of erythropoietin by administration of synthetic or human rEPO. The administration of rEPO has a pronounced effect on the aerobic performance of endurance athletes, once time is allowed for the over-stimulation of the bone marrow to have its effects. It increases the red cell count, haemoglobin, haematocrit and reticulocyte count. However, it also affects the type of red blood cell produced by the bone marrow. Casoni *et al.* (1993) noted a significant increase in the percentage of red blood cells with a mean corpuscular volume $> 120 \, fl$ and a mean corpuscular haemoglobin $< 28 \, pg$. These cells are described as macrocytic and hypochromic. This increase was not the result of simultaneous decreases in vitamin B_{12}, folic acid and/or iron, as supplements were provided to recipients of erythropoietin. Moreover, erythropoietin increases macrocytosis and hypochromasia in patients with renal disease.

The use of rEPO does have serious risks if administered to athletes. The magnitude of the increase in red blood cell production cannot be accurately gauged and the haematocrit may eventually be raised to dangerously high levels thus increasing systolic blood pressure and blood viscosity. The combination of increased blood viscosity and elevated blood pressure can lead to left ventricular hypertrophy and, ultimately, to left ventricular failure. There is also an increased possibility of thrombosis and stroke. The risk may be accentuated by haemocon-centration and dehydration during prolonged exercise. In 1990 *L'Equipe* drew attention to the long list of cyclists who had died of heart failure, either during or shortly after the end of their careers. The *Observer* (1991) cited 16 early deaths in Dutch cyclists in the preceding 20 years, of which 12 had occurred between 1987 and 1991. This coincided with the alleged advent of the illicit use of erythropoietin in sport. The evidence is circumstantial but entirely consistent with the pathophysiology of cardiac failure.

A study of Canadian swimmers at an altitude of 1.85 km provided a chance of monitoring the changes in haemoglobin and erythropoietin during the stay at the training camp and for 6 months afterwards. The increases in erythropoietin differed between endurance swimmers and sprint specialists. The results did not clarify how specific training deter-mines the erythropoietin response to altitude exposure, and there is scope here for more research (Roberts and Smith, 1992).

8.7 BLOOD DOPING CONTROL

Blood doping in any of its forms and the use of rEPO in sports are contrary to the regulations which prohibit the use of physiological substances in abnormal amounts, by abnormal methods and with the exclusive aim of obtaining an artificial or unfair increase in performance in competition. The International Olympic Committee (IOC) added 'blood doping' to its banned procedures in 1985. The potential abuse of rEPO became known later and resulted in the IOC banning its use in 1990. Methods have been developed for the detection of these abusers but the techniques are not foolproof. For example it may be possible to set a threshold for the percentage of macrocytic and hypochromic red cells above which only recipients of erythropoietin would be found. However, this would only detect 50% of erythropoietin abusers and leave the other 50% undetected (Casoni *et al.*, 1993). Acceptance of rEPO administration by some athletes and their mentors reflects the lengths to which they are prepared to go to gain a competitive advantage.

Altitude training to enhance subsequent performance capability at sea level is widely used by sea-level natives in a range of sports. Such a manoeuvre is legal and has spawned the development of training camps based at altitude resorts. The benefits of the haematological adaptation to altitude will depend on a host of factors. These include the nature of the sport, the training and nutritional state of the athlete, the duration of the sojourn, the frequency of visits to altitude and the timing of the return to sea level. The opportunity to take advantage of altitude training depends either on an accident of birth or the financial support available to the sea-level dweller. Even then, exposure to altitude demands careful attention to physiological detail so that adverse effects (such as acute mountain sickness) are avoided and the training stimulus carefully matched to the prevailing capability of the individual.

8.8 CONCLUSION

The maximal oxygen uptake of aerobically trained sportspersons is limited largely by their cardiac output and the oxygen-carrying capacity of their blood. The latter is determined by the total body haemoglobin. Since it is not possible to increase, artificially, the haemoglobin content of individual red cells, the strategy of practitioners has been to increase the total number of red cells and hence the overall quantity of haemoglobin that the 'erythron' contains. This led to the introduction of altitude training into the programmes of élite aerobic sportsmen and women. The cost in terms of time, inconvenience and money led to the search for alternative methods for augmenting the total red cell count. The first approach was to reinfuse the subjects' own packed red cells. However, the lifespan of reinfused cells was relatively brief, a couple of weeks at the most. The advent of rEPO provided a means of directly stimulating erythropoiesis without the need for withdrawal and subsequent reinfusion of red blood cells. The administration of rEPO would appear to confer an unfair advantage upon the recipient. It is contrary to the ethos of sport, is banned by the IOC and may have been linked to the death of élite professional cyclists. Unfortunately, however, blood doping cannot be detected with confidence, hence it is likely to continue until such time as detection does become foolproof or the ideal of fair play is totally restored to the competitive sport environment.

8.9 REFERENCES

Berglund, B. (1992) High altitude training: aspects of haematological adaptations. *Sports Medicine*, **14**, 289–303.

Bick, R.L., Bennett, J.M., Brynes, R.K. *et al.* (1993) *Haematology: Clinical and Laboratory Practice*, Mosby, St Louis, Missouri.

Brien, T. and Simon, T.L. (1987) The effects of red blood cell infusion on 10 km race time. *JAMA*, **257**, 2761–5.

British National Formulary. Number 29, March (1995) British Medical Association and the Royal Pharmaceutical Society of Great Britain.

British Olympic Association (1993) *The Altitude Factor in Athletic Performance.* Proceedings of International Symposium (Lilleshall), 13–15 December, BOA, London.

Casoni, I., Ricci, G., Ballarin, E. *et al.* (1993) Haematological indices of erythropoietin administration in athletes. *Int. J. Sports Med.*, **14**, 307–11.

Ganong, W.F. (1995) *Review of Medical Physiology*, 7th edn, Appleton & Lange, Connecticut, USA.

Grobler, J. and Faulmann, L. (1993) The British experience. *BOA Technical News*, **1**(5), 3–5.

Hoffbrand, A.V. and Lewis, S.M. (eds) (1989) *Postgraduate Haematology*, 3rd edn, Heineman Medical Books, Oxford.

Ingjer, F. and Myhre, K. (1992) Physiological effects of altitude training on young élite male cross-country skiers. *J. Sports Sci.*, **10**, 49–63.

International Meeting of IOC, April 1990, Lausanne, Switzerland.

Roberts, D. and Smith, D.J. (1992) Serum erythropoietin of élite swimmers training at moderate altitude, in *Biomechanics and Medicine in Swimming: Swimming Science VI*, (eds D. MacLaren, T. Reilly and A. Lees), E. and F.N. Spon, London, pp. 341–5.

Doping control in sport 9

Michele Verroken and David R. Mottram

9.1 HISTORY OF DRUG TESTING

The ingestion of substances to enhance performance in sport is probably as old as sport itself. However, the widespread use of sophisticated chemical agents began in the 1950s and 1960s in parallel with the evolution of the modern pharmaceutical industry. New drugs were being discovered through methods of chemical synthesis rather than from extraction of plant or animal sources. In parallel with this, the pharmaceutical industry developed its processes of chemical analysis in order to test its products for efficacy and safety. This evolution of sensitive methods of drug screening was vital for the subsequent quest for accurate methods of drug testing in sport.

A number of sports federations introduced drug testing in the 1950s and early 1960s. Tests were targeted at amphetamines, which were then the most widely misused performance-enhancing agents. Amphetamines had been implicated in the death of the cyclist, Knut Jensen, at the 1964 Rome Olympics (Beckett and Cowan, 1979; Voy, 1991) and of the British cyclist, Tommy Simpson, who died on the 13th day of the Tour de France in 1967. These most public examples of the use of drugs to improve performance pressured some sports organizations into action.

Early testing methods were relatively unsophisticated: the technology available to analyse an athlete's urine resulted in inaccurate findings that failed to deter the use of drugs. Athletes realized that a clearance time between drug use and testing was all that was needed to avoid traces of banned substances, particularly the metabolites of substances, being detected. At that time athletes were being tested after a competition and had little difficulty in calculating clearance times. Moreover, the detection methods were not capable of unequivocal detection of anabolic steroids, substances known to enhance the effects of training.

Drugs in Sport, 2nd edn. Edited by David R. Mottram. Published in 1996 by E & FN Spon, London. ISBN 0 419 18890 8

Although the International Olympic Committee (IOC) was amongst the first to establish rules about doping and to introduce testing, it was preceded by FIFA (Fédération Internationale de Football Association) which introduced testing at the 1966 World Cup in England and by the UCI (Union Cycliste Internationale) which formed its Medical Examination Regulations in 1967. The IOC first set up a Medical Commission in 1961, under the Chairmanship of Sir Arthur Porritt. In 1967 the IOC re-established the Medical Commission under the Chairmanship of Prince Alexandre de Merode from Belgium, a former cyclist who had been working towards the development of a doping control programme in the 1950s. The Commission has three main responsibilities:

1. for guidance and approval to the host country of an Olympic Games on medical and paramedical equipment and facilities at the Olympic Village;
2. for doping controls at the Olympic Games, for classifying the pharmacological substances and methods and for proposing sanctions to the IOC Executive Board when doping rules have been contravened;
3. for femininity control of women's sporting events at the Games and issuing certificates of femininity to those who have passed the control.

The IOC instituted its first compulsory doping controls at the Winter Olympic Games in Grenoble, France, in 1968 and again at the Summer Olympic Games in Mexico City in the same year. At that time the list of banned substances issued in 1967 included narcotic analgesics and stimulants, which comprised sympathomimetic amines, psychomotor stimulants and miscellaneous central nervous system stimulants. Although it was suspected that androgenic anabolic steroids were being used at this time (Beckett, 1981; Wade, 1972), testing methods were insufficiently developed to warrant the inclusion of anabolic steroids in the list of banned substances.

When testing took place at the Games of 1968 it was of a limited nature. One athlete was disqualified for using alcohol. The IOC itself was clear about the limits of its responsibility on doping control; the International Olympic Committee *Newsletter* of August 1968 stated:

> The function of the IOC is to alert the National Olympic Committees and the international federations and promote an education campaign. The International Olympic Committee has its rule and has defined dope and it should see that provisions are made by the Organising Committee for testing but the actual testing is left in the hands of others. This is a responsibility that the International Olympic Committee is not prepared to take.

Subsequently, the IOC extended its responsibilities for accrediting laboratories and for the testing programme at the Olympic Games. It takes no responsibility for testing outside the Games, despite a clear involvement because of its accredited laboratories and its publication of a list of doping classes and methods adopted by the majority of sports.

The first full-scale testing of Olympic athletes occurred at the 1972 Summer Olympics in Munich, Germany (de Merode, 1979). Again, tests were limited to narcotic analgesics and to the three classes of stimulants; however testing was much more comprehensive, with 2079 samples being analysed. Seven athletes were disqualified, one athlete having already been disqualified at the Winter Games in Sapporo.

9.1.1 INTRODUCTION OF TESTS FOR ANABOLIC STEROIDS

At St Thomas's Hospital, London, Professor Raymond Brooks had been developing methods for detecting anabolic steroids in the early 1970s. Unofficial tests for these substances were undertaken at the 1972 Munich Games. The test for anabolic steroids at that time was based on radio-immunoassay (Brooks, Firth and Sumner, 1975). Using this method it was possible to carry out sufficient tests over a short period of time to allow the method to be adopted at a major sporting event. The IOC therefore added anabolic steroids to the list of banned substances in 1975.

The first official tests for anabolic steroids were carried out at the Montreal Olympic Games in Canada in 1976 (Hatton and Catlin, 1987). Of the samples collected, 15% (some 275 samples) were tested for anabolic steroids at these Games, and of the 11 athletes disqualified, eight had been using anabolic steroids. Similar tests were conducted at the Moscow Olympic Games in 1980; however no incidence of drug taking was reported. The Chairman of the IOC Medical Commission told a press conference that technical difficulties in testing for testosterone cast doubt on the findings (Sydney *Morning Herald*, 18 August 1980, quoted in *Drugs in Sport: An Interim Report of the Senate Standing Committee on Environment, Recreation and the Arts,* 1989).

Some anabolic steroids were not detectable through radioimmunoassay. A new assay based on gas chromatography/mass spectrometry (GC-MS) was, however, being developed. This method that identified banned substances in the urine in minute quantities (one part per billion) by molecular weight, also permitted the detection of the naturally occurring steroid, testosterone. The adoption of the GC-MS method for testing androgenic anabolic steroids and testosterone at the 1983 Pan-American Games in Caracas, Venezuela, led to the disqualification of 19 athletes. However, many athletes withdrew from the Games, presumably to avoid the testing programme. At the 1984 Olympic Games in Los Angeles, of the 1510 samples taken, 12 were found to contain anabolic steroids or testosterone (Catlin *et al.*, 1987). At the Seoul Olympic Games in 1988, there were 10 positive drug tests, of which four were for anabolic steroids. An additional six cases were reported by the laboratory as containing a substance from a banned pharmacological class, but the IOC Medical Commission decided that these cases should not be considered as positive (IOC Laboratory Statistics, 1991). The Barcelona Games of 1992 were more indicative of the increased level of testing to disqualify athletes before they compete in the Olympics. Although screening programmes are regarded as unethical, the enhanced level of testing that precedes a major event revealed a number of athletes prepared to take the risk and use drugs. At the Games itself, there were only five positive tests reported. Testing at the Winter Olympic Games in Albertville (1992) and Lillehammer (1994) revealed no reports of drug abuse.

The fight against doping has not been one which sport has had to face alone – there have been other significant developments that have involved governments and international sports and health organizations. Progress and major landmarks are described more fully in section 9.4 on testing programmes in this chapter.

9.1.2 OUT-OF-COMPETITION TESTING

Testing was originally scheduled after a competition had taken place. Athletes having taken part in an event knew there was a possibility that they could be selected for testing. To counter this, athletes started to reschedule their drug use to the training period and to calculate clearance times in the body. It was evident that the testing programmes themselves would have to develop. Testing out of competition was trialled and found to be a useful deterrent as athletes could be tested at any time; moreover the testing coincided more closely with athletes' drug regimes.

Norway was the first country to conduct out-of-competition controls; starting in 1977, the programme was increased to 75% of the total programme by 1988. In the UK, out-of-competition testing was introduced in the early 1980s. In 1985, the Sports Council financed a pilot scheme for out-of-season testing of British track and field athletes eligible for international selection. The (then) British Amateur Athletic Board began a programme of random out-of-competition testing from a register of eligible athletes (Bottomley, 1988).

The experiences of these early testing programmes were significant in shaping the present day systems. Additional measures have been introduced to extend this testing programme abroad, wherever the athlete may be, and to make non-availability for testing (by failure to notify the sport's governing body if the athlete is absent from the notified address for a period of 5 days or longer) a doping offence. The key principle of out-of-competition testing is to give the athlete short or no notice of the test, to reduce any opportunity to manipulate the procedure. Although other countries and organizations have introduced out-of-competition testing, it is not carried out world-wide.

9.2 IOC ACCREDITED LABORATORIES

Testing of body fluids for the presence of pharmacological substances is routinely carried out in laboratories throughout the world. For major sporting events and for the programmes of doping control in sport, this testing is carried out by laboratories accredited by the IOC. Such laboratories receive accreditation by complying with written guidelines regarding the equipment to be available, the general analytical procedures to be followed and a code of ethics by which the laboratory must operate.

Accreditation began in 1976, although the proposal to create accredited laboratories was not formally adopted until 1980 (Royal Society of New Zealand, 1990). The first accredited laboratories were those that had already analysed samples from international competitions, namely Cologne, Kriescha, Moscow, Montreal and London. Re-accreditation was introduced in 1985, primarily to avoid legal challenges to the operating standards of these laboratories (Dubin, 1990). Through an increased volume of testing and further development of the laboratory accreditation process, an internationally acknowledged standard has been obtained.

An accredited laboratory must allow itself to be subjected to periodic, 4-monthly, testing by the IOC and must seek re-accreditation each year. Initial accreditation requires the successful identification of three sets of 10 samples over a period of 6–12 months. Supported by documentation, a similar analytical test on accreditation is carried out in the presence of a delegate of the IOC Sub-commission on Doping and Biochemistry. Re-accreditation involves analysis of up to 10 control samples within a specified time limit (IOC, 1990).

IOC accredited laboratories currently analyse urine samples, although the use of blood samples as a supplementary form of evidence is presently under investigation. Analysis of blood may provide the evidence of blood doping (or boosting) and may indicate more clearly the levels of endogenous (naturally occurring) substances. For major sporting events, the laboratories must be able to report on results within 24 to 48 hours of receiving the sample.

The requirements for Accreditation and Good Laboratory Practice, version 5 (Dugal and Donike, 1988) were published as an appendix to the International Olympic Charter against Doping in Sport. These requirements were intended to specify the competence levels of laboratories, to standardize the quality of the analytical methods and to identify the essential equipment, such as:

- gas chromatography;
- high pressure liquid chromatography;

- thin layer chromatography;

- mass spectrometry in combination with gas chromatography and computer evaluation;

- access to immunoassay equipment.

The accreditation process came under close scrutiny during the Dubin Inquiry, when it became known that the members of the IOC Sub-commission who are responsible for accreditation are also heads of IOC laboratories seeking re-accreditation. In correspondence quoted regarding the loss of accreditation of the Calgary laboratory, it was noted: 'The structure of the Sub-commission, which permits your members to be the professionals who act as consultants, then accreditors, subsequently adjudicators, and also the appeal group while maintaining a monopoly commercial interest, defies common standards of public accountability' (Dubin, 1990).

The location of accredited laboratories follows the sites of major events such as the Olympic Games.

Table 9.1 IOC accredited laboratories 1994

Athens	Greece	Phase II	
Barcelona	Spain		
Beijing	People's Republic of China		
Cologne	Germany		
Copenhagen	Denmark	Phase II	
Ghent	Belgium		
Helsinki	Finland		
Huddinge	Sweden		
Indianapolis	USA	Phase II	
Kreischa	Germany		
Lausanne	Switzerland		
Lisbon	Portugal		
London	UK		
Los Angeles	USA		
Madrid	Spain		
Montreal	Canada		
Moscow	URS	Phase I	
Oslo	Norway		
Paris	France		
Prague	The Czech and Slovak Republics		
Rome	Italy		
Seoul	South Korea		Phase II
Sydney	Australia	Phase II	
Tokyo	Japan	Phase II	

9.2.1 IOC ACCREDITED LABORATORIES 1994

In 1994, 24 laboratories were accredited by the IOC: 17 have full accreditation and the remainder are subject to the Phase I and Phase II restrictions listed in Table 9.1.

Phase I   The laboratory is temporarily suspended from international testing. At the national level (samples originating from the country in which the laboratory is located), the laboratory may perform screening procedures, but analytical positive A-samples must be confirmed by another IOC accredited laboratory. The corresponding B-sample will also be analysed in the accredited laboratory which has provided confirmation of the A-sample.

Phase II The laboratory is temporarily suspended from confirmation of analytically positive A-samples and analysing B-samples. Confirmation of the A-sample and analysis of the B-sample will be performed in another IOC accredited laboratory.

9.2.2 CODE OF ETHICS FOR IOC ACCREDITED LABORATORIES

1. **Competition testing** The laboratories should only accept and analyse samples originating from known sources within the context of doping control programmes conducted in competitions organized by national and international sports governing bodies. This includes national and international federations, national Olympic committees, national associations, universities and other similar organizations. This rule applies to Olympic and non-Olympic sports. Laboratories should ascertain that the programme calls for specimens collected according to IOC (or similar) guidelines. This includes collection, under observation, of A and B samples, appropriate sealing conditions, athletes' declarations with appropriate signatures, formal chain of custody conditions and adequate sanctions.

2. **Out-of-competition testing** The laboratories should accept samples taken during training (or out of competition) only if the following conditions are simultaneously met:

- the samples have been collected and sealed under the conditions generally prevailing in competitions themselves as in (1) above;

- the collection is a programme of a national or international sport governing body as defined in (1) above;

- appropriate sanctions will follow a positive case.

Thus laboratories should not accept samples from individual athletes on a private basis or from individuals acting on their behalf.

Laboratories should, furthermore, not accept samples, for the purposes of either screening or identification, from commercial or other sources when the conditions in the above paragraph are not simultaneously met. These rules apply to Olympic and non-Olympic sports.

3. **Other situations** If the laboratory is required to analyse a sample for a banned drug allegedly coming from a hospitalized or ill person in order to assist a physician in the diagnostic process, the laboratory director should explain the pre-testing issue to the requester and agree subsequently to analyse the sample only if a letter accompanies the sample and explicitly certifies that the sample is not from an athlete. The letter should also explain the medical reason for the test.

Finally, the heads of laboratories and/or their delegates will not discuss or comment to the media on individual results. Laboratory directors will not provide counsel to athletes or others regarding the evasion of a positive test.

Where a country is hosting a major international sporting event and does not have an IOC accredited laboratory, that country may apply to have an IOC accredited laboratory temporarily installed to a non-accredited laboratory/facility for the duration of the event. The host city must provide the analytical facilities but the procedures are, partly, staffed and conducted by personnel from the IOC accredited laboratory, with its director being responsible for all results. The accreditation is temporary for the duration of the event.

9.3 GOVERNMENT ACTION AND POLICY

International sports federations and the IOC were the first to introduce testing as a means to control the use of drugs in sport. However, governments were also expressing concern and seeking action about the use of drugs by sportsmen and women. In 1967, prior to the first Olympic testing, the Committee of Ministers of the Council of Europe adopted a resolution on doping in sport. The resolution gave a broad definition of doping, including doping methods as well as the misuse of drugs. It stressed the moral and ethical principle at stake for sport and the health dangers for athletes; more specifically, doping was referred to as cheating. Governments were recommended to persuade sports organizations to take the necessary steps to have proper and adequate regulations and to penalize offenders. The resolution also recommended that governments take action themselves if the sports organizations did not act sufficiently within 3 years. Anti-doping legislation and action was taken by several European countries.

The Council of Europe continued to monitor the situation and, in 1978, sports ministers adopted a resolution that called for governments to provide a coordinated policy and an overall framework in which the doping controls of sports organizations could take place. Meetings of anti-doping experts under the Chairmanship of Prince Alexandre de Merode (then Chairman of the IOC Medical Commission) led to the drafting of a European Anti-Doping Charter in 1984. The Charter was a statement of principles, anti-doping strategies and policies that received support from international sports organizations. It was, however, not binding upon governments, but would have 'moral, political and practical impact' (Council of Europe, 1989).

Progress towards a uniform international anti-doping policy took a further step forward when the IOC, international sports organizations and national governments came together at the First Permanent World Conference on Anti-Doping in 1988. The outcome of this conference was the development of the International Olympic Charter against Doping in Sport (1990). This important document identified the policies and practices required to counter doping. Its adoption as an IOC Charter was crucial to its success and influence.

Eager to keep up the momentum, the Council of Europe Committee of Ministers pressed for testing without warning outside competition, more significantly to secure a commitment to international harmonization not only between sports but also between countries. In 1989, sports ministers agreed to an Anti-Doping Convention. The key significance of such a document is the recognition of political will to counter doping. The Convention provides for common standards – legislative, financial, technical and educational – for implementation by governments themselves and by government in support of sports organizations. In June 1994, there were 23 contracting parties and nine signatory states, including countries outside Europe. The Convention is binding on contracting governments.

The response of governments and international organizations to the whole issue of doping in sport has been significant and interesting. Government initiated enquiries in Australia, Canada, New Zealand and the UK have acted as a catalyst for progress in anti-doping activities. There has also been criticism of the lack of action by sports organizations themselves to address the problem seriously from within. In the UK, the report by Moynihan and Coe in 1987 noted: 'Within the present arrangements there appear to be too many loopholes, and perhaps insufficient security for satisfactory levels of effectiveness and confidence to be achieved ... there is too much potential for evasion, leading to public concern and also to frustration among administrators and sportsmen and women.'

Similarly the Commission of Inquiry into the Use of Drugs and Banned Practices Intended to Increase Athletic Performance in Canada pointed to the failure of leadership amongst sports organizations and to the involvement and compliance of officials in drug use. 'The evidence of those witnesses at this inquiry who admitted their use of banned substances was in large part instrumental in uncovering the scandalous and pervasive practice of doping in sport that until then was hidden from public view, although not from the view of national and international sports federations' Dubin (1990).

The action taken by sport itself, whilst an important contribution, can only be strengthened by a concerted world-wide effort. Regrettably, there have been incidents of testing programmes actually being used to cover up drug misuse. Testing of athletes prior to a major event to determine whether they would pass the competition test has been admitted in several former Eastern Bloc countries. Covering up results from major competitions has also been revealed. Robert Voy, formerly Chief Medical Officer to the United States Olympic Committee explained how problematic this is: 'Allowing National Governing Bodies (NGBs), International Federations (IFs) and National Olympic Committees (NOCs) such as the United States Olympic Committee to govern the testing process to ensure fair play in sport is terribly ineffective. In a sense it is like having the fox guard the hen house' (Voy, 1991). Independence of the testing programmes and an openness of information would seem to be the only way forward if public confidence and, in particular, the confidence of athletes is to be restored.

The Chairman of the IOC Medical Commission has acknowledged this strategy to be the most effective. In an article published in 1992, he stated: 'A commonly accepted international policy is necessary for the elimination of doping in sport. Such a policy would lead to an improved and more consistent approach and would contribute to equality and equity in the international sporting community. Both public authorities and the independent sports organisations have separate but complementary responsibilities and should work together for this purpose at all levels' Sports Council (1992).

9.4 THE TESTING PROGRAMMES

Competitors may now be subject to testing at any time, both in and out of competition. At a national level, there is an increase in programmes of testing that are supplemented in some sports by testing programmes operated by the individual international sports federations. Regrettably there is no coordination or documentation of the testing undertaken so that in some sports a competitor may be subject to testing under the authority of a country's law, of an open championship, of an international federation and within a national programme. On the other hand, in some sports and in some countries testing is not as comprehensive. An announcement in January 1994, following a meeting of the IOC and international sports federations (IOC, 1994) indicates the commitment of these organizations to intensify and coordinate action. At this meeting the following principles were agreed:

- to unify their anti-doping rules and procedures for the controls they perform both during and out of competition (unannounced tests);

- to adopt, each year, as a basic document the list of banned classes and methods established by the IOC Medical Commission and to undertake the necessary controls for each sport;

- to accelerate unification of the minimum sanctions provided for by the IOC Medical Commission for violations of the anti-doping regulations and to ensure their application at both international and national level;

- to recognize the sanctions imposed by another international federation;

- to use the laboratories accredited by the IOC for all international competitions and for out-of-competition tests;

- to develop the cooperation between the IOC, international sports federations, national Olympic committees, national federations and governmental or other organizations concerned in order to organize and carry out doping controls and to combat the trafficking of doping substances in sport;

- to set up a special financial assistance programme for those international sports federations that need it, in order to help them intensify their anti-doping controls;

- to provide that sports included in the Olympic programme must be governed by international federations that agree to comply with the above mentioned principles.

9.4.1 PROCEDURES FOR DRUG TESTING

However a competitor is selected, as a winner, randomly or as part of a programme of out-of-competition testing, the sample collection procedure should follow the same principles. If such principles and policies are not sound and adhered to they become the target of lawsuits (Uzych, 1991).

The general procedure for drug testing in competition is outlined in Figure 9.1. This process follows the recommended procedure of the Anti-Doping Convention of the Council of Europe and is accepted by the majority of countries and sports federations.

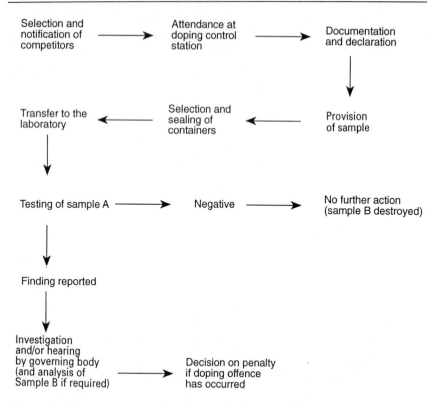

Figure 9.1 General procedure for drug testing in competition.

Selection of competitors

The policy for selection of competitors at an event where testing is being carried out should clearly define who will be selected. The selection policy is normally specified in the doping regulations that govern the event. This may involve those competitors who are placed in the first three or four of an event, additional randomly selected competitors, all team members or a combination of these. For example at Olympic competition the usual format is to select the first four competitors in each event, with one or two other randomly selected competitors. Sports that have record performances, such as track and field athletics, swimming and weightlifting, can require negative tests to ratify a record.

For out-of-competition testing, the selection and notification procedures vary slightly from those of competition testing. Selection may be from a register of eligible competitors or from a targeted group within the register. Eligibility depends upon the criteria laid down by the authorizing body, such as ranking, membership of the national team or potential selection for a representative team.

Notification

An official from the sample collection team will notify the competitor, in writing, that they have been selected for testing. The sampling official is responsible for accompanying the competitor at all times until it is practical to escort him/her to the doping control station. There may be considerable delay between the end of the event and attendance at the doping control station because of award ceremonies, press conferences, treatment for injury, etc. It is therefore vital that the chaperoning of competitors is effective, to ensure there has not been an opportunity for urine manipulation or substitution. The competitor may be accompanied to the doping control station by a coach or other team official.

Documentation

At the doping control station the competitor's identity and time of arrival are recorded. At a convenient point during the testing procedure, the competitor is invited to declare any medications or other substances taken recently (usually in the previous week). Such a declaration is not obligatory but it is in the competitor's interest. Where possible, the name of the substance, its dose and when it was last taken should be recorded. Competitors are reminded that they should declare not only prescription medications but also preparations which may have been obtained from a pharmacy, health food shop or other outlet.

Providing the sample

At the end of most events, the competitor may be dehydrated. A significant period of time may elapse before a urine sample is produced. The competitor is invited to consume drinks from supplies available at the doping control station; these are individually sealed, non-alcoholic and caffeine-free. Such precautions are taken to negate allegations of spiking of drinks. When the competitor is ready to provide a urine sample, he/she is invited to select a collection vessel that should be individually sealed in a plastic wrapping to prevent prior contamination. Collection of the urine takes place under the direct observation of a sampling officer of the same sex. Normally, the competitor must produce a sample of at least 75 ml.

The competitor may then select two, pre-sealed glass bottles, labelled A and B, and two bottle containers. The urine sample is divided between these bottles; normally two-thirds of the sample is placed in bottle A and one-third in bottle B. Both bottles are closed and sealed with numbered seals.

Sometimes regulations require that the pH and specific gravity of the urine are measured at the site of collection, using a small residue of the sample in the collection vessel. The pH should be between 5 and 7 and the specific gravity should read at least 1.01. If the sample does not meet these specifications, a further sample may be required.

Once the samples have been sealed, the documentation is completed and agreed by the sampling officer, the competitor and any accompanying official. A copy of the form is given to the competitor. Another copy that does not include the name of the competitor but records the sex of the competitor, the volume of urine, the bottle and seal numbers and any medications declared is enclosed with the samples that are sent to the laboratory.

Transfer to the laboratory

The sealed bottles are transported in secure, sealed transit bags to a laboratory along with the laboratory copies of documentation. The chain of custody for the transport of the samples from the doping control station to the laboratory must be documented to ensure integrity of the samples. On arrival at the laboratory the seal numbers are checked and recorded. Any irregularity is noted and the analysis of the sample may be suspended until the integrity can be confirmed. The A sample is prepared for analysis whilst the B sample is stored at low temperatures (the IOC recommend 4°C or less) pending the result of the analysis of the A sample.

Laboratory testing procedures

There are several analytical techniques that are used, alone or in combination, for the detection of drugs in urine. Techniques are selected according to the procedure being adopted. In general, drug-testing procedures are divided into two categories: screening and confirmatory. The additional volume placed in the A bottle enables the full range of screens to be applied and, if necessary, further investigations prior to reporting findings. If required, the analysis of the B sample will specifically target those substances found in the A sample.

The IOC list of doping substances represents a large and diverse group of chemical substances. Furthermore some sports ban additional substances. Testing procedures must be capable of detecting each of these chemical substances. The problem is compounded by the fact that many of these drugs are metabolized within the body, therefore detection techniques must be capable of identifying these metabolites. The screening procedures are used to isolate and detect the presence of drugs and their metabolites in urine. This initial screen often merely identifies the general class of chemical substance that is present. The second testing procedure is confirmatory in that it re-analyses the sample with the aim of positively identifying the precise nature of the drug or metabolite.

The laboratory techniques employed include thin-layer chromatography (TLC), gas chromatography, either alone or in combination with mass spectrometry, high performance liquid chromatography (HPLC) and immunoassay.

9.4.2 TLC

There are several types of chromatography, of which thin-layer was one of the earliest to be developed. In general, all chromatographic techniques employ a medium which allows chemicals to become absorbed on to its surface as the sample passes through. Different chemicals are bound to the medium with different strengths and will therefore move through the medium at different rates. This technique can be used to separate mixtures of chemicals, and their characteristic retention properties can also be used as a means of identification.

In the case of TLC, the medium is a layer of alumina or silica which is applied to a glass plate. A drop of the sample is placed at one end of the plate which is then placed in a shallow bath of solvent. As the solvent slowly rises up the plate the chemicals within the sample are carried along with the solvent but travel at different rates depending on how firmly they bind to the silica or alumina. After a period of time, the plates are removed from the solvent and the distance the solvent front has reached is marked on the plate. The plate is then dried, after which it is sprayed with marking agents which highlight the chemicals on the plate. Their position, relative to the solvent front, can be used to identify the type of chemical involved.

Whilst TLC provides rapid results at relatively little cost and can be used to screen a broad spectrum of drugs (Gold and Dackis, 1986), it lacks sophistication and therefore sensitivity. It is now rarely used in IOC laboratories and is restricted to the initial screening process.

9.4.3 HPLC

In HPLC, the matrix on which the drugs are adsorbed is packed in a column and the solvent is forced through the column under high pressure. Mixtures of chemicals will be driven through at different rates and each drug can be identified by the retention time within the column.

In addition, many drugs are detected as they leave the column by ultraviolet light. By selecting appropriate wavelengths, the detector can characterize and quantify the drug present in the urine.

9.4.4 GAS CHROMATOGRAPHY

In gas chromatography, the matrix on which the drugs are adsorbed is again packed in a capillary column through which a gas, such as helium or hydrogen, is driven. The column is heated and when the drug reaches the temperature at which it becomes too volatile to remain on the matrix it will be carried by the gas to a detector. The detectors are able to show the presence of certain atoms, such as nitrogen or phosphorus. Gas chromatography is, therefore, a technique which merely indicates the presence of drugs in urine. In order to identify precisely the drug in question, gas chromatography must be accompanied by mass spectrometry.

9.4.5 MASS SPECTROMETRY

Mass spectrometry is a technique which enables the tester to identify the specific drug which is present in the urine. The procedure involves breakdown of the parent drug or its metabolite(s) into its constituent parts by subjecting it to bombardment by a beam of electrons. The machine then measures the levels of the component parts which are plotted graphically. This mass spectrum is unique for any particular drug.

The combination of gas chromatography and mass spectrometry provides a method for positive identification of drugs in urine which is considered by many to be foolproof. Mass spectrometry can be used as a confirmatory test following any chromatographic or immunoassay screening technique.

9.4.6 IMMUNOASSAY

Immunoassay is a technique which is based on the body's allergic response to foreign material within the body. Foreign material is known as an antigen and the immune system produces antibodies to recognize and bind to these antigens. Drugs are a class of antigens. Specific antibodies which selectively bind to particular drugs may be produced in the laboratory. These antibodies normally involve radioactive iodine (radioimmunoassay, RIA) or the enzyme glucose-6-phosphate dehydrogenase (enzyme immunoassay, EIA). Urine samples may be exposed to these antibodies and if the drug, which the antibody is designed to recognize, is present in the urine it will be bound to the antibody. This drug/antibody complex can be isolated and identified by one of a number of assay procedures.

9.5 PROBLEMS IN DRUG DETECTION

9.5.1 LIMITATIONS TO THE TESTING PROCEDURES

In addition to the inherent problems associated with the selection of athletes, the processes in obtaining a urine sample, maintaining accurate documentation and ensuring the accuracy and validity of the testing procedures, Uzych (1991) has identified a number of limitations to the testing procedures:

1. A positive test result merely indicates that the athlete providing the urine specimen was exposed to the drug. Whether this was voluntary or involuntary remains open to question.
2. McBay (1987) has shown that errors may occur in the identification of the specimen or in the analytical procedures. In addition, the presence of a drug or a metabolite in the urine sample provides no scientific basis for determining when, how often or in what dose the drug was taken.
3. In general, a positive test result cannot be used to determine the effects of a drug on an individual and, most critically, the effects on performance.

Rule makers have responded to these limitations by making doping an absolute offence, then allowing for an investigative stage at which any justification, explanation or other information may be considered. The question of whether a substance would, in fact, improve performance in a particular sport is one that has not been addressed to date. It would be difficult to justify ethically the use of substances in the quantities detected in some athletes for research purposes. Moreover, performance improvement is not the only reason why substances are used, there might also be performance or health maintenance. There is a very fine line between treating a minor ailment to 'return health to normal' and the use of substances to improve performance. Some of the benefits that an athlete might derive from the use of a substance (real or placebo) may be psychological. This in itself could influence performance measurements. The limitations identified by Uzych often emerge in a legal challenge to a doping infraction.

9.5.2 ANABOLIC STEROIDS AND STEROID PROFILING

Detection of anabolic steroid misuse poses particular problems, since the steroids can be taken prior to competition, allowing a 'wash-out' period before competing. Clearly, out-of-competition testing provides one means for overcoming this problem. However, this is not uniformly adopted internationally.

An alternative approach to determine anabolic steroid use involves steroid profiling. One technique proposes that blood samples are taken to determine the amount and endocrine status of endogenous steroids, such as androsterone, etiocholanolone, 11-hydroxy-androsterone and 11-hydroxy-etiocholanolone. These endogenous steroids have been shown to be changed when exogenous anabolic steroids are taken, either orally or by injection.

Donike *et al.* (1989) have described the long-term influence of anabolic steroid misuse on the steroid profile, and conclude:

1. Taking anabolic steroids decreases the concentrations of endogenous steroids.
2. In steroid users there is a change in the ratios of endogenous isomer steroids like *cis*-androsterone.
3. The decrease in concentration and excretion of endogenous anabolic steroids can be observed even if the exogenous anabolic steroid can no longer be detected in the urine.

Although endocrine profiling has its critics in the scientific community (because of the lack of scientific studies to determine normal and abnormal levels of substances), the International Weightlifting Federation has publicly announced that it will use this process to identify drug users in the sport (Yesalis, 1993).

More recently, Lukas (1993) has suggested that other biochemical markers may be used to determine anabolic steroid use. Such markers could include liver function tests (e.g. lactate dehydrogenase), muscle enzymes (e.g. creatine phosphokinase), blood biochemistry (e.g. high density/low density lipoprotein ratios and haematocrit levels) and sperm count and motility. It is suggested that any suspected abnormalities in blood chemistry profiles could be followed with a urine screen for positive identification of the anabolic steroid involved. This could provide a more cost-effective approach. However, these alternative techniques for identifying anabolic steroid misuse require blood samples. This would represent a radical new approach to drug testing and would be subject to ethical approval.

9.5.3 TESTOSTERONE

Determination of the ratio of testosterone to epitestosterone (T/E ratio) in the urine is used to detect the administration of testosterone by competitors. Under the 1993 IOC list of doping classes, a T/E ratio greater than 10 was considered as evidence of an offence. If the ratio was greater than 6 and not greater than 10 the IOC Medical Commission recommended that further tests be conducted before considering the result positive or negative. Such investigations included:

- a review of previous tests;

- endocrinological investigations;

- unannounced testing over several months.

In 1994 the IOC revised this rule, reducing the reporting level to 6:1 with a mandatory investigation before the sample is declared positive. In the absence of previous test data, unannounced testing over a period of 3 months is required.

Testosterone abuse can be difficult to substantiate; published scientific data on the validity of the 6:1 ratio is sparse (Yesalis, 1993) and control of an endogenous substance requires agreement on the 'normal' endogenous level in the population.

It has been acknowledged that some males may have unusually high levels of endogenous testosterone, and T/E ratios between 6 and 9 have been recorded (Catlin and Hatton, 1991). It has been found that the anti-fungal drug, ketoconazole, inhibits testosterone biosynthesis in men (Pont et al., 1982). This observation has led to the development of a testing procedure, using ketoconazole, to differentiate between competitors with unusually high endogenous testosterone levels and those using testosterone as a performance-enhancing agent (Kicman et al., 1993). The results of this study showed that ketoconazole caused a differential suppression of the urinary excretion rates of testosterone and epitestosterone. The administration of ketoconazole to an athlete with a naturally above-normal T/E ratio results in a decrease in the ratio, but causes the ratio to increase in normal men who have received exogenous testosterone. This difference in response indicates that ketoconazole could be used to distinguish between male athletes with naturally large T/E ratios and those who have large ratios due to testosterone administration.

The use of this test as part of the drug-testing procedures is feasible, since only urine samples are required and the changes in T/E ratios, following ketoconazole administration, occur within 6–8 hours. The IOC and international sports federations have yet to adopt this procedure formally as a recognized detection method. Moreover, athletes themselves would need to be agreeable to the administration of ketoconazole and are likely to question its safety.

9.5.4 BLOOD DOPING

Blood doping was added to the IOC list of banned substances and methods after the 1984 Olympic Games, contrary to the policy of not banning anything for which an unequivocal testing procedure is not available.

Berglund (1988) describes the development of techniques for the detection of blood doping in sport. Whilst it is possible to demonstrate that an individual has undergone blood doping, there are several factors which must be considered, not least of which is that the method requires a blood rather than urine sample. Furthermore, since the test relies on changes in blood parameters over a period of time, two blood samples must be taken with a minimal interval of 1 to 2 weeks. If these criteria are met, then alteration in the levels of at least two parameters, such as haemoglobin, serum iron, bilirubin and serum erythropoietin, during that period is indicative of blood doping.

Despite the current lack of an unequivocal method for the detection of blood doping, it is unlikely that blood doping will become more widespread for a number of reasons:

- Where a subject reinfuses their own blood (autologous transfusion), this requires the help of skilled personnel and a period of storage for 4–5 weeks in a blood bank which increases the risk of detection.

- Where a subject uses blood from a matching donor (heterologous transfusion), they run the risk of mismatch of blood possibly leading to anaphylactic shock or the possibility of contracting blood-borne diseases such as AIDS or hepatitis B.

- For either technique, the risk of introducing an infection at the site of infusion, leading to a septicaemia, is ever present.

9.5.5 PEPTIDE HORMONES

The IOC introduced the new doping class of 'Peptide Hormones and Analogues' in 1989, again despite the lack of unequivocal tests for these agents. Currently, this class includes human growth hormone, human chorionic gonadotrophin and adrenocorticotrophic hormone, including all releasing factors for these hormones. The list also includes erythropoietin.

Kicman and Cowan (1992) have reviewed the misuse and detection of this class of doping agents. The standard methods of chemical analysis for drugs, using gas chromatography and mass spectroscopy, are unsuitable for the detection of the peptide hormones at the present time. The only currently available method is that of immunoassay; however, the IOC does not accept the use of immunoassay alone without a confirmatory test being applied. Research is continuing in order to refine extraction techniques, such as ultrafiltration, in order to gain IOC approval for a suitable testing procedure for this class of doping agents.

9.6 BLOOD TESTING IN DOPING CONTROL

In 1993, the IOC decided to recommend that in the 1994 Winter Olympics in Lillehammer blood tests as prescribed by the International Ski Federation (FIS) should be carried out. Blood samples were taken at the 1994 Winter Olympic Games as part of the doping control procedures for the first time in Olympic history.

The purpose of blood tests is to detect blood doping and to develop more sophisticated methods to combat other doping methods in sports. The FIS approved guidelines for blood sampling included the following:

1. The doping control notification shall state whether the competitor is required to undergo blood sampling in addition to urine sampling. The procedures for selection and notification are the same as for urine sampling.
2. Blood sampling may be performed before or after the urine sampling procedure. All blood sampling shall be taken by qualified personnel.
3. The same type of equipment will be used to store and transport blood as for urine samples.
4. Only a small amount of blood (4 ml) will be taken. The blood will be taken from a superficial vein in the elbow region and 2 ml will be used for each of sample A and B.
5. The competitor shall declare to the doping control officer any blood transfusion(s) he or she may have received in the preceding 6 months, with details, including the reason for such transfusions.
6. As soon as possible after arrival at the doping control laboratory, the blood samples shall be tested for the presence of foreign blood cells.
7. Refusal to submit to a blood sample may have the same consequences as failure to submit to a urine sample.

The IOC Medical Commission also decided to support any similar initiatives taken by other international sports federations. FIS was the only international federation to agree to the collection of blood samples in Lillehammer. The International Amateur Athletic Federation (IAAF) have also adopted compulsory blood testing as part of the requirements at the 'Golden Four' meetings. As further information has become available, variations to the original FIS procedures have been made. The IAAF have ruled for the collection of up to 25 ml of blood; tests at the Olympic Games involved 'up to but not more than 25 ml' (IAAF, 1994). The collected blood was centrifuged on site to prepare it for analysis.

9.6.1 STATISTICS FROM IOC LABORATORIES

The IOC laboratories provide annual statistics on the number and nature of identified substances in the A samples tested. Table 9.2 summarizes the identified substances from the samples analysed by IOC accredited laboratories over the period 1986 to 1991. Statistics beyond this period have not been published.

Table 9.2 Numbers of substances identified by IOC accredited laboratories 1986–1991

	1986	1987	1988	1989	1990	1991
Anabolic steroids	439	521	791	611	579	552
Stimulants	177	299	420	508	340	221
Narcotics	23	55	58	76	62	72
Beta blockers	31	32	8	6	8	10
Diuretics	2	9	57	45	37	47
Masking agents	NT	24	19	10	6	1
Peptide hormones	NT	NT	NT	NT	1	1
Totals	672	940	1353	1256	1033	1004

NT = Not tested.
In addition to the substances listed, a number of related substances, not included on the IOC list, were identified each year.
Source: IOC statistics.

It is clear from looking at the IOC statistics (Table 9.2) that anabolic steroids and stimulants are the classes of drugs most frequently detected and, by implication, most frequently misused in sport. However the type of testing programmes undertaken and the sports involved may have influenced these statistics. The year-on-year trend, particularly for steroids and stimulants, shows a distinct peak in the years 1988 and 1989 (Figure 9.2). This begs the question as to whether the misuse of drugs in

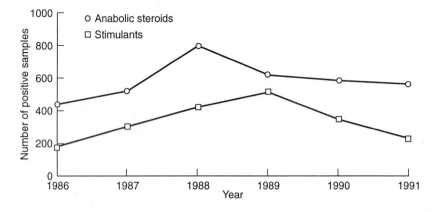

Figure 9.2 Trends in IOC positive samples for stimulants and steroids.

sport has peaked and will now decline or whether the downward trend reflects a deterioration in the ability to detect drug misusers, perhaps linked with an increased ability to avoid detection.

9.7 PROBLEMS WITH OVER-THE-COUNTER (OTC) DRUGS

The data presented in Table 9.2 merely give an overview of the situation regarding numbers of positive samples detected. It is acknowledged that competitors have and will continue to experience problems when purchasing from a pharmacy OTC preparations which contain banned substances. The two areas of particular difficulty are with regard to stimulants and narcotic analgesics since members of these groups of drugs are available OTC, particularly in cough and cold preparations and as painkillers.

The stimulants in question involve sympathomimetic amines which are present in some cough and cold preparations. The pharmacological rationale for their inclusion in such preparations to reduce nasal secretions. If we look at the IOC statistics for 1991, specifically for stimulants, we see that 46.1% of the substances identified were for sympathomimetics available OTC (Table 9.3).

Table 9.3 IOC sample analysis for stimulants, 1991

Total number of stimulants identified:	221
Number of stimulants identified which can be purchased OTC:	
Ephedrine	22
Pseudoephedrine	57
Phenylpropanolamine	23
Total	102

(Therefore the number of stimulants identified which can be purchased OTC represent 46.1% of the total stimulants identified.)

Similarly, for the narcotic analgesics there were 72 positive samples in 1991. Of these, 36 (50%) were for codeine which is a relatively mild narcotic analgesic available in many OTC preparations.

There are several issues raised in considering these figures:

• Should these particular types of drugs be included at all on the list of banned drugs? After all they are, relatively speaking, pharmacologically less active than other members within their respective groups of drugs. In fact, in the March 1993 IOC list of banned substances, codeine was removed from the list of banned narcotics and reclassified as a permitted substance for therapeutic use, provided a declaration is made if a competitor is selected for testing. In 1994, dihydrocodeine was also reclassified by the IOC as a permitted substance.

- If these drugs are to remain on the list, should there be a published maximum permitted urine level, as presently occurs for caffeine?
- There is an urgent need to educate competitors on the dangers of taking OTC preparations which contain banned substances.

These concerns about OTC drugs were expressed by élite athletes who were administered a questionnaire on various aspects of drug misuse in sport (Radford, 1992a). The athletes were clearly concerned that OTC drugs could be taken in error, and two out of three athletes questioned believed that the penalty for the first offence in these circumstances should be no more than a warning.

In addition to OTC medicines which are known to contain banned substances, there are many preparations which may possibly contain certain banned drugs. These include food supplements where there is no legal requirement for manufacturers to list the content of the food supplement, therefore making it difficult to determine whether taking such a preparation would contravene the doping regulations. Similarly, various 'natural' products, such as herbal preparations, may, and in some cases frequently do, contain banned substances. These include Ma Huang (Chinese ephedra) which is a plant which contains ephedrine, and ginseng, which itself does not contain banned substances in its natural form of ginseng root, but in preparations such as tablets, solutions, teas, etc., other ingredients, such as anabolic steroids, ephedrine and other stimulants, may be present.

It must be remembered that because a product is termed 'natural' or 'herbal' it is not devoid of potential adverse side-effects. Many drugs, whether or not banned by the IOC, are derived from plant sources. It is the dose of the product taken which is the principal determinant of whether the drug will be toxic, coupled with the sensitivity of the individual to a particular substance.

9.8 REPORTING TEST RESULTS

Reports are prepared by the analysing laboratory and relayed in confidence to the relevant governing body. In some countries, there is a requirement for the reporting to be directed via a national anti-doping organization or independent body who oversee the management of the results. If the test result is negative, the governing body should advise the competitor of the result and the B sample will be destroyed by the laboratory.

In the case of a positive result, it is the responsibility of the governing body to act in accordance with their own particular anti-doping policy. The competitor is notified of the finding and may be suspended from competition for the duration of the investigation. The competitor is invited to explain the finding and will be invited to attend and/or be represented at the analysis of the B sample, which will take place in the same laboratory as the A sample finding (subject to the accreditation restrictions). In most circumstances, a representative of the governing body must also be present at the B sample analysis.

A governing body hearing is arranged at which the analytical report and possible breach of the doping regulations are considered. The competitor and/or a representative is invited to attend and will be given an opportunity to present their case.

Following the hearing, decisions are made about the disciplinary action to be taken and the penalties that will apply. The competitor has the right to appeal, with recourse to law if it is deemed appropriate.

Where a country has a national anti-doping organization, the results of the analysis and subsequent action can be monitored. Reports issued directly to international sports federations may not be subject to the same scrutiny, and publication of the information is in the hands of the individual organization.

Irregularities in the sample collection procedure, such as refusal or failure to provide a sample, follow the same investigation and disciplinary procedures. The report originates from the organization responsible for the collection.

9.8.1 SANCTIONS

Sanctions are determined by each governing body in accordance with its regulations. The current IOC list of sanctions is presented in Table 9.4. There are many critics of the sanctions imposed by the IOC Medical Commission, who believe that they are not severe enough. Some federations operate their own sanctions appropriate to the career profile of their sport. National rules and legislation can also mean different sanctions: in Greece an anabolic steroid finding can mean two years' imprisonment, Canada applies a 4-year ban for a first offence and a life ban for a second offence.

Views concerning the need for testing and the effectiveness of sanctions are varied. Certainly one group of élite British athletes was in favour of strong action (Radford, 1992a). Virtually all (98.3%) of those questioned considered there should be a testing strategy in their particular sport. The current system of doping control in Britain was thought to be effective by 79.3%, and 82.6% thought that out-of-competition testing is a better deterrent than competition testing. With regard to penalties, although a more lenient approach to positive results involving OTC drugs was recommended, over half of those questioned considered that the penalty for a positive result involving steroids, amphetamines or blood doping should be a life ban.

Table 9.4 IOC recommended sanctions for positive cases in doping control (March 1993)

Androgenic anabolic steroids, amphetamine-related and other stimulants, caffeine, diuretics, beta blockers, narcotic analgesics and designer drugs:

- 2 years for the first offence
- life ban for the second offence

Ephedrine, phenylpropanolamine (when administered orally as a cough suppressant or painkiller in association with decongestants and/or antihistamines):

- a maximum 3 months for the first offence
- 2 years for the second offence
- life ban for the third offence

The IOC Medical Commission recommends that before a final decision is made on a particular case, a fair hearing be granted for the athlete (and possibly the other persons concerned). Such a hearing should take into consideration the circumstances (extenuating or not) and the known facts of the case. During the hearing, it is recommended that the head of the IOC accredited laboratory who reported the results be consulted.

The Medical Commission also recommends to sport authorities that even more severe sanctions have to be taken against all persons, other than the athlete involved in the doping case, if the guilt of such persons can be unequivocally established.

A survey carried out by the Australian Sports Drug Agency (ASDA) in 1994 concluded: 85% of Australian athletes (n = 616) believed the ASDA's drug-testing programme would deter Australian athletes from using prohibited drugs; 73% indicated that the sanctions imposed on the athletes testing positive should be made public; 71% believed the names of athletes testing positive should be made public by their national sporting organization. However, only 11% believed this should be the case if the positive test was the result of inadvertent use (inadvertent use defined as unknowing use of a banned substance contained in a common drug preparation, for example a cough or cold medicine).

Investigations of findings may help to identify the source of supply of some of the more serious substances, such as steroids, amphetamines, cocaine etc., and in these cases action can then be taken for 'non-use infractions'. In Canada and elsewhere, there are penalties for coaches and administrators who support and encourage the use of drugs.

9.9 EDUCATION

Clearly, despite the shortcomings and expense involved, the control of drug misuse in sport requires an effective testing programme and associated deterrent sanctions. However, testing alone is not likely to control the use of drugs. Equal, if not greater, attention and resources should be directed towards an effective education policy and programme. A surprisingly high percentage (94.2%) of competitors questioned in the Radford survey (1992a) thought that an anti-doping education programme aimed at young competitors would be effective in reducing drug use in the future.

The International Olympic Charter against Doping in Sport (IOC, 1990) recognizes that drug education is a fundamental element of any anti-doping programme. As part of a comprehensive anti-doping strategy, an education programme can help to develop healthy and discerning attitudes towards sports performance and the use of drugs and other substances.

More use should be made of coaches, nutritionists, pharmacists and other health professionals involved with drugs to help and advise competitors, particularly at the start of their sporting career, to identify the psychosocial factors that could lead to drug use and to be aware of how to deal with them. Coaches and officials also need to be educated about their role (passive or active) in advocating drug-free sport.

Whilst there is a role for information dissemination in raising awareness, the expectation that this will bring about a negative attitude towards drug use is naive. Knowledge may increase, but attitudes and behaviours are unlikely to be affected. As Tricker and Cook (1990) point out: 'One-shot presentations given by strangers probably prepared athletes to deal with drug education issues as thoroughly as one training session per year would prepare them adequately for the national championships'. An integrated approach to athlete education, including drugs education, is more likely to achieve results. Set in the context of principles of sports performance, nutrition, psychology, training programmes, competition schedules and dealing with injury and delivered by individuals familiar with the athlete, drug education is likely to be more successful. Above all, the messages should be consistent and relevant to the athlete.

9.10 REFERENCES

Beckett, A.H. (1981) Use and abuse of drugs in sport. *J. Biosoc. Sci. (Suppl)*, **7**, 163–70.

Beckett, A.H. and Cowan, D.A. (1979) Misuse of drugs in sport. *Br. J. Sports Med.*, **12**, 185–94.

Berglund, B. (1988) Development of techniques for the detection of blood doping in sport. *Sports Medicine*, **5**, 127–35.

Bottomley, M. (1988) Report, in *Second International Athletic Foundation World Symposium on Doping in Sport: Official Proceedings*, (eds P. Bellotti, G. Benzi and A. Lungqvist), International Athletic Foundation, Monte Carlo, pp. 209–11.

Brooks, R.V., Firth, R.G. and Sumner, N.A. (1975) Detection of anabolic steroids by radioimmunoassay. *Br. J. Sports Med.*, **9**, 89–92.

Catlin, D.H. and Hatton, C.K. (1991) Use and abuse of anabolic and other drugs for athletic enhancement. *Adv. Intern. Med.*, **36**, 399–424.

Catlin, D.H., Kammerer, R.C., Hatton, C.K. *et al.* (1987) Analytical chemistry at the games of the XXIIIrd Olympiad in Los Angeles, 1984. *Clin. Chem.*, **33**, 319–27.

Council Of Europe (1989) Anti-Doping Convention, Strasbourg, France.

de Merode, A. (1979) Doping tests at the Olympic Games in 1976. *J. Sports Med.*, **19**, 91–6.

Donike, M., Geyer, H., Kraft, M. and Rauth, S. (1989) Long-term influence of anabolic steroid misuse on the steroid profile, in *Second International Athletic Foundation World Symposium on Doping in Sport: Official Proceedings*, (eds P. Bellotti, G. Benzi and A. Ljungqvist), International Athletic Foundation, Monte Carlo, pp. 107–16.

Dubin, L. (1990) Commission of *Inquiry into the Use of Drugs and Banned Practices Intended to Increase Athletic Performance*, Ministry of Supply and Services, Ottawa, Canada.

Dugal, P. and Donike, M. (1988) Requirements for accreditation and good laboratory practice. IOC Medical Commission document, October.

Gold, M.S. and Dackis, C.A. (1986) Role of the laboratory in the evaluation of suspected drug abuse. *J. Clin. Psychiat.*, **47**(1), 17–23.

Hatton, C.K. and Catlin, D.H. (1987) Detection of androgenic anabolic steroids in urine. *Clinics in Laboratory Medicine*, **7**, 655–68.

International Olympic Committee (1994) Preventing and fighting against doping in sport. IOC, Lausanne, January.

IAFF (1994) IAAF regulations, April, Mondro.

IOC (1968) International Olympic Committee Newsletter, Lausanne, Switzerland.

IOC (1990) International Olympic Charter against Doping in Sport. IOC. Lausanne.

IOC Laboratory Statistics (1991). In *Sports Council Doping Control Information Booklet*, No. 3, Sports Council, London.

Kicman, A.T. and Cowan, D.A. (1992) Peptide hormones and sport: misuse and detection. *Br. Med. Bull.*, **48**, 496–517.

Kicman, A.T., Oftebro, H., Walker, C. *et al.* (1993) Potential use of ketoconazole in a dynamic endocrine test to differentiate between biological outliers and testosterone use by athletes. *Clin. Chem.*, **39**(9) 1798–1803.

Lukas, S.E. (1993) Current perspectives on anabolic–androgenic steroid abuse. *Trends. Pharmacol. Sci.*, **14**, 61–8.

McBay, A.J. (1987) Drug analysis technology – pitfalls and problems of drug testing. *Clin. Chem.*, **33**, 33B–40B.

Moynihan, C. and Coe, S. (1987) *The Misuse of Drugs in Sport*, Department of the Environment, London.

Pont, A., Williams, P.L., Azhar, S. *et al.* (1982) Ketoconazole blocks testosterone synthesis. *Arch. Intern. Med.*, **142**, 2137–40.

Radford, P. (1992a) Drug testing and drug education programs. *Sports Medicine*, **12**, 1–5.

Royal Society of New Zealand (1990) *Drugs and Medicine in Sport*, Royal Society of New Zealand, Wellington.

Sports Council (1992) *Relay, The Magazine of the British International Sports Committee*, p. 12.

Tricker, R. and Cook, D.L. (1990) Athletes at Risk – Drugs and Sport, W.M.C. Brown, USA.

Uzych, L. (1991) Drug testing of athletes. *Br. J. Addiction*, **86**, 25–31.

Voy, R. (1991) Drugs in sport and politics.

Wade, N. (1972) Anabolic steroids: doctors denounce them, but athletes aren't listening. *Science*, **176**, 1399–1403.

Yesalis, C. (1993) *Anabolic Steroids in Sport and Exercise*, Human Kinetics Publishers Inc., Champaign, Illinois, USA.

9.11 FURTHER READING

de Merode, A. (1992) The moral authority of the IOC. *Relay*, Issue 7, Winter.

Merdink, J. and Woolley, B. (1990) Drug testing: history, philosophy and rationale, in *Athletes at Risk: Drugs and Sport*, (ed. W.C. Brown and B. Woolley), Dubuque, Iowa, pp. 161–71.

Olympic Review (1991) Dope control laboratories accredited by the IOC.

Olympic Review, Lausanne, Switzerland, **284**, 279–82.

Radford, P. (1992b) The fight against doping in sport: the last five years. *Sport and Leisure*, May/June.

Raynaud, E., Audrant, M., Pegas, J. Ch. *et al.* (1993) Determination of urinary testosterone and epitestosterone during pubertal development: a cross-sectional study in 141 normal male subjects. *Clin. Endoc.*, **38**, 353–9.

Sports Council Doping Control Information Booklet No. 3, November 1991. Sports Council, London.

Verroken, M. (1993) The testing process. *Coaching Focus*, No. 23, 21–3.

Index